T0073797

Osteoarthritis

Editor

DAVID J. HUNTER

CLINICS IN GERIATRIC MEDICINE

www.geriatric.theclinics.com

May 2022 • Volume 38 • Number 2

ELSEVIER

1600 John F. Kennedy Boulevard • Suite 1800 • Philadelphia, Pennsylvania, 19103-2899

http://www.theclinics.com

CLINICS IN GERIATRIC MEDICINE Volume 38, Number 2
May 2022 ISSN 0749–0690, ISBN-13: 978-0-323-98707-3

Editor: Katerina Heidhausen
Developmental Editor: Hannah Almira Lopez

Clinics in Geriatric Medicine (ISSN 0749-0690) is published quarterly by Elsevier Inc., 360 Park Avenue South, New York, NY 10010-1710. Months of issue are February, May, August, and November. Business and Editorial Offices: 1600 John F. Kennedy Blvd., Suite 1800, Philadelphia, PA 191023-2899. Periodicals postage paid at New York, NY, and additional mailing offices. Subscription prices are $303.00 per year (US individuals), $901.00 per year (US institutions), $100.00 per year (US & Canadian student/resident), $330.00 per year (Canadian individuals), $928.00 per year (Canadian institutions), $431.00 per year (international individuals), $928.00 per year (international institutions), and $195.00 per year (international student/resident). Foreign air speed delivery is included in all *Clinics* subscription prices. All prices are subject to change without notice. POSTMASTER: Send address changes to *Clinics in Geriatric Medicine*, Elsevier Health Sciences Division, Subscription Customer Service, 3251 Riverport Lane, Maryland Heights, MO 63043. **Telephone: 1-800-654-2452 (U.S. and Canada); 314-447-8871 (outside U.S. and Canada). Fax: 314-447-8029. E-mail:** journalscustomerservice-usa@elsevier.com **(for print support)** or journalsonlinesupport-usa@elsevier.com **(for online support).**

Reprints. For copies of 100 or more, of articles in this publication, please contact the Commercial Reprints Department, Elsevier Inc., 360 Park Avenue South, New York, New York 10010-1710. Tel.: 212-633-3874; Fax: 212-633-3820, E-mail: reprints@elsevier.com.

Clinics in Geriatric Medicine is covered in *MEDLINE/PubMed (Index Medicus), EMBASE/Excerpta Medica, Current Contents/Clinical Medicine (CC/CM),* and the *Cumulative Index to Nursing & Allied Health Literature.*

Contributors

EDITOR

DAVID J. HUNTER, MBBS, MSc (Clin Epi), M SpMed, PhD, FRACP (Rheum)
Florance and Cope Chair of Rheumatology, Rheumatology Department, Royal North Shore Hospital, Institute of Bone and Joint Research, Kolling Institute, Faculty of Medicine and Health, The University of Sydney, Sydney, New South Wales, Australia; Clinical Research Centre, Zhujiang Hospital, Southern Medical University, Guangzhou, China

AUTHORS

KELLI ALLEN, PhD
Thurston Arthritis Research Center, The University of North Carolina at Chapel Hill, Chapel Hill, North Carolina, USA

TAMARA ALLISTON, PhD
Department of Orthopaedic Surgery, University of California, San Francisco, San Francisco, California, USA

NAOMI SIMICK BEHERA, MPhys
The University of Sydney, Sydney, New South Wales, Australia

KIM BENNELL, PhD
Centre for Health, Exercise and Sports Medicine, The University of Melbourne, Victoria, Australia

SITA M.A. BIERMA-ZEINSTRA, PhD
Department of General Practice and Orthopedics & Sports Medicine, Erasmus MC University Medical Center Rotterdam, Rotterdam, the Netherlands

JOCELYN L. BOWDEN, BLA, BHMSc, BSc(Hons), PhD
Institute of Bone and Joint Research, Kolling Institute, Faculty of Medicine and Health, University of Sydney, Department of Rheumatology, Royal North Shore Hospital, Sydney, New South Wales, Australia

ANDREW M. BRIGGS, BSc(Physiotherapy)Hons, PhD, FACP
Professor, Curtin School of Allied Health, Curtin University, Perth, Western Australia, Australia

SAMANTHA BUNZLI, PhD
Department of Surgery, The University of Melbourne, St Vincent's Hospital, Melbourne, Victoria, Australia

ANNETTE BURGESS, PhD, MMedEd, MEd, MBiothics, MBT
Sydney Medical School, Faculty of Medicine and Health, The University of Sydney, Sydney, Australia

LEIGH F. CALLAHAN, PhD
Professor, Division of Rheumatology, Allergy and Immunology, Thurston Arthritis Research Center, The University of North Carolina at Chapel Hill, Chapel Hill, North Carolina, USA

MURILLO DÓRIO, MD, PhD
Division of Rheumatology, Hospital das Clínicas da Faculdade de Medicina da Universidade de São Paulo, São Paulo, São Paulo, Brazil

ZHAOLI DAI, PhD, MS, MA
Sydney Pharmacy School and the Charles Perkins Centre, Faculty of Medicine and Health, The University of Sydney, Centre for Health Systems and Safety Research, Australian Institute of Health Innovation, Macquarie University, Sydney, New South Wales, Australia

LETICIA A. DEVEZA, MD, PhD
Rheumatology Department, Royal North Shore Hospital, Institute of Bone and Joint Research, Kolling Institute, The University of Sydney, Sydney, New South Wales, Australia

MICHELLE M. DOWSEY, BHealthSci (Nursing), MEpi, PhD
Department of Surgery, The University of Melbourne, St Vincent's Hospital, Melbourne, Victoria, Australia

VICKY DUONG, DPT
Department of Rheumatology, Institute of Bone and Joint Research, Kolling Institute, Royal North Shore Hospital, Northern Clinical School, The University of Sydney, Sydney, Australia

JILLIAN P. EYLES, BAppSc(Physiotherapy), PhD
Institute of Bone and Joint Research, Kolling Institute, Faculty of Medicine and Health, The University of Sydney, Department of Rheumatology, Royal North Shore Hospital, Sydney, New South Wales, Australia

MAY ARNA GODAKER RISBERG, PhD
Norwegian School Sport Sciences, Oslo, Norway

SANDRA GRACE, BA, MSc, PhD
Faculty of Health, Southern Cross University, Lismore, New South Wales, Australia

BIMBI GRAY, BClinSci, BNat, MOstMed
Institute of Bone and Joint Research, Kolling Institute, The University of Sydney, Department of Rheumatology, Royal North Shore Hospital, Sydney, New South Wales, Australia

FRANCIS GUILLEMIN, MD, PhD
Professor, APEMAC, Université de Lorraine, Nancy, France

GILLIAN A. HAWKER, MD, MSc
Sir John and Lady Eaton Professor and Chair, Department of Medicine, University of Toronto, Toronto, Ontario, Canada

RANA S. HINMAN, BPhysio (Hons), PhD
Centre for Health, Exercise and Sports Medicine, The University of Melbourne, Victoria, Australia

MELANIE HOLDEN, PhD
Primary Care Centre Versus Arthritis, School of Medicine, Keele University, Keele, Staffordshire, United Kingdom

DAVID J. HUNTER, MBBS, MSc (Clin Epi), M SpMed, PhD, FRACP (Rheum)
Florance and Cope Chair of Rheumatology, Rheumatology Department, Royal North Shore Hospital, Institute of Bone and Joint Research, Kolling Institute, Faculty of Medicine and Health, The University of Sydney, Sydney, New South Wales, Australia; Clinical Research Centre, Zhujiang Hospital, Southern Medical University, Guangzhou, China

MOHIT KAPOOR, PhD
Department of Surgery and Laboratory Medicine and Pathobiology, Schroeder Arthritis Institute, Krembil Research Institute, University Health Network, University of Toronto, Toronto, Ontario, Canada

JENNIFER L. KENT, BSc (Environmental Science), MEnvPl, PhD
School of Architecture, Design and Planning, The University of Sydney, Sydney, New South Wales, Australia

LAUREN K. KING, MD, MSc
Department of Medicine, University of Toronto, Toronto, Ontario, Canada

SARAH KOBAYASHI, BLAS, PhD
Kolling Institute, Faculty of Medicine and Health, The University of Sydney, Sydney, New South Wales, Australia

CHRISTOPHER B. LITTLE, BVMS, PhD
Raymond Purves Bone and Joint Research Laboratories, Kolling Institute, The University of Sydney, Faculty of Medicine and Health, Royal North Shore Hospital, Sydney, New South Wales, Australia

RICHARD F. LOESER, MD
Department of Medicine, Division of Rheumatology, Allergy and Immunology, Thurston Arthritis Research Center, The University of North Carolina at Chapel Hill, Chapel Hill, North Carolina, USA

ANNE-MARIE MALFAIT, MD, PhD
Department of Internal Medicine, Division of Rheumatology, Rush University Medical Center, Chicago, Illinois, USA

KAKA MARTINA, RN, BN, GradDip (Clinical Teaching)
Rheumatology Department, Royal North Shore Hospital, Institute of Bone and Joint Research, Kolling Institute, The University of Sydney, Mater Hospital Sydney, North Sydney Orthopedic and Sports Medicine Center, Sydney, New South Wales, Australia

RACHEL E. MILLER, PhD
Department of Internal Medicine, Division of Rheumatology, Rush University Medical Center, Chicago, Illinois, USA

TUHINA NEOGI, MD, PhD
Professor, Department of Medicine, Section of Rheumatology, Boston University School of Medicine, Boston, Massachusetts, USA

PHILIPPA J.A. NICOLSON, PhD
Department of Rheumatology, Institute of Bone and Joint Research, Kolling Institute, Royal North Shore Hospital and Northern Clinical School, The University of Sydney, Sydney, New South Wales, Australia; Nuffield Department of Orthopaedics, Rheumatology and Musculoskeletal Sciences, University of Oxford, Oxford, United Kingdom

WIN MIN OO, MD, PhD
Department of Physical Medicine and Rehabilitation, Mandalay General Hospital, University of Medicine, Mandalay, Mandalay, Myanmar; Rheumatology Department, Royal North Shore Hospital, Institute of Bone and Joint Research, Kolling Institute, The University of Sydney, Sydney, New South Wales, Australia

NINA ØSTERÅS, BSc Physiotherapy, MSc, PhD
Division of Rheumatology and Research, Diakonhjemmet Hospital, Oslo, Norway

JONATHAN QUICKE, BSc(Hons) Physiotherapy, MSc, PhD
School of Medicine/Impact Accelerator Unit, Keele University, Keele, Staffordshire, United Kingdom

JUSTIN P. ROE, MBBS, FRACS
North Sydney Orthopedic and Sports Medicine Center, University of New South Wales, Sydney, New South Wales, Australia

JOS RUNHAAR, PhD
Department of General Practice, Erasmus MC University Medical Center Rotterdam, Rotterdam, the Netherlands

LUCY J. SALMON, BAppSci (Physio), PhD
North Sydney Orthopedic and Sports Medicine Center, University of Notre Dame, Sydney, New South Wales, Australia

DIEUWKE SCHIPHOF, BSc Physiotherapy, MSc, PhD
Department of General Practice, Erasmus MC University Medical Center, Rotterdam, the Netherlands

SAURAB SHARMA, PhD
Centre for Pain IMPACT, Neuroscience Research Australia (NeuRA), University of New South Wales, Sydney, New South Wales, Australia

MARTIN J. THOMAS, PhD, MCSP
Primary Care Centre Versus Arthritis, School of Medicine, Keele University, Haywood Academic Rheumatology Centre, Midlands Partnership NHS Foundation Trust, Haywood Hospital, Burslem, Staffordshire, United Kingdom

LINDA TROEBERG, PhD
University of East Anglia, Norwich Medical School, Norwich, United Kingdom

MARTIN VAN DER ESCH, PhD
Amsterdam University of Applied Sciences, Faculty of Health, Reade, Centre for Rehabilitation and Rheumatology, Amsterdam, the Netherlands

TONIA L. VINCENT, MD, FRCP, PhD
Centre for Osteoarthritis Pathogenesis Versus Arthritis, Kennedy Institute of Rheumatology, University of Oxford, Oxford, United Kingdom

NI WEI, PhD, MS
Department of Rheumatology, Dongfang Hospital, Beijing University of Chinese Medicine, Beijing, China

MATTHEW J. WOOD, PhD
Department of Internal Medicine, Division of Rheumatology, Rush University Medical Center, Chicago, Illinois, USA

Contents

The Burden of Osteoarthritis in Older Adults   181

Gillian A. Hawker and Lauren K. King

Osteoarthritis (OA) is the most common form of arthritis and a leading cause of disability among older people. One in 3 people over age 65, and disproportionately more women than men, are living with OA. The prevalence of OA is rising related to an increasing prevalence of OA risk factors, including aging and obesity. In older adults, OA frequently exists alongside other common chronic conditions and may increase the risk for worse outcomes from these conditions. Given the growing burden and impact of OA, enhanced effort is required to deliver effective and safe treatments to those living with the disease.

Osteoarthritis Pathophysiology: Therapeutic Target Discovery may Require a
Multifaceted Approach   193

Tonia L. Vincent, Tamara Alliston, Mohit Kapoor, Richard F. Loeser, Linda Troeberg, and Christopher B. Little

Molecular understanding of osteoarthritis (OA) has greatly increased through careful analysis of tissue samples, preclinical models, and large-scale agnostic "-omic" studies. There is broad acceptance that systemic and biomechanical signals affect multiple tissues of the joint, each of which could potentially be targeted to improve patient outcomes. In this review six experts in different aspects of OA pathogenesis provide their independent view on what they believe to be good tractable approaches to OA target discovery. We conclude that molecular discovery has been high but future transformative studies require a multidisciplinary holistic approach to develop therapeutic strategies with high clinical efficacy.

The Genesis of Pain in Osteoarthritis: Inflammation as a Mediator of Osteoarthritis
Pain   221

Matthew J. Wood, Rachel E. Miller, and Anne-Marie Malfait

Chronic pain is a substantial personal and societal burden worldwide. Osteoarthritis (OA) is one of the leading causes of chronic pain and is increasing in prevalence in accordance with a global aging population. In addition to affecting patients' physical lives, chronic pain also adversely affects patients' mental wellbeing. However, there remain no pharmacologic interventions to slow down the progression of OA and pain-alleviating therapies are largely unsuccessful. The presence of low-level inflammation in OA has been recognized for many years as a major pathogenic driver of joint damage. Inflammatory mechanisms can occur locally in joint tissues, such as the synovium, within the sensory nervous system, as well as systemically, caused by modifiable and unmodifiable factors. Understanding how inflammation may contribute to, and modify pain in OA will be instrumental in identifying new druggable targets for analgesic therapies. In this narrative review, we discuss recent insights into inflammatory mechanisms in OA pain. We discuss how local inflammation in the joint can contribute to mechanical sensitization and to the structural neuroplasticity of joint nociceptors, through pro-inflammatory factors such as nerve growth factor, cytokines, and chemokines. We consider the role of synovitis, and the amplifying mechanisms of neuroimmune interactions. We then explore emerging evidence around the role of neuroinflammation in the dorsal root ganglia and dorsal horn. Finally, we discuss how systemic inflammation associated with obesity may modify OA pain and suggest future research directions.

Osteoarthritis Flares

Martin J. Thomas, Francis Guillemin, and Tuhina Neogi

The phenomenon of flares is a common feature in the daily life of people with osteoarthritis (OA). Characterized by episodes of sudden-onset increases in signs and symptoms, their impact can often be distressing and disabling. Despite their potential to have both short-term and long-term consequences for patients across the whole course of the condition, their occurrence and optimal management are not fully understood. This article provides a contemporary perspective on defining OA flares and their potential triggers, and offers suggestions for how health professionals might explore flare patterns with patients in clinical practice and frame timely best-practice treatment approaches.

The Challenges in the Primary Prevention of Osteoarthritis

Jos Runhaar and Sita M.A. Bierma-Zeinstra

In the absence of disease-modifying drugs and small to moderate efficacy of symptom relieving therapies, the primary prevention of osteoarthritis (OA) is important. The current review addresses some of the key challenges for primary OA prevention. Identification of the target group, the design of the intervention, and aspects of the effect evaluation are all discussed from an OA prevention perspective. Although OA prevention is still in its infancy, it holds great potential. Given the enormous burden of OA for patients and society, primary OA prevention should be a high priority in the field of OA research.

Phenotypes in Osteoarthritis: Why Do We Need Them and Where Are We At?

Murillo Dório and Leticia A. Deveza

This article is part of the Osteoarthritis issue for the Clinics in Geriatric Medicine journal. It covers the main aspects related to research and clinical practice of osteoarthritis phenotyping, including the concepts, the rationale for studies of OA phenotypes and their history, the approaches to OA phenotyping, recent advances in this area, and future directions.

populations, there is less research examining alternative interventions, or in the hand OA population. This problem is complicated by the lack of gold-standard measurement of adherence for core osteoarthritis treatments. The predictors of treatment adherence are not well understood, and findings are contradictory. Strategies incorporating behavior change techniques should be implemented to improve and maintain long-term adherence.

Osteoarthritis (OA) is a leading cause of disability. Clinical practice guidelines recommend education on OA management, exercise, and weight control. However, many people with OA do not receive this recommended OA care. Some health care professionals (HCPs) lack the knowledge and skills to deliver recommended OA care. This article presents a framework to guide the development and evaluation of education and training for HCPs in the delivery of evidence-based OA care including: (1) Overarching principles for education and training; (2) Core capabilities for the delivery of best evidence OA care; (3) Theories of learning and preferences for delivery; (4) Evaluation of education and training.

This narrative review highlights the prevalence of osteoarthritis as a chronic disease that directly contributes to the ever-growing health care expenditure to treat this condition. The increasing demand of total joint arthroplasty globally is explained in conjunction with the importance of understanding candidate suitability for arthroplasty surgery in order to maximize surgical outcomes and self-reported patient satisfaction after the surgery. Rehabilitation care following total hip arthroplasty and total knee arthroplasty, particularly the inappropriate use of inpatient rehabilitation service, is also explained, in addition to the enhanced recovery after surgery.

Osteoarthritis (OA) causes a massive disease burden with a global prevalence of nearly 23% in 2020 and an unmet need for adequate treatment, given a lack of disease-modifying drugs (DMOADs). The author reviews the prospects of active DMOAD candidates in the phase 2/3 clinical trials of drug development pipeline based on key OA pathogenetic mechanisms directed to inflammation-driven, bone-driven, and cartilage-driven endotypes. The challenges and possible research opportunities are stated in terms of the formulation of a research question known as the PICO approach: (1) population, (2) interventions, (3) comparison or placebo, and (4) outcomes.

Improving the health and well-being of people with osteoarthritis (OA) requires effective action beyond health service delivery. Integration of the different contexts and settings in which people live, work, and socialize, also known as the social determinants of health (SDH), with health care has the potential to provide additional benefits to health and well-being outcomes compared with traditional OA care. This article explores how SDH can impact the lives of people with OA, how SDH intersect at different stages of OA progression, and opportunities for integrating SDH factors to address the onset and management of OA across the life course.

CLINICS IN GERIATRIC MEDICINE

FORTHCOMING ISSUES

August 2022
COVID-19 in the Geriatric Patient
Francesco Landi, *Editor*

November 2022
Polypharmacy
Edward Schneider and Brandon K. Koretz,
Editors

February 2023
**Practical Aspects of Cognitive Impairment
and the Dementias**
Philip B. Gorelick and Farzaneh Sorond,
Editors

RECENT ISSUES

February 2022
**Alcohol and Substance Abuse in Older
Adults**
Rita Khoury and George T. Grossberg,
Editors

November 2021
Women's Health
Karen A. Blackstone and
Elizabeth L. Cobbs, *Editors*

August 2021
Sleep in the Elderly
Steven H. Feinsilver and Margarita Oks,
Editors

SERIES OF RELATED INTEREST

Primary Care: Clinics in Office Practice
https://www.primarycare.theclinics.com/
Immunology and Allergy Clinics
http://www.immunology.theclinics.com/

THE CLINICS ARE AVAILABLE ONLINE!
Access your subscription at:
www.theclinics.com

Preface

Developing a Deeper Understanding of Osteoarthritis: Care to Joint Us?

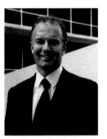

David J. Hunter, MBBS, MSc (Clin Epi), M SpMed, PhD, FRACP (Rheum)
Editor

It gives me great pleasure to introduce this thematic issue for *Clinics in Geriatric Medicine* with a brief overview of what you can anticipate learning more about by reading further. I have had the enviable privilege of being the Guest Editor for a number of previous themed issues, and I am pleased to say that the content compiled herein is unsurpassed in my experience. All credit for this goes to the authors of the individual articles, who have compiled insightful and critical iterations of complex and important topics. I sincerely thank them for their invaluable contributions.

This is an exciting time to be involved in what is characteristically a much-maligned disease. Our understanding of many important concepts is rapidly evolving, and our therapeutic armamentarium is continuing to expand. The importance of this thematic issue is underpinned by the huge burden of this highly prevalent, disabling disease affecting more than 500 million people worldwide.[1] This substantial prevalence is accompanied by tremendous individual and socioeconomic burden. It is this impact that provides a solid motivation to make a difference for the millions of people who are affected.

Osteoarthritis (OA) was historically regarded as a degenerative disorder resulting from cartilage damage, but our modern understanding of this whole joint disease involves structural alterations in hyaline articular cartilage, subchondral bone, synovium, ligaments, capsule, and periarticular muscles. Consistent with the complex underlying pathogenesis is a remarkably detailed route to symptom onset and pain progression. It is important to understand that the majority of people who present with pain characteristically have this as an episodic phenomenon, which we otherwise describe as "flares."[2] Many irreversible management decisions are made during these flare episodes, and it's important to understand their finite natural history and the typical pattern of resolution within days.

For most of the millions of people affected by OA, its development can be linked to multiple risk factors. For knee OA, which accounts for approximately 85% of the burden attributable to OA,[3] the leading risk factors are eminently modifiable, namely, obesity and joint injury. As there is currently no cure for OA, this is of paramount importance, and we hope to see increasing public health interventions to stem disease onset.[4]

OA is an umbrella diagnosis referring to a multifaceted and heterogeneous syndrome rather than one single disease.[5] Recent literature describes subgrouping of OA and characterization based on differences in prognosis, therapeutic response, or disease mechanisms. The commonly described identifiable predisposing factors (possible mechanistic phenotypes) for most forms of OA include hormonal, metabolic syndrome, posttraumatic, mechanical overload, inflammatory, genetic, and aging.

The initial assessment for OA should include a complete history and physical examination, including ascertaining the effect of OA on function, quality of life, occupation, mood, sleep, social interactions, ability to engage within the community, and leisure activities.[6,7] A number of recent studies have demonstrated that the majority of patients do not receive appropriate care[8] and have further highlighted the areas where we are not serving our patients well by underutilizing efficacious, evidence-based lifestyle and behavioral management, particularly exercise and weight loss.[9]

Active, nonpharmacologic interventions are the mainstay of OA management and should be tried first, followed by or in concert with medications to relieve pain when necessary.[10] These core treatments (often referred to as nonpharmacologic/conservative therapies) include education, weight management/diet, promotion of physical activity, strengthening exercises, and behavior change support.[11] Optimal uptake of recommendations and adherence to behavior change modifications are key elements of OA treatment and can be enhanced by education, establishing treatment goals, and regular monitoring. Referral of patients with end-stage OA to a surgeon should be considered when all appropriate conservative options, delivered for a reasonable period, have failed.

It is my sincere hope that you enjoy reading and learning from the wonderful content compiled in this issue. The authors have been a pleasure to work with, and I am sure you will see from their respective contents an abundance of insight and thoughtful appraisals of complicated and evolving fields.

DISCLOSURES

D.J.H. provides consulting advice on scientific advisory boards for Pfizer, Lilly, TLCBio, Novartis, Tissuegene, and Biobone.

David J. Hunter, MBBS, MSc (Clin Epi), M SpMed, PhD, FRACP (Rheum)
Kolling Institute
Level 10, 10 Westbourne Street
St Leonards, NSW 2064, Australia

E-mail address:
david.hunter@sydney.edu.au

REFERENCES

1. Hunter DJ, March L, Chew M. Osteoarthritis in 2020 and beyond: a Lancet Commission. Lancet 2020;396(10264):1711–2.
2. Bowden JL, Kobayashi S, Hunter DJ, et al. Best-practice clinical management of flares in people with osteoarthritis: a scoping review of behavioral, lifestyle and adjunctive treatments. Semin Arthritis Rheum 2021;51(4):749–60.
3. Disease GBD. Injury I, Prevalence C. Global, regional, and national incidence, prevalence, and years lived with disability for 310 diseases and injuries, 1990-2015: a systematic analysis for the Global Burden of Disease Study 2015. Lancet 2016;388(10053):1545–602.
4. Runhaar J, Zhang Y. Can we prevent OA? Epidemiology and public health insights and implications. Rheumatology (Oxford) 2018;57(suppl_4):iv3–9.
5. Deveza LA, Loeser RF. Is osteoarthritis one disease or a collection of many? Rheumatology (Oxford) 2018;57(suppl_4):iv34–42.
6. National Institute for Health and Care Excellence (NICE). Osteoarthritis: care and management. Clinical guideline (CG177). UK: National Institute for Health and Care Excellent; 2014.
7. Hunter DJ. Guideline for the management of knee and hip osteoarthritis. 2nd edition. Melbourne (Australia): RACGP; 2018.
8. Runciman WB, Hunt TD, Hannaford NA, et al. CareTrack: assessing the appropriateness of health care delivery in Australia. Med J Aust 2012;197(2):100–5.
9. Basedow M, Esterman A. Assessing appropriateness of osteoarthritis care using quality indicators: a systematic review. J Eval Clin Pract 2015;21(5):782–9.
10. Bowden JL, Hunter DJ, Deveza LA, et al. Core and adjunctive interventions for osteoarthritis: efficacy and models for implementation. Nat Rev Rheumatol 2020;16(8):434–47.
11. McAlindon TE, Bannuru RR, Sullivan M, et al. OARSI guidelines for the non-surgical management of knee osteoarthritis. Osteoarthritis Cartilage 2014;22(3): 363–88.

The Burden of Osteoarthritis in Older Adults

Gillian A. Hawker, MD, MSc[a,b,*], Lauren K. King, MD, MSc[a,b]

KEYWORDS

- Osteoarthritis - Prevalence - Incidence - Risk factors - Economic burden

KEY POINTS

- OA is a serious, disabling condition that disproportionately affects older women and individuals with obesity.
- The coprevalence of symptomatic OA in older individuals with other common chronic conditions is high because of common risk factors, for example, aging and obesity.
- Untreated painful OA impacts sleep quality, causes fatigue, limits mobility and physical activity, and contributes to depressed mood, all of which reduce individuals' quality of life and the effective management of comorbid conditions.
- Enhanced efforts to diagnose and treat symptomatic OA among older adults are needed.

INTRODUCTION

Osteoarthritis (OA) is a serious disease. The most common form of arthritis,[1] OA typically affects the hips, knees, hands, feet, and spine, and multijoint involvement is common.[2] OA affects 1 in 3 older adults and women more so than men.[1,3] Risk factors for OA include aging, obesity, prior joint injury, genetics, sex, and anatomic factors related to joint shape and alignment.[4,5] As longevity and obesity increase, so, too, has the prevalence of OA.[4,6,7]

OA is both a disease, with pathologic changes in the joint tissues (articular cartilage, subchondral bone, menisci, ligaments, etc.)[8] and an illness (ie, symptomatic OA), characterized by joint pain and functional limitations.[9–12] There is imperfect concordance between the disease and the illness; many people with structural changes on imaging will not develop symptoms, whereas the illness may occur before

Disclosure: G.A. Hawker has received research support as the Sir John and Lady Eaton Professor and Chair of Medicine, Department of Medicine, University of Toronto; all other authors declare no other relationships or activities that could appear to have influenced the submitted work.
^a Department of Medicine, University of Toronto, 6 Queen's Park Crescent West, 3rd Floor, Toronto, Ontario M5S 3H2, Canada; ^b Women's College Research Institute, 76 Grenville Street, 6th Floor, Toronto, Ontario, M5S 1B2, Canada
* Corresponding author.
E-mail address: g.hawker@utoronto.ca

Clin Geriatr Med 38 (2022) 181–192
https://doi.org/10.1016/j.cger.2021.11.005
0749-0690/22/© 2021 Elsevier Inc. All rights reserved.

radiographic changes are evident. It is the illness that drives affected individuals to seek care. OA-related joint pain causes functional limitations, fatigue, depressed mood, and loss of independence, and is the primary indication for joint replacement surgery.[9,10,12] Addressing the illness of OA is crucial to reduce the enormous individual and societal burden of OA.[13]

Although effective evidence-based treatments exist for OA,[14] competing health care demands,[15] due to comorbidities and widespread societal beliefs that OA is an inevitable part of aging for which nothing can be done, often lead to underdiagnosis and undertreatment of OA. A new narrative that reflects current evidence is needed.

INCIDENCE AND PREVALENCE OF SYMPTOMATIC OA

Estimates of the incidence and prevalence of OA vary depending on the definition (disease vs illness) and joints considered. Irrespective of the definition, the number of people living with symptomatic OA is on the rise. From the Global Burden of Diseases, Injuries, and Risk Factors Study, the age-standardized annual incidence rates for symptomatic hip and knee OA rose 8.2% between 1990 and 2017.[16] In 2019, it was estimated that more than 500 million people or roughly 7% of the global population were living with OA (knee, hip, hand, and other sites).[17] Of these, nearly 70% had knee OA, compared with 6% hip OA and 27% hand OA.[17] From population-based studies, the prevalence of OA in persons over 40 years of age is about 22%.[18] From prospective population-based studies, the rates of doctor-diagnosed hand, knee, and hip OA increase with age, peaking in the 70s overall, but somewhat earlier for hand OA, while prevalence continues to rise.[19]

The prevalence of multijoint OA is high. From the US Osteoarthritis Initiative and multicenter OA (MOST) studies, 80% of individuals with bilateral knee pain had remote site pain, including low back pain.[20] In a cohort of individuals undergoing primary, elective knee replacement for knee OA, 25.9% had concomitant low back pain; 23.95% had pain, aching, and stiffness in one or both hips; and 50.3% reported these symptoms in both knees.[21]

RISK FACTORS FOR OA

As noted earlier, there are many risk factors for OA. Of these, *aging* is the most prominent (**Fig. 1**).[6,16,19] However, OA is not an inevitable consequence of aging. From the US National Health Interview Survey (NHIS), the prevalence of diagnosed knee OA among those aged 85 years and older ranged from ~13% in men without obesity to 32% in women with obesity.[22]

The relationship between aging and OA is complex. As joints age, their ability to withstand insult lessens.[23] Increased cellular stresses in OA joint tissues, mitochondrial dysfunction, and dysfunction in energy metabolism associated with aging may contribute to cellular damage and disturbance of homeostatic physiologic cell signaling. Age-related changes in the extracellular matrix of cartilage reduce their ability to sense and respond to joint loading, increasing the risk for joint injury. A proinflammatory, catabolic state that, in the context of increased susceptibility to cell death and defective repair of the damaged matrix, leads to joint tissue destruction.[23]

Irrespective of age, OA disproportionately affects *women* (see **Fig. 1**) and those with *obesity*.[16,24] As for aging, the relationship between OA and sex/gender is complex. Systematic sex/gender differences in exposure to OA risk factors likely contribute to higher incidence and prevalence of OA in women than men. The incidence of OA rises among women around the time of menopause. Thus, many studies have investigated the potential impact of hormonal factors on risk for OA though findings remain

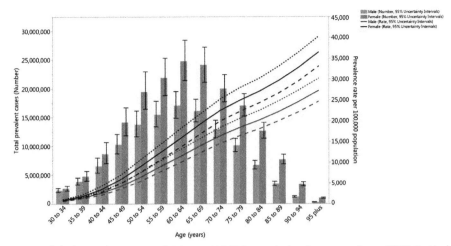

Fig. 1. Global prevalence rate of OA per 100,000 population by age and sex, 2017. Dotted and dashed lines indicate 95% upper and lower uncertainty intervals, respectively. Generated from data available from http://ghdx.healthdata.org/gbd-results-tool. (*From* Safiri S, Kolahi A, Smith E, et al. Global, regional and national burden of osteoarthritis 1990-2017: a systematic analysis of the Global Burden of Disease Study 2017 Ann Rheum Dis. 2020;79(6):819-28; with permission. (Figure 1 in original).)

inconclusive.[25] Systematic sex/gender differences in muscle strength, mechanical joint load, bone mass/bone turnover, metabolic factors, and nutritional differences may also contribute to higher incidence and prevalence of symptomatic OA in women than men.[26,27] Gender differences in financial resources, social support, and gender biases in access to OA diagnosis and treatment may also contribute to these differences.[28,29]

Obesity is the most important modifiable risk factor for the development and progression of OA, more so for knee OA than for OA in other joints. In a meta-analysis of 14 prospective studies, Zheng and colleagues found that overweight and obesity were associated with significantly higher knee OA risks (relative risk [RR] 2.45, 95% confidence interval [CI] 1.88–3.20, and RR 4.55, 95% CI 2.90–7.13, respectively); the risk of knee OA increased by 35% (95% CI 18%–53%) per 5 kg/m^2 increase in body mass index (BMI).[30] The lifetime risk of symptomatic knee OA has been estimated to be approximately 3 times higher among individuals with BMI $\geq$ 30 kg/m^2 and 5 times higher among individuals with BMI $\geq$ 35 kg/m^2 compared with individuals with BMI less than 25 kg/m^2 (**Fig. 2**).[31] BMI is also strongly predictive of lifetime risk for hip or knee joint replacement surgery.[32,33]

THE RELATIONSHIP BETWEEN SOCIAL DETERMINANTS OF HEALTH AND OA

Race/ethnicity, socioeconomic status, and geographic variations in the prevalence and severity of knee and hip OA are well established. This variation likely reflects person-level differences in risk for OA, for example, due to obesity, physical inactivity, and joint injury, and health system variability in access and outcomes of care. For example, OA prevalence is higher in high-income than lower-income countries (**Fig. 3**).[16,18] Compared with other countries, the United States had the highest age-standardized prevalence of OA in 2017 (6128.1 per 100,000) and had experienced the greatest increase in prevalence (23.2%) over the period 1990 to 2017.[16] Within

Incidence of knee OA
(1,000/ persons-year)

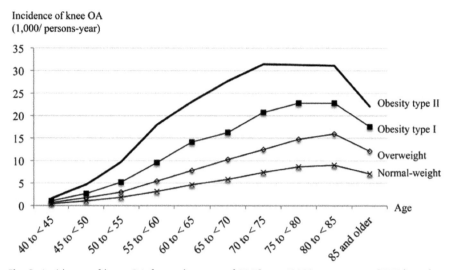

Fig. 2. Incidence of knee OA for each range of BMI[a] per 1000/persons-year. [a]BMI based on WHO definitions: normal-weight (<25 kg/m^2), overweight (25 to <30 kg/m^2), obesity I (30 to <35 kg/m^2), and obesity II (35 kg/m^2 and over). (*From* Reyes C, Leyland KM, Peat G, Cooper C, Arden NK, Prieto-Alhambra D. Association Between Overweight and Obesity and Risk of Clinically Diagnosed Knee, Hip, and Hand Osteoarthritis: A Population-Based Cohort Study. Arthritis Rheumatol 2016;68:1869-75; with permission. (Figure 1 in original).)

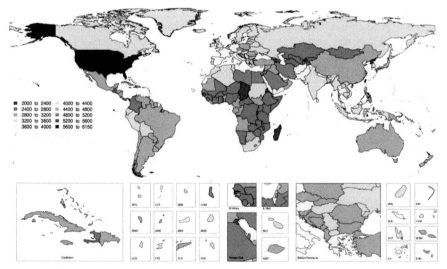

Fig. 3. Age-standardized prevalence estimates of OA per 100,000 population in 2017, by country. Generated from data available from http://ghdx.healthdata.org/gbd-results-tool. (*From* Safiri S, Kolahi A, Smith E, et al. Global, regional and national burden of osteoarthritis 1990-2017: a systematic analysis of the Global Burden of Disease Study 2017. Ann Rheum Dis. 2020;79(6):819-28; with permission. (Figure 2 in original).)

the United States, both lower socioeconomic status and African Americans have been found to have higher incidence, prevalence, and severity of OA than US whites.[34]

IMPACT OF OA ON OTHER CONDITIONS AND MORTALITY

Older age and obesity are risk factors for OA and many other chronic conditions. Thus, most older people living with symptomatic OA have at least one other chronic condition,[35] typically cardiometabolic conditions such as type 2 diabetes mellitus (T2DM) and cardiovascular (CV) diseases.[36] For example, in a meta-analysis of more than 1 million individuals, the risk of T2DM was 40% higher in individuals with versus without OA and 30% of individuals with T2DM had OA.[37]

Symptomatic hip and knee OA have also been linked to higher risk for incident cardiometabolic conditions, such as diabetes and heart disease,[7,38] and both CV-related and all-cause mortality.[39] Across multiple cohorts, and after controlling for potential confounders, a meta-analysis found that individuals with hip and knee OA were at 21% higher risk for CV-related death (hazard ratio [HR] 1.21, 95% CI 1.10–1.34) and 18% increased risk of all-cause death (HR 1.18, 95% CI 1.08–1.28) compared with those without.[40] These relationships appear to be due, at least in part to OA-related walking disability and resultant physical inactivity.[40–42]

LIVING WITH OA

Pain is the top concern for people living with OA. The pain associated with joint discomfort is highly variable and evolves over time. From qualitative studies, people describe early-stage OA pain as worse with joint use and improving with rest.[8,43] As the disease progresses, the pain may become more constant, punctuated increasingly with short episodes of a more intense, often unpredictable, and emotionally draining pain, leading to avoidance of social and recreational activities.[43] Consistent with this, clinical studies suggest that early-stage OA pain is largely nociceptive in nature, emanating from richly innervated joint tissues, including the subchondral bone and periosteum.[44] As OA progresses, neuroplastic changes in the peripheral and central nervous systems may occur, resulting in pain sensitisation[44,45] Pain in OA can be best considered using a biopsychosocial model (**Fig. 4**).[46]

The downstream effects of OA-related joint pain are considerable. From a community-based longitudinal study of more than 500 people with hip and knee OA, OA pain is causally related to fatigue[10,47] and functional limitations.[48] Fatigue and functional limitations, in turn, increase individuals' risk for depressed or anxious mood,[9,12] which leads to worsening of OA pain and disability and increased risk for loss of independence (**Fig. 5**).[9,48,49]

Fatigue and Sleep

From 35% to 41% of adults with OA report clinically significant fatigue, similar to that seen among adults with rheumatoid arthritis.[50,51] The high prevalence of fatigue in OA may be due, at least in part, to OA pain-related sleep disturbances.[52,53] OA pain is associated with delayed sleep onset, bedtime anxiety, and altered sleep architecture, resulting in sleep deprivation and disruption of slow-wave sleep.[54] These effects are exacerbated by a high prevalence of comorbid sleep disturbances, including restless legs syndrome and obstructive sleep apnea.[52,53] Thus, among older people with symptomatic OA, there is a high prevalence of poor sleep. In a community cohort of more than 600 individuals with symptomatic hip/knee OA (mean age 78 years), 70% reported poor sleep (Pittsburgh Sleep Quality Index >5).[10]

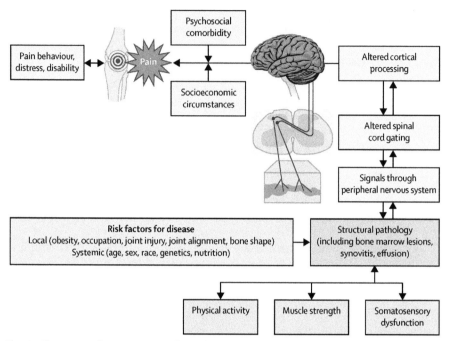

Fig. 4. The cause of pain in OA within a biopsychosocial model. (*From* Hunter DJ, Bierma-Zeinstra S. Osteoarthritis. Lancet 2019;393:1745–59; with permission. (**Figure 3** in original). Reprinted with permission of Elsevier.)

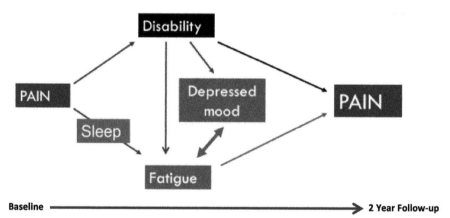

Fig. 5. Longitudinal relationships between OA-related pain, sleep, fatigue, mood, and disability, over time and adjusting for covariates[a]. [a]A path analysis was performed to test interrelationships among pain, depression, fatigue, and disability for more than 500 community-cohort participants with symptomatic hip or knee OA. Controlling for psychosocial and demographic factors, it was found that female gender, older age, pain catastrophizing, poor coping behaviors, lower social support, worse general health status, and greater number of other chronic conditions negatively influenced these relationships over time. (*Adapted from* Hawker GA, Gignac MA, Badley E, et al. A longitudinal study to explain the pain-depression link in older adults with osteoarthritis. Arthritis Care Res (Hoboken). 2011;63(10):1382-1390; with permission. (Figure 2 in original).)

Mental Health

The prevalence of anxiety and depression is significantly higher in people with versus without OA. A systematic review reported a pooled prevalence of symptoms of depression of ~20% and symptoms of anxiety of ~21% among people with symptomatic OA.[55] Greater OA symptom severity increases the likelihood of developing depressed or anxious mood. Among individuals with painful OA, the presence of depressed or anxious mood is associated with greater health care use and worse outcomes.[9,56,57]

Activity Limitations and Participation Restrictions

Hand OA is the most common disease affecting hand function in the elderly. Symptomatic hand OA is associated with reduced grip and pinch strength,[58] resulting in difficulty lifting, dressing, and eating.[59] Lower extremity OA is associated with activity limitations, contributing to physical inactivity, participation restrictions, and loss of independence.[7,60,61] Inadequate treatment of OA pain also contributes, as people learn to manage their symptoms by avoiding physical activities, like walking, that exacerbate their pain.[38,62,63] In a Canadian cohort of ~30,000 people aged 55 years or older,[60] the estimated probability of difficulty walking for an 80-year-old middle-income woman rose from 11% (no OA, no health conditions) to 52% with hypertension, heart disease, and a prior hip fracture, compared with 65% with 2 hips or knee affected by symptomatic OA (**Fig. 6**). If she had hypertension, heart disease, a prior hip fracture, and OA, the probability of difficulty walking was 99%.

CONTEXTUAL FACTORS INFLUENCING THE DOWNSTREAM IMPACT OF PAINFUL OA

Individuals' ability to cope with OA pain is influenced by their attitudes and tolerance of the pain (pain catastrophizing), efforts expended on coping, and level of social support. Greater pain catastrophizing, poor coping, and lower social support have consistently been found to negatively influence the impact of OA pain on sleep, fatigue, disability, and mood, and thus on OA-related quality of life over time.[9,10,12]

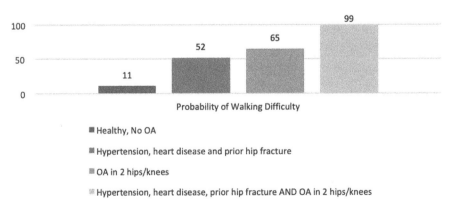

Fig. 6. Estimated probability of difficulty walking for an 80-year-old middle-income woman without obesity by the presence of comorbid conditions and hip/knee OA. (*Adapted from* King LK, Kendzerska T, Waugh EJ, Hawker GA. Impact of Osteoarthritis on Difficulty Walking: A Population-Based Study. Arthritis Care Res (Hoboken) 2018;70:71-9; with permission.)

Table 1 Economic costs of OA		
Direct Costs	**Indirect Costs**	**Intangible Costs**
Costs of surgery	Loss of productivity	Pain and suffering
Hospital resources	Absenteeism	Decreased quality of life
Caregiver time	Premature mortality	Potential depression/
Pharmacologic and nonpharmacologic treatments	Disability payments/ benefits	anxiety
Costs of side effects from treatments		
Research		

From Chen A, Gupte C, Akhtar K, Smith P, Cobb J. The Global Economic Cost of Osteoarthritis: How the UK Compares. Arthritis. 2012;2012:698709; with permission. (Table 1 in original)

ECONOMIC IMPACT OF OA

Musculoskeletal conditions, including OA, have a substantial contribution to health care costs, accounting for an estimated 1.0% to 2.5% of the gross domestic product in the United States, Canada, the United Kingdom, France, and Australia.[64] Approximately 80% of the costs owing to musculoskeletal conditions are estimated to be related to symptomatic OA, including direct costs to the health care system, indirect costs to individuals living with OA, and the intangible costs of living with a chronic disabling condition (**Table 1**).[65] Greater health care use and associated costs are strongly related to OA pain severity.[66] The largest contributor to direct health care costs for OA is joint replacement surgery.[67] As the incidence and prevalence of symptomatic OA rises, so too do the societal costs. The aggregate expenses paid for the treatment of knee OA increased by $1 billion from 2009 to 2014.

SUMMARY

Symptomatic OA is associated with substantial, persistent morbidity impacting day-to-day functioning. The pain, fatigue, depressed or anxious mood, and disability, including loss of mobility, that characterizes symptomatic OA present major barriers to healthy aging. The burden of symptomatic OA is increasing worldwide and disproportionately among women, those with lower education levels, and the socially disadvantaged. Although there is currently no cure for OA, many treatments exist to improve the OA-related quality of life of older adults. It is time to recognize that OA is a serious disease. It warrants far greater attention by health care providers and the health care system.

CLINICS CARE POINTS

- OA is a serious, disabling condition that disproportionately affects older women and individuals with obesity
- The coprevalence of symptomatic OA in older individuals with other common chronic conditions is high because of common risk factors, for example, aging and obesity
- Untreated painful OA impacts sleep quality, causes fatigue, limits mobility and physical activity, and contributes to depressed mood, all of which reduce individuals' quality of life and the effective management of comorbid conditions
- The burden and impact of OA is rising
- Enhanced efforts to diagnose and treat symptomatic OA among older adults are needed

REFERENCES

1. Global, regional, and national incidence, prevalence, and years lived with disability for 301 acute and chronic diseases and injuries in 188 countries, 1990-2013: a systematic analysis for the Global Burden of Disease Study 2013. Lancet 2015;386:743–800.
2. Badley EM, Wilfong JM, Yip C, et al. The contribution of age and obesity to the number of painful joint sites in individuals reporting osteoarthritis: a population-based study. Rheumatology (Oxford) 2020;59:3350–7.
3. Murphy L, Schwartz TA, Helmick CG, et al. Lifetime risk of symptomatic knee osteoarthritis. Arthritis Rheum 2008;59:1207–13.
4. Vina ER, Kwoh CK. Epidemiology of osteoarthritis: literature update. Curr Opin Rheumatol 2018;30:160–7.
5. Felson DT, Lawrence RC, Dieppe PA, et al. Osteoarthritis: new insights. Part 1: the disease and its risk factors. Ann Intern Med 2000;133:635–46.
6. Silverwood V, Blagojevic-Bucknall M, Jinks C, et al. Current evidence on risk factors for knee osteoarthritis in older adults: a systematic review and meta-analysis. Osteoarthr Cartil 2015;23:507–15.
7. Herbolsheimer F, Schaap LA, Edwards MH, et al. Physical activity patterns among older adults with and without knee osteoarthritis in six European Countries. Arthritis Care Res (Hoboken) 2016;68:228–36.
8. Vincent TL. Peripheral pain mechanisms in osteoarthritis. Pain 2020;161(Suppl 1): S138–46.
9. Hawker GA, Gignac MA, Badley E, et al. A longitudinal study to explain the pain-depression link in older adults with osteoarthritis. Arthritis Care Res (Hoboken) 2011;63:1382–90.
10. Hawker GA, French MR, Waugh EJ, et al. The multidimensionality of sleep quality and its relationship to fatigue in older adults with painful osteoarthritis. Osteoarthr Cartil 2010;18:1365–71.
11. Hawker GA. Osteoarthritis is a serious disease. Clin Exp Rheumatol 2019; 37(Suppl 120):3–6.
12. Sale JE, Gignac M, Hawker G. The relationship between disease symptoms, life events, coping and treatment, and depression among older adults with osteoarthritis. J Rheumatol 2008;35:335–42.
13. Whittaker JL, Runhaar J, Bierma-Zeinstra S, et al. A lifespan approach to osteoarthritis prevention: narrative review, part of the series. Osteoarthr Cartil 2021. https://doi.org/10.1016/j.joca.2021.06.015.
14. Bannuru RR, Osani MC, Vaysbrot EE, et al. OARSI guidelines for the non-surgical management of knee, hip, and polyarticular osteoarthritis. Osteoarthr Cartil 2019; 27:1578–89.
15. Christiansen MB, White DK, Christian J, et al. "It ... doesn't always make it [to] the top of the list": primary care physicians' experiences with prescribing exercise for knee osteoarthritis. Can Fam Phys 2020;66:e14–20.
16. Safiri S, Kolahi AA, Smith E, et al. Global, regional and national burden of osteoarthritis 1990-2017: a systematic analysis of the Global Burden of Disease Study 2017. Ann Rheum Dis 2020;79:819–28.
17. Global burden of disease study 2019 results. Available at: http://ghdx.healthdata.org/gbd-results-tool.
18. Cui A, Li H, Wang D, et al. Global, regional prevalence, incidence and risk factors of knee osteoarthritis in population-based studies. EClinicalMedicine 2020;29-30: 100587.

19. Prieto-Alhambra D, Judge A, Javaid MK, et al. Incidence and risk factors for clinically diagnosed knee, hip and hand osteoarthritis: influences of age, gender and osteoarthritis affecting other joints. Ann Rheum Dis 2014;9:1659–64.
20. Suri P, Morgenroth DC, Kwoh CK, et al. Low back pain and other musculoskeletal pain comorbidities in individuals with symptomatic osteoarthritis of the knee: data from the osteoarthritis initiative. Arthritis Care Res (Hoboken) 2010;62:1715–23.
21. Hawker GA, Conner-Spady BL, Bohm E, et al. Patients' preoperative expectations of total knee arthroplasty and satisfaction with outcomes at one year: a prospective cohort study. Arthritis Rheumatol 2021;73:223–31.
22. Losina E, Weinstein AM, Reichmann WM, et al. Lifetime risk and age at diagnosis of symptomatic knee osteoarthritis in the US. Arthritis Care Res (Hoboken) 2013; 65:703–11.
23. Loeser RF, Collins JA, Diekman BO. Ageing and the pathogenesis of osteoarthritis. Nat Rev Rheumatol 2016;12:412–20.
24. Srikanth VK, Fryer JL, Zhai G, et al. A meta-analysis of sex differences prevalence, incidence and severity of osteoarthritis. Osteoarthr Cartil 2005;13(9): 769–81.
25. Wluka AE, Cicuttini FM, Spector TD. Menopause, oestrogens and arthritis. Maturitas 2000;35:183–99.
26. Nicolella DP, O'Connor MI, Enoka RM, et al. Mechanical contributors to sex differences in idiopathic knee osteoarthritis. Biol Sex Differ 2012;3:28.
27. Ferre IM, Roof MA, Anoushiravani AA, et al. Understanding the observed sex discrepancy in the prevalence of osteoarthritis. JBJS Rev 2019;7:e8.
28. Hawker GA, Wright JG, Coyte PC, et al. Differences between men and women in the rate of use of hip and knee arthroplasty. N Engl J Med 2000;342:1016–22.
29. Borkhoff CM, Hawker GA, Kreder HJ, et al. Influence of patients' gender on informed decision making regarding total knee arthroplasty. Arthritis Care Res (Hoboken) 2013;65:1281–90.
30. Zheng H, Chen C. Body mass index and risk of knee osteoarthritis: systematic review and meta-analysis of prospective studies. BMJ Open 2015;5:e007568.
31. Reyes C, Leyland KM, Peat G, et al. Association between overweight and obesity and risk of clinically diagnosed knee, hip, and hand osteoarthritis: a population-based cohort study. Arthritis Rheumatol 2016;68:1869–75.
32. Lohmander LS, Gerhardsson de Verdier M, Rollof J, et al. Incidence of severe knee and hip osteoarthritis in relation to different measures of body mass: a population-based prospective cohort study. Ann Rheum Dis 2009;68:490–6.
33. Wang Y, Simpson JA, Wluka AE, et al. Relationship between body adiposity measures and risk of primary knee and hip replacement for osteoarthritis: a prospective cohort study. Arthritis Res Ther 2009;11:R31.
34. Callahan LF, Cleveland RJ, Allen KD, et al. Racial/ethnic, socioeconomic, and geographic disparities in the epidemiology of knee and hip osteoarthritis. Rheum Dis Clin North Am 2021;47:1–20.
35. Muckelt PE, Roos EM, Stokes M, et al. Comorbidities and their link with individual health status: a cross-sectional analysis of 23,892 people with knee and hip osteoarthritis from primary care. J Comorb 2020;10. 2235042x20920456.
36. Swain S, Sarmanova A, Coupland C, et al. Comorbidities in osteoarthritis: a systematic review and meta-analysis of observational studies. Arthritis Care Res (Hoboken) 2020;72:991–1000.
37. Louati K, Vidal C, Berenbaum F, et al. Association between diabetes mellitus and osteoarthritis: systematic literature review and meta-analysis. RMD Open 2015;1: e000077.

38. van Dijk GM, Veenhof C, Schellevis F, et al. Comorbidity, limitations in activities and pain in patients with osteoarthritis of the hip or knee. BMC Musculoskelet Disord 2008;9:95.

39. Hawker GA, Croxford R, Bierman AS, et al. All-cause mortality and serious cardiovascular events in people with hip and knee osteoarthritis: a population based cohort study. PLoS One 2014;9:e91286.

40. Veronese N, Cereda E, Maggi S, et al. Osteoarthritis and mortality: a prospective cohort study and systematic review with meta-analysis. Semin Arthritis Rheum 2016;46:160–7.

41. Wang H, Bai J, He B, et al. Osteoarthritis and the risk of cardiovascular disease: a meta-analysis of observational studies. Sci Rep 2016;6:39672.

42. Nuesch E, Dieppe P, Reichenbach S, et al. All cause and disease specific mortality in patients with knee or hip osteoarthritis: population based cohort study. BMJ 2011;342:d1165.

43. Hawker GA, Stewart L, French MR, et al. Understanding the pain experience in hip and knee osteoarthritis–an OARSI/OMERACT initiative. Osteoarthr Cartil 2008;16:415–22.

44. Neogi T. Structural correlates of pain in osteoarthritis. Clin Exp Rheumatol 2017; 35(Suppl 107):75–8.

45. Arendt-Nielsen L. Pain sensitisation in osteoarthritis. Clin Exp Rheumatol 2017; 35(Suppl 107):68–74.

46. Hunter DJ, Bierma-Zeinstra S. Osteoarthritis. Lancet 2019;393:1745–59.

47. Power JD, Badley EM, French MR, et al. Fatigue in osteoarthritis: a qualitative study. BMC Musculoskelet Disord 2008;9:63.

48. Gignac MA, Cott C, Badley EM. Adaptation to chronic illness and disability and its relationship to perceptions of independence and dependence. J Gerontol B Psychol Sci Soc Sci 2000;55:P362–72.

49. Neogi T. The epidemiology and impact of pain in osteoarthritis. Osteoarthr Cartil 2013;21:1145–53.

50. Hackney AJ, Klinedinst NJ, Resnick B, et al. A review and synthesis of correlates of fatigue in osteoarthritis. Int J Orthop Trauma Nurs 2019;33:4–10.

51. Cross M, Lapsley H, Barcenilla A, et al. Association between measures of fatigue and health-related quality of life in rheumatoid arthritis and osteoarthritis. Patient 2008;1:97–104.

52. Wilcox S, Brenes GA, Levine D, et al. Factors related to sleep disturbance in older adults experiencing knee pain or knee pain with radiographic evidence of knee osteoarthritis. J Am Geriatr Soc 2000;48:1241–51.

53. Moldofsky H. Sleep and pain. Sleep Med Rev 2001;5:385–96.

54. Lavigne GJ, Nashed A, Manzini C, et al. Does sleep differ among patients with common musculoskeletal pain disorders? Curr Rheumatol Rep 2011;13:535–42.

55. Stubbs B, Aluko Y, Myint PK, et al. Prevalence of depressive symptoms and anxiety in osteoarthritis: a systematic review and meta-analysis. Age Ageing 2016; 45:228–35.

56. Gleicher Y, Croxford R, Hochman J, et al. A prospective study of mental health care for comorbid depressed mood in older adults with painful osteoarthritis. BMC Psychiatry 2011;11:147.

57. Sharma A, Kudesia P, Shi Q, et al. Anxiety and depression in patients with osteoarthritis: impact and management challenges. Open Access Rheumatol 2016;8: 103–13.

58. Bagis S, Sahin G, Yapici Y, et al. The effect of hand osteoarthritis on grip and pinch strength and hand function in postmenopausal women. Clin Rheumatol 2003;22:420–4.
59. Dillon CF, Hirsch R, Rasch EK, et al. Symptomatic hand osteoarthritis in the United States: prevalence and functional impairment estimates from the third U.S. National Health and Nutrition Examination Survey, 1991-1994. Am J Phys Med Rehabil 2007;86:12–21.
60. King LK, Kendzerska T, Waugh EJ, et al. Impact of osteoarthritis on difficulty walking: a population-based study. Arthritis Care Res (Hoboken) 2018;70:71–9.
61. Petursdottir U, Arnadottir SA, Halldorsdottir S. Facilitators and barriers to exercising among people with osteoarthritis: a phenomenological study. Phys Ther 2010;90:1014–25.
62. Hawker GA, Croxford R, Bierman AS, et al. Osteoarthritis-related difficulty walking and risk for diabetes complications. Osteoarthr Cartil 2017;25:67–75.
63. Reeuwijk KG, de Rooij M, van Dijk GM, et al. Osteoarthritis of the hip or knee: which coexisting disorders are disabling? Clin Rheumatol 2010;29:739–47.
64. March LM, Bachmeier CJ. Economics of osteoarthritis: a global perspective. Baillieres Clin Rheumatol 1997;11:817–34.
65. Chen A, Gupte C, Akhtar K, et al. The global Economic cost of osteoarthritis: How the UK Compares. Arthritis 2012;2012:698709.
66. Rejas-Gutierrez J, Llopart-Carles N, García-López S, et al. Disease burden on health care by pain severity and usual analgesic treatment in patients with symptomatic osteoarthritis: a Spanish nationwide health survey. Expert Rev Pharmacoecon Outcomes Res 2021;21:711–9.
67. Ackerman IN, Bohensky MA, Zomer E, et al. The projected burden of primary total knee and hip replacement for osteoarthritis in Australia to the year 2030. BMC Musculoskelet Disord 2019;20:90.

Osteoarthritis Pathophysiology
Therapeutic Target Discovery may Require a Multifaceted Approach

Tonia L. Vincent, MD, FRCP, PhD[a], Tamara Alliston, PhD[b],
Mohit Kapoor, PhD[c], Richard F. Loeser, MD[d], Linda Troeberg, PhD[e],
Christopher B. Little, BVMS, PhD[f],*

KEYWORDS

- Osteoarthritis • Pathophysiology • Treatment targets • Bone • Cartilage
- Inflammation • Aging • Fibrosis

KEY POINTS

- Osteoarthritis is a complex disease affecting multiple tissues and involving multiple cellular processes. These are rarely all studied by a single research group.
- Target discovery therefore requires a holistic multidisciplinary approach to ensure that targets are valid across multiple tissues and relevant to the patient population.
- Good groundwork has been laid for the next phase in OA research, which will ensure that the right targets are tested to deliver translational benefit for patients.

INTRODUCTION

Osteoarthritis (OA) is the single most common painful joint condition; knee OA alone currently affects greater than 250 million people globally, and it is one of the fastest increasing health conditions worldwide.[1,2] The individual impact of OA includes pain

NOTE: All authors contributed equally to this research.
[a] Centre for Osteoarthritis Pathogenesis Versus Arthritis, Kennedy Institute of Rheumatology, University of Oxford, Oxford OX3 7FY, UK; [b] Department of Orthopaedic Surgery, University of California San Francisco, San Francisco, CA 94143, USA; [c] Department of Surgery and Laboratory Medicine and Pathobiology, Schroeder Arthritis Institute, Krembil Research Institute, University Health Network, University of Toronto, Toronto, Canada; [d] Department of Medicine, Division of Rheumatology, Allergy and Immunology and the Thurston Arthritis Research Center, University of North Carolina, Chapel Hill, NC, USA; [e] University of East Anglia, Norwich Medical School, Norwich NR4 7UQ, UK; [f] Raymond Purves Bone and Joint Research Laboratories, Kolling Institute University of Sydney Faculty of Medicine and Health at Royal North Shore Hospital, St. Leonards, New South Wales 2065, Australia
* Corresponding author.
E-mail address: christopher.little@sydney.edu.au

Clin Geriatr Med 38 (2022) 193–219
https://doi.org/10.1016/j.cger.2021.11.015
0749-0690/22/© 2021 Elsevier Inc. All rights reserved.

and loss of mobility and independence, 25% of patients being unable to carry out normal activities of daily life.[3,4] OA's societal burden is enormous, with current annual direct health care costs of knee OA alone estimated at up to $15 billion in the United States.[5] This figure is dwarfed by indirect costs of work absenteeism, early retirement, and loss of productivity associated with OA and associated medication use.[6] OA remains one of the major unresolved medical conditions, with no registered therapies that halt structural damage, and symptom-modifying interventions having only moderate long-term effect at best.[7]

It is clear that developing new, safe, effective OA treatments is an international health care and socioeconomic priority. A key underpinning requirement for therapeutic advancement in OA, as it is for all diseases, is knowledge of the cellular and molecular pathophysiology.[8] There has been an extraordinary increase in understanding of human-relevant OA biomolecular mechanisms over the last 15 years.[9–11] This has been associated with the recognition of OA as a joint-wide disease affecting and involving molecular and mechanical crosstalk between multiple tissues, and these with systemic processes and pathways. The complexity and breadth of new knowledge in OA pathophysiology, means the task of summarizing the key pathways is immense and crosses diverse mechanobiologic domains. In the current review, we have therefore taken the approach to ask individuals with expertise in six different aspects of OA pathogenesis (cartilage matrix degradation, inflammation, fibrosis, failed cartilage repair, bone remodeling, and aging), to provide a brief narrative review of what they consider the key disease mechanisms in their domain, with a lens to focus on those that may that offer the most promise for therapeutic targeting. The essays were written independently to avoid unintended collusion bias and are presented below, followed by a brief conclusion written after collation of the individual sections. We hope this approach not only provides a different, interesting, and more approachable review on a daunting topic but also allows identification of pathways and mechanisms that cross multiple aspects of OA and that contribute to the changing crosstalk between joint tissues as disease progresses.

TARGETING CARTILAGE DEGRADATION TO TREAT OSTEOARTHRITIS: LINDA TROEBERG

Degradation of the cartilage extracellular matrix (ECM) is appreciated to be an important feature of OA pathogenesis that, together with bone remodeling, leads to progressive joint damage and structural failure. Breakdown of type II collagen and aggrecan are thought to be most important, because these are the two most abundant cartilage matrix biomolecules and their loss reduces tensile strength and resistance to compression. A large body of evidence supports the conclusion that matrix metalloproteinases (MMPs) mediate type II collagen degradation, whereas related metalloproteinases, the adamalysins with thrombospondin motifs (ADAMTSs) are responsible for the degradation of aggrecan (**Fig. 1**).

Type II collagen is a stable molecule whose triple helical structure can only be cleaved by a handful of proteases, including cathepsin K and 4 collagenolytic MMPs (ie, MMP1, 8, 13, and 14). Collagen degradation occurs progressively in osteoarthritic cartilage,[12,13] and is blocked by metalloprotease inhibitors in vitro,[14,15] suggesting that the collagenolytic MMPs play a central role in this catabolic process. Two key papers support the assertion that MMP13 is a key collagenase in OA. First, transgenic mice overexpressing MMP-13 in cartilage exhibited increased collagen degradation by 5 months of age, along with increased cartilage erosion and joint pathology.[16] Second, *Mmp13*-null mice developed significantly less cartilage erosion

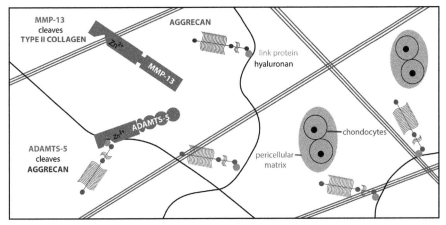

Fig. 1. MMPs and ADAMTSs metalloproteases cleave type II collagen and aggrecan in the OA cartilage extracellular matrix. Chondrocytes secrete metalloproteases that degrade the cartilage extracellular matrix in OA. Studies on transgenic mice suggest that MMP13 is the key collagenase in cartilage, whereas ADAMTS5 is the main aggrecanase.

8 weeks after surgical induction of OA.[17] Expression of MMP13 is increased in human and murine OA cartilage, and is highly inducible in vitro by inflammatory cytokines. The catalytic domains of MMPs are structurally homologous, so it has historically been difficult to design inhibitors that effectively target a single MMP without undesirable side effects. This is thought to be the reason that metalloproteinase inhibitors failed as cancer therapies,[18] despite clear evidence showing the important roles of MMPs in cancer metastasis and progression. MMP13, however, is unusual among MMPs in that it has deep pockets in its active site, so attempts have been made to design MMP13 inhibitors as potential OA therapies. These fared well in preclinical models,[19] but have not progressed further at present, most likely because of lingering concerns about lack of specificity and consequent toxicity.

The sequence of events in early OA is difficult to ascertain, but in vitro studies indicate that collagen breakdown starts late in the pathogenesis of OA, whereas breakdown of aggrecan occurs earlier.[20,21] Importantly, aggrecan loss in these models is reversible, whereas collagen loss is not. For many years, MMPs were thought to be responsible for the pathologic degradation of collagen and aggrecan in OA cartilage, but this view was challenged by Sandy and colleagues,[22] who showed that aggrecan fragments released into the synovial fluid of patients with OA had been cleaved at the $Glu^{373} \sim Ala^{374}$ bond, which is not targeted by MMPs. This sparked considerable interest in identifying the aggrecanases or enzymes responsible for pathologic breakdown of aggrecan, as targets for development of OA therapies. The first aggrecanase was purified from interleukin (IL)-1-stimulated bovine cartilage by Tortorella and colleagues,[23] and named A Disintegrin And Metalloproteinase with Thrombospondin motifs 4 (ADAMTS4) based on its homology to ADAMTS1. Another aggrecanase, ADAMTS5, was cloned shortly afterward,[24,25] and subsequent studies indicated this is the main murine aggrecanase, because mice lacking *Adamts5* were protected against aggrecan degradation and cartilage damage in two preclinical models of OA.[26,27] ADAMTS5 may also be the primary human aggrecanase,[28] although ADAMTS4 may also play a role.

Aggrecanase inhibitors have been designed by several groups, with some of these showing promising efficacy in preclinical models.[29] For example, Galapagos and Servier developed an ADAMTS5 catalytic domain inhibitor, GLPG1972/s201086, with good selectivity for ADAMTS5 and efficacy in preclinical rat and mouse OA models.[30,31] However, this inhibitor failed to meet its primary outcome (reduction in cartilage loss over 1 year by quantitative Magnetic Resonance Imaging (MRI)) or secondary outcomes, including pain and structural progression in a clinical trial (https://clinicaltrials.gov, NCT03595618). Some groups have taken the approach of designing inhibitors that target the noncatalytic domains of ADAMTSs, to reduce the potential for cross reactivity and off-target inhibition of homeostatic MMPs and related metalloproteases, such as ADAMs. For example, Santamaria and colleagues[32] recently generated small molecule exosite inhibitors of ADAMTS5, and Merck generated a cross-domain bispecific nanobody with good efficacy in a murine OA model.[33] However, a word of caution was raised by GlaxoSmithKline,[34] who found that their antibody against ADAMTS5 caused cardiac abnormalities in cynomolgus monkeys, which they suggest may relate to expression of ADAMTS5 in cardiovascular tissue. ADAMTS5 also has homeostatic roles in other tissues (reviewed by Santamaria[35]), suggesting further challenges for inhibitor design.

TARGETING INFLAMMATION TO TREAT OSTEOARTHRITIS: CHRISTOPHER B. LITTLE

Historically OA was considered a noninflammatory degenerative-joint-disease, and alternative names, such as osteoarthrosis, were proposed. However, just as the concept of passive wear-and-tear OA cartilage loss has been replaced with an understanding of a dynamic balance between biocellular repair and destruction (see sections by Troeberg and Vincent), the presence of synovial inflammation is now a well-recognized and consistent finding in patients with OA and preclinical animal models.[10,11,36,37] OA synovium, even in early stage disease, displays focal hyperplasia and hypertrophy of synovial lining cells, subintimal accumulation of inflammatory cells (macrophages, lymphocytes, plasma cells), and increased vascularity,[38,39] along with progressive fibrosis of the joint capsule (see section by Kapoor). In the OA knee, the infrapatellar fat pad as part of the functional synovial unit also has increased inflammatory cells and fibrotic changes, although with some unique characteristics compared with other synovial tissues.[40–42]

Synovial inflammation in OA is associated not only with symptoms but structural disease severity and progression in patients.[43–47] Beyond simply being a secondary response to late-stage joint tissue breakdown, synovial inflammatory mediators are more elevated acutely after OA-inducing joint injury[48] and in early compared with late OA.[38,45,49,50] Importantly, synovitis/joint effusion is associated not only with faster progression of established disease, but also more incident OA[43] and increased risk of post-traumatic OA following joint injury.[51] In light of this, it seems clear that the "itis" in OA is indeed appropriate, not only from the perspective of correctly describing the presence of synovial inflammation but also its potential pathophysiologic role in initiation and progression of structural and symptomatic disease.

Activation of the innate inflammatory/immune response in OA has been well-described and may be triggered by mechanical injury directly, as has been proposed for articular cartilage.[52] It is characterized by the influx of blood-derived monocytes and macrophages, which may contribute directly to increases in cytokines, growth factors, and pathologically relevant enzymes (eg, IL1, IL6, tumor necrosis factor [TNF], transforming growth factor [TGF]-β, MMP1, MMP13, ADAMTS4, ADAMTS5).[53–55] Lymphocytes, particularly CD4 and CD8 T cells, are also increased in OA synovium even in early disease stages, these cells producing cytokines, chemokines, and enzymes implicated in disease progression (eg, IL8, IL17, TNF, Chemokine (C-C motif) ligand 2 (CCL2), MMP1, MMP3, MMP9).[38,40,42,56–58] Stromal cells in the synovium and other joint tissues (eg, injured cruciate ligament) also increase synthesis of cytokines and chemokines,[59–61] and OA chondrocytes themselves increase expression of procatabolic cytokines (eg, IL8, IL12, IL17) that may act in an autocrine or paracrine manner to promote cartilage degradation.[62] Finally, systemic inflammation, particularly circulating cytokines (eg, IL6, TNF) and activated monocytes (eg, associated with obesity/metabolic-syndrome), further contribute to the proinflammatory milieux and complex cellular crosstalk that may initiate, perpetuate, and exacerbate joint-wide OA structural pathology and pain (**Fig. 2**).[53,63–66]

The previous discussion provides a glimpse of the burgeoning evidence for upregulation of a multitude of inflammatory pathways locally and systemically in OA, involving innate and adaptive immune cells, and numerous cytokines, chemokines, and growth factors. Dysregulation does not equal causality, however, so are there data supporting the therapeutic potential of targeting "inflammation" in OA, and which if any of the pathways may hold the most promise? Notwithstanding that samples are predominantly from late-stage disease, unbiased genome-wide mRNA expression and network analyses of different human joint tissues have identified highly relevant/hub genes and/or inflammatory processes in OA.[53,56,59,62,67] Although there are, not surprisingly, some differences between joint-tissue compartments and even cells with a given tissue, the commonly identified dysregulated inflammatory pathways in OA include: IL1, IL6, IL8, IL12, IL17, TNF, CCL2, M1/M2 macrophage polarization, and Th1 and Th17 CD4 T cells. There is supporting evidence from preclinical tissue culture and/or animal models that inhibiting or ablating any of the previously mentioned identified inflammatory pathways can modify onset, progression, and/or severity of various aspects of joint-wide structural and/or symptomatic OA.[10,11]

Despite the previously mentioned evidence, clinical trials targeting some of these pathways in patients with OA have been disappointing.[68,69] Does this mean inflammation is not as important an OA-therapeutic target as it appeared? In answering this, it is noteworthy that variable outcomes are reported in different OA disease models and

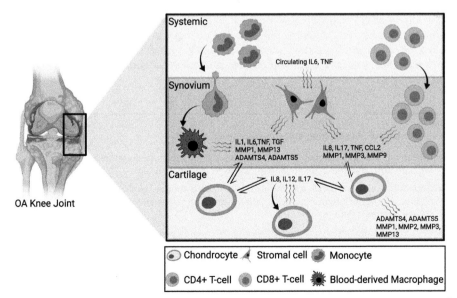

Fig. 2. Schematic image depicting the key inflammatory cells and soluble mediators and pathways implicated in osteoarthritis pathogenesis.

model systems, such as IL1 in monoiodoacetate-, meniscal destabilization-, meniscectomy-, and collagenase-induced OA[70–73]; and IL6 in post-traumatic and age-associated OA.[74,75] These preclinical data suggest that the specific inflammatory pathways involved and therefore usefully therapeutically targeted, may differ depending on the disease model, that is, it is disease-phenotype-dependent. This is consistent with human OA patient data showing differences in inflammatory dysregulation, such as in hip versus knee OA,[76] in knee OA in males versus females,[77] and the cytokines that correlate with different aspects of knee OA pain.[45,78] Even within a given OA population, distinct inflammatory cell/cytokine patient clusters can be identified, such as in those presenting for knee replacement.[79]

This OA inflammatory heterogeneity may, at least in part, explain the poor outcomes from clinical trials.[69] Just as in recognized inflammatory arthropathies,[80,81] a more nuanced approach to anti-inflammatory therapy in OA may be needed, such as selecting patients with a more inflammatory clinical phenotype, or potentially using biomarker analysis to identify particular inflammatory molecular endotypes within OA subpopulations. This is supported by serendipitous data from a large trial of IL1β inhibition for myocardial infarction in patients with elevated C-reactive protein, that demonstrated a significant reduction of incident or worsening OA symptoms and rates of total knee and hip replacement.[82] Although not designed with OA-relevant structure and symptom outcomes, this study strongly suggests that targeting the right inflammatory pathways in the right patients at the right time may make significant inroads to successfully treating OA (**Box 1**). As with many of the potential OA therapeutic approaches based on targeting pathophysiologic pathways, developing biomarkers to identify different patient cohorts is a key research imperative.

TARGETING SYNOVIAL FIBROSIS TO TREAT OSTEOARTHRITIS: MOHIT KAPOOR

The synovial membrane is a thin membrane that surrounds articular joints and comprises two main layers: a cellular intima and underlying collagen I–rich subintima.[83,84] The synovium is required to maintain joint integrity, lubrication, and homeostasis. Although most OA research has focused on mechanisms associated with articular cartilage degeneration, it is now believed that changes in the synovium may play an active role in driving OA pathogenesis. During OA, synovium presents with different synoviopathies, including inflammatory (see preceding section), hyperplastic, fibrotic, and detritus-rich forms.[85]

Box 1
Evidence in favor of targeting inflammation in osteoarthritis

- Human and preclinical animal model data consistently show upregulation and activation of inflammatory and immune pathways in the joint and systemically.

- Data from selective preclinical in vitro and in vivo models confirm that genetically or pharmacologically inhibiting specific inflammatory cytokines and immune cells can reduce structural and/or symptomatic OA.

- High priority, and potentially joint-tissue and OA-phenotype specific inflammatory pathways identified from unbiased genome-wide human OA expression studies.

- Many efficacious therapeutics already developed, approved, and in clinical use in other diseases could be repurposed for specific OA phenotypes.

- Treating systemically with an inhibitor of IL1β (canakinumab) shows disease modification in patients with a systemic inflammatory phenotype.

Synovial fibrosis is characterized by excessive ECM deposition and contributes to the joint stiffness and pain associated with OA. Underlying endogenous mechanisms associated with synovial fibrosis are not well characterized and several critical questions remain to be answered. (1) Why and how does synovial fibrosis occur? (2) Which cell types are responsible for the initiation and progression of synovial fibrosis? (3) How can one control fibrosis to reduce structural and symptomatic OA?

Fibrosis is speculated to occur because of uncontrolled tissue repair responses, prolonged inflammatory insults, and crosstalk between a variety of endogenous profibrotic molecular and cellular mechanisms. The synovium consists of cells including, but not limited to, fibroblast-like synoviocytes (FLS) and macrophages. FLS are the key cell type of the synovium that is responsible for maintaining homeostatic functions and promoting inflammatory and fibrogenic responses (reviewed in Ref.[86]). FLS respond to a wide array of stimuli in the OA joint microenvironment resulting in increased proliferation, migratory capacity, and acquiring a myofibroblast-like phenotype (**Fig. 3**), all contributing toward increased ECM deposition and fibrogenic responses in the synovium. Some of the key triggers associated with FLS activation include TGFβ, cartilage wear products, Wnt/β-catenin signaling pathway, and hypoxia inducible factor-1α,[87–93] among others. TGFβ is a major profibrotic mediator known to activate FLS and induce their transition to highly contractile myofibroblast-like cells that are believed to be involved in excessive ECM accumulation in the synovium.[94] Targeting TGFβ and its signaling to achieve antifibrotic effects has proved to be complex because of its homeostatic roles in other joint tissues, such as the articular cartilage.[95,96]

At this point, clinical evidence to support efficacy of antifibrotic therapies to minimize the degree of joint destruction during OA requires further investigation. One could speculate that controlling inflammation during early stages of OA initiation and development could indirectly minimize the profibrotic events and associated pathologic mechanisms. Another potential therapeutic modality may include the simultaneous targeting of inflammation and fibrosis using a combination of anti-inflammatory and antifibrotic agents. In this context, pirfenidone, an anti-inflammatory and antifibrotic drug currently approved for the treatment of idiopathic

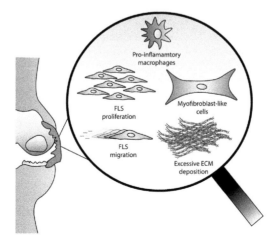

Fig. 3. FLS and macrophages are key cell types present in the synovium. FLS exhibit increased proliferation and migration, and also acquire a myofibroblast-like phenotype, resulting in the excessive ECM deposition in the synovium during osteoarthritis.

pulmonary fibrosis,[97] has been shown to attenuate synovial fibrosis and delay the progression of OA in a preclinical model.[98] Future clinical trials would help determine the therapeutic efficacy of such drugs and agents in reducing fibrosis and minimizing the degree of joint destruction during OA.

The Wnt family of proteins are also involved in OA pathogenesis[99–101] and have drawn significant attention in the OA field. For instance, a phase II study of lorecivivint (SM04690) an inhibitor of intranuclear kinases CDC-like kinase 2 (CLK2) and dual-specificity tyrosine phosphorylation-regulated kinase 1A (DYRK1A) that modulates the Wnt pathway, shows initial efficacy in improving pain, function, and joint space narrowing in patients with unilateral moderate to severe symptomatic knee OA,[102] with phase III trials currently underway.[103] Preclinical studies using SM04690 shows cartilage protective effects in vivo.[104] It would therefore be of interest to investigate the potential of SM04690 to reduce synovial inflammation and fibrosis in preclinical animal models and in clinical trials. In this context, intra-articular injection with XAV-939, a small-molecule inhibitor of Wnt/β-catenin signaling, reduces the degree of synovitis and cartilage degeneration in a mouse model of knee OA in vivo, and reduces proliferation and collagen synthesis of FLS treated with XAV-939 in vitro[89]; however, it remains to be determined if XAV-939-induced cartilage protective effects are driven by reductions in synovitis or vice versa.

Research on synovium as a key driver of OA pathogenesis is garnering significant attention in the OA field. To better understand the contribution of synovium and to devise adequate therapeutic strategies to control processes, such as synovial fibrosis and inflammation in joint destruction, it is essential to identify and understand the roles of individual synovial cell types and subpopulations that are involved in the initiation and progression of OA. The emergence of single cell sequencing, high throughput omics technologies, and advanced bioinformatics provides an excellent opportunity to deep dive into the role of the synovium in OA pathogenesis. Applying these technologies to investigations using preclinical animal models and well characterized human OA synovial samples will allow for the identification of putative therapeutic targets that may limit pathologic processes in OA, including synovial fibrosis.

TARGETING REGENERATION OF CARTILAGE TO TREAT OSTEOARTHRITIS: TONIA L. VINCENT

OA textbooks frequently describe OA as a disease determined by the balance between catabolic and anabolic pathways activated within the tissue. Historically this was based on the observation that some chondrocytes seemed to display an exuberant synthetic response in OA tissue when measuring uptake of radiolabeled sulfate (indicative of synthesis of sulfated proteoglycans), whereas other chondrocytes were in regions of the matrix completely devoid of proteoglycan.[105] Later evidence was based on transcriptomic analyses where evidence of new matrix synthesis was often upregulated alongside catabolic enzymes and other inflammatory molecules.[106,107] The textbooks shied away from describing the anabolic response as evidence for regenerative activities, because the pervasive view had been that articular cartilage was incapable of repairing itself.

Mounting evidence in the past 10 years indicates that this paradigm is incorrect. Not only is there evidence from careful prospective arthroscopy studies that many focal cartilage lesions heal spontaneously (reviewed in[108]), but also that established OA can repair if the hostile mechanical environment of the joint is corrected, such as by joint distraction, using an external frame attached above and below the joint, or by high tibial osteotomy.[109,110] Such studies demonstrate MRI-proven regeneration of cartilage-like tissue even where the erosion was down to the underlying bone.[111] In the case of joint distraction, which is typically in situ for 6 weeks, this tissue seems to be maintained up to 2 years after removal of the frame and is associated with a sustained clinical benefit over longer periods.[112] Whether the tissue that is produced is true hyaline cartilage with newly synthesized type II collagen or fibrocartilage (type I collagen rich) is unclear. This fact may also be irrelevant so long as it shows resilience over time with associated symptom improvement. Several studies point to minimal type II collagen incorporation after skeletal maturity, which does not seem to change with OA.[113,114]

Molecular mechanisms that underlie regenerative activities in articular cartilage are being revealed. These fall into two broad areas: the identity, control, and activity of progenitor cells in the joint that mediate cartilage repair; and tissue factors that signal the injury and activate the tissue repair response. Meachim famously described two distinct repair responses in articular cartilage; one that was intrinsic to the cartilage, mediated by cells that resided within the substance of the tissue; and a second that was mediated by cells migrating from the underlying bone marrow (especially where the osteochondral junction had been breached), which he called extrinsic repair. Intrinsic repair was thought to be mechanically superior, producing excellent integrated hyaline cartilage compared with the fibrocartilaginous response elicited by extrinsic bone marrow–derived cells. He concluded that, because extrinsic repair was rapid, one needed to suppress this to enable intrinsic repair to occur (reviewed in[115]). Several groups since this time have described pluripotent progenitor cells that can be expanded in vitro from cells derived from the articular cartilage.[116–118] Repair cells have also been identified in the synovium, periosteum, and synovial fluid taken from human OA joints.[119–121] Such cells may be distinct from classical mesenchymal stem cells derived from the bone marrow. For instance, synovial-derived cells are marked by being GDF5-positive, arising from those cells that originated from the joint interzone during development.[122] Collectively these results are consistent with Meachim's idea that intrinsic repair cells are distinct from those derived from the bone marrow. It also raises the possibility that orthopedic procedures, such as Pridie drilling, may be encouraging extrinsic repair by stimulating bone marrow–derived mesenchymal stem cells, and this may not be in the long-term interests of the tissue.

The tissue injury signals likely originate from the cartilage matrix itself. The pericellular matrix, a region immediately surrounding individual chondrocytes in the tissue, is rich in the proteoglycan perlecan, on whose heparan sulfate chains are attached several heparin-binding growth factors.[123] Four such growth factors were identified by proteomic analysis, including Figroblast Growth Factor 2 (FGF2), Cellular Communication Network Factor 2 (CCN2) bound to latent TGFβ, hepatoma-derived growth factor, and CCN1.[124,125] These are released immediately in response to mechanical injury of the tissue by a mechanism that involves a localized increase in sodium concentration as water is squeezed out of the compressed tissue.[126] This is sufficient to displace the growth factors from their pericellular matrix binding sites and allow their binding to high-affinity cell surface receptors (**Fig. 4**). In OA, when proteolytic activity causes loss of the negatively charged aggrecan from the tissue, the sodium is no longer held in the tissue and mechanical compression is unable to generate the concentration of sodium required to release growth factors.[126] These results indicate that proteolytic loss of aggrecan in OA suppresses intrinsic repair just at the time it is most needed. FGF2 and TGFβ are the best described of these molecules and are known chondroprotective and chondrogenic molecules in preclinical and in vitro studies.[127–129] They are also implicated in repair responses in other tissues, such as the skin.[130]

The clinical relevance of TGFβ and FGF family members in cartilage repair is strongly supported by agnostic evidence arising from recent genome-wide

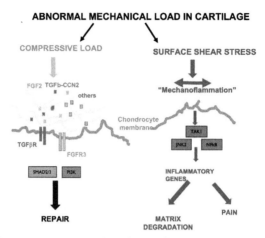

Fig. 4. Balance of proregenerative and mechanoinflammatory responses in articular cartilage with abnormal mechanical load. Compressive load leads to sodium-dependent release of pericellular matrix growth factors, which drive repair and chondroprotection through a variety of intracellular signaling pathways. Surface shear stress (perpendicular to compressive load) leads to activation of TGFβ-activated kinase 1 (TAK1) dependent inflammatory signaling and results in nerve growth factor regulation (driving pain) and matrix degradation.

association studies in OA. To date, polymorphic variants associated with expression of eight members of the TGFβ family (TGFβ1, TGFβ2, LTBP1, LTBP3, GDF5, SMAD3, ACVR1, BMP5) and two members of the FGF family (FGF18, FGFR3) have been documented.[131–135] Where described, these are hypomorphic variants associated with increased OA, thus confirming their chondroprotective role in human OA. Other growth factor families also emerge, such as the Wnts (DOT1L; WNT9a, WNT1, WNT10a) and TGFα, a ligand for the epidermal growth factor receptor. Few recognizable inflammatory genes are identified in these analyses raising the possibility that OA could be viewed primarily as a disease of failed repair (**Box 2**).

Will this change the approach to disease modification in OA? Evidence to support this concept is already emerging. To date, the only successful structure-modifying pharmacologic trial is that using intra-articular injections of sprifermin, a truncated form of FGF18. In this extended 3-year trial (the study was originally 2 years[136]), there

---

Box 2
Evidence in favor of targeting cartilage regeneration in osteoarthritis

- Experimental data in preclinical models show that articular cartilage makes a strong synthetic response after injury and in some instances can repair.

- Human data show spontaneous cartilage repair, especially when the hostile mechanical environment in OA is corrected.

- Articular cartilage matrix is full of chondroprotective growth factors that are released on tissue injury. This response is lost in OA when the tissue loses aggrecan.

- Growth factor families arise from large-scale agnostic genome-wide association studies in OA.

- Delivery of a growth factor (sprifermin, modified FGF18) intra-articularly shows disease modification in phase II clinical trials.

was evidence of a delay in cartilage loss in the sprifermin group and increased carti-lage thickness measured in the affected and unaffected regions of the joint.[137] Although not reaching its primary end point for symptoms, a recent post hoc analysis, considering a subgroup at risk of progression (defined by lower joint space width and higher pain at baseline), was able to demonstrate structural and symptomatic improvement over the study period.[138] Collectively these data seem to represent a striking U-turn for molecular pathogenesis and target discovery in OA.

TARGETING BONE REMODELING TO TREAT OSTEOARTHRITIS: TAMARA ALLISTON

In the healthy joint, subchondral bone provides mechanical and vascular support to overlying avascular cartilage.[139] Given this vital role in joint structure, function, and shape, it is not surprising that subchondral bone is thought to be a target and a driver of OA progression.

Human imaging studies demonstrate that changes in the subchondral bone compartment precede and predict degradative changes in overlaying cartilage, with the effects of OA apparent on the thin subchondral bone plate, subchondral trabecular bone, and the surrounding bone marrow. First, subchondral bone loss early in OA, because of increased bone remodeling by osteoclasts and osteoblasts, is followed by radiographic detection of sclerosis, or thickening, of the subchondral bone plate and trabecular bone.[140,141] Second, machine learning analyses of MRI in the Osteoar-thritis Initiative identify changes in subchondral bone shape as one of the earliest known predictors of OA, and joint pain.[142] Third, the appearance of bone marrow le-sions in clinical MRI is associated with joint pain and increased cartilage loss.[143] His-tologically, bone marrow lesions are associated with greater cartilage degeneration, increased marrow vasculature, fibrosis, and edema, and increased osteoid deposition and osteocyte density.[144,145] Bone marrow lesions seem to be a response to sub-chondral bone microdamage, resulting from traumatic injury or mechanical insuffi-ciency of subchondral bone. Therefore, the bony sclerosis, changes in joint shape, and bone marrow lesions in OA subchondral bone are diagnostically and clinically sig-nificant because they are detected early in OA and can predict OA progression and joint pain.

These changes in subchondral bone motivate bone-targeting therapies to prevent or treat OA, some of which have been tested clinically, but still with limited success. To abrogate the hyperactive subchondral bone remodeling that occurs early in OA, osteoclast-inhibitory bisphosphonates have been evaluated in clinical trials for OA. Bisphosphonates may indeed be therapeutically beneficial in a subset of nonover-weight individuals with early stage OA,[146] even though this clinical benefit was not observed in a meta-analysis of randomized control trials.[147] In clinical trials, cathepsin K inhibitors, which suppress bone remodeling, prevent changes in subchondral bone and cartilage, but were ineffective for treating OA pain.[148] Other bone-targeting agents with potential to impact OA progression, including estrogen, Parathyroid Hormone (PTH), TGFβ antagonists, and calcitonin, show benefits in preclinical studies, but have yet to be tested in randomized clinical trials, or to show reproducible clinical ben-efits in diverse human cohorts.[139]

Discrepancies between the success of preclinical and clinical studies still limit the clinical application of bone-targeting agents to treat OA. A more precise stratification of OA subtypes, perhaps with the help of new genetic, serum, and imaging bio-markers, could improve the identification of patients who would benefit from bone-targeting therapies. Another possibility is that bone-targeting therapies for OA are still missing a critical cellular target: osteocytes.

The cellular mechanisms by which changes in subchondral bone propel cartilage degeneration have largely been attributed to osteoblasts and osteoclasts. However, the contribution of osteocytes, the most abundant bone cell type, in OA has been overlooked until recently.[139] Over the past 10 years, the dynamic role of bone-embedded osteocytes in bone homeostasis has become clearer. Osteocytes couple mechanical demands to bone resorption and deposition by osteoclasts and osteoblasts through mechanosensitive secretion of Rank ligand (RANKL; TNFSf11) and sclerostin, respectively.[149–151] Furthermore, through the process of perilacunar/canalicular remodeling (PLR), osteocytes directly resorb their local ECM by secreting acid and proteases, such as MMP13 and cathepsin K, and then later deposit new ECM. PLR maintains systemic mineral homeostasis, bone quality, and the intricate lacuno-canalicular network (LCN), which enables osteocytes to communicate with one another and the vascular supply.[152–154] Because cartilage relies on subchondral bone for mechanical and vascular support, understanding the impact of OA on osteocytes, and vice versa, became a critical question.

Several lines of evidence support a causal role for osteocytes in the progression of OA. Relative to non-OA cadaveric control subjects, subchondral bone from human OA surgical retrieval specimens shows several hallmarks of deregulated osteocyte function, including LCN degeneration, collagen disorganization, and heterogeneous mineralization.[155] Furthermore, osteocyte-intrinsic defects in genetically modified mice were sufficient to exacerbate cartilage degeneration and mimic several features of human OA subchondral bone. Specifically, mice with an osteocyte-targeted ablation of the PLR enzyme MMP13 exhibit cartilage degeneration, accompanied by sclerotic subchondral bone with degenerated LCN, disorganized collagen, and heterogeneous mineralization.[155] Similar results are observed on osteocyte-intrinsic inhibition of TGFβ signaling through targeted ablation of the TGFβ type II receptor (TβRII$^{ocy-/-}$).[156] Recently, several genes in the osteocyte transcriptome were shown to have significant associations with OA in a human genome-wide association study, including MEPE, TSKU, SEMA3F, SEMA3G, and SEMA7A, which are expressed in osteocytes but not in chondrocytes.[157] Thus, data from human clinical and genetic studies, and from mouse models with osteocyte-intrinsic mutations, support a causal role of osteocyte dysfunction in OA.

Although the mechanisms by which osteocytes affect cartilage remain to be determined, the importance of their participation in subchondral bone and cartilage homeostasis, and joint disease, is clear. Computational modeling predicts that degeneration of the osteocyte LCN in aged or TβRII$^{ocy-/-}$ mouse bone, relative to young or control bone, is sufficient to compromise bone mechanosensitivity and solute transport.[158] Either of these mechanisms could compromise cartilage integrity. Uncoupling bone remodeling from mechanical stimuli could contribute to subchondral bone sclerosis. LCN degeneration could interfere with the ability of bone vasculature to support cartilage. The downregulation of osteocytic TGFβ signaling and MMP13 is a common feature in human OA subchondral bone, the TβRII$^{ocy-/-}$ mouse model, aging mouse bone, and wild-type mouse bone following meniscal ligamentous injury (**Table 1**).[155,156,158] Determining whether the relationship between OA and osteocytic TGFβ signaling and MMP13 is correlative or causal in aging requires further investigation. Either way, these observations highlight the need to consider the joint compartment–specific effects of each factor. For example, agents that suppress MMP13 may protect cartilage from proteolytic degradation, while simultaneously interfering with osteocyte functions required for cartilage homeostasis. Unfortunately, diagnostic markers of osteocyte function, or osteocyte-specific therapies, currently do not exist. Although the osteocyte transcriptome identifies genes that are specific

Table 1
Osteocyte-intrinsic inhibition of MMP13 or TGFβ signaling is sufficient to mimic several hallmarks of human osteoarthritis

	Human OA	MMP13$^{ocy-/-}$	TβRII$^{ocy-/-}$
Cartilage degeneration	✔	✔	✔
Subchondral sclerosis	✔	✔	✔
Thickened subchondral plate	✔	✔	✔
Collagen disorganization	✔	✔	
Mineral heterogeneity	✔	✔	
Degenerated osteocyte LCN	✔	✔	✔
Impaired mechanosensitivity			✔
Altered TGFβ signaling	✔		✔
Altered MMP13 activity	✔	✔	✔

to osteocytes, relative to other skeletal cell types, more work is needed.[157] Continued efforts to understand osteocyte function and regulation, in the healthy skeleton and in aging and disease, are needed to develop new strategies to monitor and target subchondral bone to prevent or treat joint disease.

TARGETING AGING AND CELL SENESCENCE TO TREAT OSTEOARTHRITIS: RICHARD F. LOESER

There is no doubt that aging processes, systemic and within joint tissues, contribute to the pathophysiology of OA. The prevalence of radiographic and symptomatic OA in all the commonly affected joints, including hands, hips, knees, and spine, increases with increasing age.[159] The prevalence of OA and the pain and loss of function associated with it make OA one of the leading causes of disability in older adults worldwide.[160] What is not clear is precisely how aging promotes the development of OA or if targeting aging processes would slow or halt OA progression. This section focuses on cell senescence in OA and addresses the question of whether targeting senescent cells would be of therapeutic benefit.

Nine hallmarks of aging have been proposed that include genomic instability, telomere attrition, epigenetic alterations, loss of proteostasis, deregulated nutrient sensing, mitochondrial dysfunction, stem cell exhaustion, altered intercellular communication, and perhaps most importantly, cellular senescence.[161] Many, if not all these aging hallmarks have been investigated in the context of joint tissue aging, with most of the published work focused on articular cartilage and its resident cell, the chondrocyte.[162] A common denominator to the hallmarks of aging is cell senescence, because the other hallmarks can either lead to senescence or result from the senescent state.

The literature to date strongly supports cell senescence as a major factor contributing to age-related diseases including OA.[163,164] Cell senescence is defined as a state of growth arrest that prevents further cell division and results in typical phenotypic changes.[161,163] Importantly, cell senescence is not just a phenomenon seen after replicating cells have stopped dividing because of telomere shortening. Senescent cells contribute to tissue development during embryogenesis, tissue repair during wound healing, and suppress tumor formation by preventing the propagation of damaged cells.[163,165] Cell senescence can result from multiple chronic stresses that result in an accumulation of cellular damage, many of which are relevant to factors thought to contribute to OA (**Fig. 5**). DNA damage is a central mediator of cell

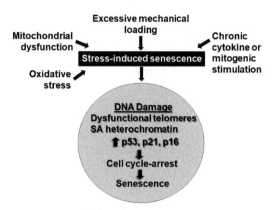

Fig. 5. Factors that promote stress-induced senescence.

senescence and has been shown to induce senescence in chondrocytes.[166] The OA joint has often been referred to as a "chronic wound" with irreparable damage, the type of environment that can promote cell senescence. Chronic signaling from inflammatory factors, such as cytokines, has been proposed to result in stress-induced senescence resulting from a feed forward loop.[167] This could be a relevant mechanism for senescence in the joint.

A central mechanism by which senescence contributes to disease is through the production of inflammatory cytokines and matrix-degrading enzymes, referred to as the senescence-associated secretory phenotype (SASP).[163] Many of the proinflammatory mediators and matrix-degrading enzymes considered to be SASP factors (**Table 2**) are found in the OA joint[53,168,169] and may directly contribute to the tissue changes seen in OA. Increased expression of p16^{INK4a}, a cell cycle inhibitor, is considered one of the most reliable markers of cell senescence.[163] p16^{INK4a} mRNA expression was found to be significantly increased with age in murine cartilage and in primary human chondrocytes from cadaveric tissue donors and this correlated with expression of the SASP transcripts IGFBP3, MMP1, and MMP13.[170] However, deletion of p16^{INK4a} in chondrocytes of adult mice did not mitigate SASP expression and did not alter the severity of age-related OA, suggesting the effects of chondrocyte senescence on OA are most likely driven by the production of SASP factors and not by the loss of chondrocyte replicative function that occurs with increased p16^{INK4a}.

It has been suggested that senescent progenitor cells may be present in aged cartilage and release inflammatory mediators, including IL8, to promote the SASP.[171] Transplantation of senescent cells into mouse knee joints was shown to promote OA-like changes.[172] Nuclear factor-κB is considered a key regulator of the SASP[163] and a recent study found activation of nuclear factor-κB signaling in mice promoted age-related OA and production of SASP factors.[173] Other important regulators of the SASP include C/EBPβ, STAT3, and GATA4, whereas the SASP may be inhibited by activity of FOXOs.[163,165] Importantly, all these mediators have also been implicated in OA pathogenesis,[174–178] providing further support for a strong connection between SASP regulation and the development of OA.

Perhaps the strongest evidence for a causal role of senescent joint tissue cells in OA comes from studies that have demonstrated reduced OA severity in the anterior cruciate ligament transection model of post-traumatic OA and in age-related OA in mice treated with small molecules called senolytics to selectively kill senescent cells or using a molecular approach to kill senescent cells expressing p16.[179,180] However,

Table 2
Senescence-associated secretory phenotype factors most relevant to OA

Class	Component
Cytokines	IL1, IL6, IL7, IL13, IL15, IL17, OSM
Chemokines	IL8 (CXCL15), GRO (CXCL1), MCP1 (CCL2), MIP1α (CCL3), ENA78 (CCXL5)
Other inflammatory molecules	TGFβ, MIF
Growth factors, regulators	EGF, FGF2, HGF, VEGF, SDF1 (CXCL12), NGF, IGFBP2, IGFBP3, IGFBP4, IGFBP6, IGFBP7
Proteases and regulators	MMP1, MMP3, MMP10, MMP12, MMP13, MMP14, TIMP1, TIMP2, PAI1 (SERPINE1), PAI2 (SERPINEB2), CTSB
Receptors and ligands	OPG (TNFRSF11 B), sTNFRI (TNFRSF1B), sTNFRII (TNFRSF1A), FAS, uPAR (PLAUR), EGFR
Nonprotein molecules	PGE2, nitric oxide, reactive oxygen species
Insoluble factors	Fibronectins, collagens

Abbreviations: bFGF, basic fibroblast growth factor; EGF, epidermal growth factor; EGFR, epidermal growth factor receptor; ENA, epithelial neutrophil-activating peptide; GRO, growth-related onco-gene; HGF, hepatocyte growth factor; IGFBP, insulin-like growth factor binding protein; MCP, monocyte chemotactic protein; MIF, macrophage inhibitory factor; MIP, macrophage inflammatory protein; NGF, nerve growth factor; OPG, osteoprotegerin; OSM, oncostatin M; PAI, plasminogen activator inhibitor; PGE2, prostaglandin E_2; SDF, stromal cell–derived factor; sTNFR, soluble tumor necrosis factor receptor; TIMP, tissue inhibitor of metalloproteinases; uPAR, urokinase-type plasminogen activator receptor; VEGF, vascular endothelial growth factor.
Adapted from Gorgoulis V, Adams PD, Alimonti A, et al. Cellular Senescence: Defining a Path Forward. Cell. 2019;179(4):813–827. doi:10.1016/j.cell.2019.10.005; with permission.

translation of this preclinical work to the treatment of human OA has not yet been realized. The senolytic compound UBX0101 that reduced OA severity in mice, did not achieve a significant reduction in WOMAC knee pain compared with a placebo when tested as an intra-articular therapy in a 12-week phase 2 clinical study in humans (UNITY Biotechnology Announces 12-week data from UBX0101 Phase 2 Clinical Study in Patients with Painful Osteoarthritis of the Knee|Unity Biotechnology).

There are many possible reasons why a single injection of a senolytic drug would fail in a short-term trial with pain as the outcome. Clearly, further work is needed to: (1) define an OA phenotype that may be more responsive to an intervention targeting senescent cells by discovering one or more biomarkers of joint tissue senescence, (2) decide on the timing in the disease course of when such an intervention would be most useful, (3) establish how many doses of the senolytic would be needed, and (4) determine what outcome measures in early phase studies would best predict efficacy. Alternatives to killing senescent joint tissue cells with a senolytic also need to be developed, such as senomorphics that target the production of SASP factors.[181] Although the link between aging and the development of OA is well established, and the underlying mechanisms are becoming clearer, the field is still not at the point where targeting a specific aging process to slow OA progression and improve symptoms is possible.

SUMMARY

Molecular pathogenesis is a new scientific discipline in OA. The scientific community has needed to overcome significant hurdles associated with working with matrix-rich paucicellular tissues, and to develop preclinical models of disease that are accepted as being clinically informative. In recent years, additional molecular insights have emerged from agnostic "-omic" studies, such as genome-wide association studies. Being a highly prevalent condition, such studies can be performed in large numbers to elucidate common pathways associated with OA risk.[134] As demonstrated, there has been a rapid expansion of cellular and molecular pathogenic understanding across multiple tissues of the OA joint. But how likely is it that this knowledge will deliver translational success?

Epidemiology, perhaps the oldest discipline in OA research, has much to teach us. It reminds us that mechanical strain remains a principal driver of OA development and progression.[182] It also teaches us that the disease is heterogeneous, having a variable course and symptoms.[183] Using all sources of data available, clinicians should be able to improve chances of success but as independently highlighted by the authors of the individual sections, there are key questions that need constant reinforcement if one is to translate the ever more detailed understanding of OA pathophysiology to treatment and patient care.

- Which of the pathways are targetable?
- If targetable, do they deliver a clinically meaningful effect?
- Does the target have benefits across all tissues of the joint or is it tissue-specific (see discussion on conflicting roles of MMP13 in bone and cartilage)?
- Do several targets need to be delivered in combination?
- Will treatments work when the adverse mechanical environment of the joint is uncorrected?
- Are the described processes active in all patients at all stages of disease, or will patient stratification be necessary?

Clinicians do not have all the answers yet, but progress has been rapid; there is a recognized urgency across funders and patient groups; and as this review demonstrates, the scientific community is working collaboratively and imaginatively to combat this challenging disease.

CLINICS CARE POINTS

Pearls:
- Research into OA pathophysiology is broad and has greatly enhanced the molecular knowledge of disease.
- Prospects for OA target discovery is high with real hope for patients in the future.

Pitfalls:
- Research tends to be conducted in silos and a multidisciplinary approach in this next phase will greatly increase the chance of finding meaningful treatments for patients.

FUNDING

The research of the authors related to the specific topics explored in this review were supported by funding from numerous sources: T.L. Vincent Center for OA Pathogenesis versus Arthritis (grant no. 20205 and 21,621); M. Kapoor Tier 1 Canada Research Chair Award (#950–232237) and Tony and Shari Fell Platinum Chair in Arthritis Research; R.F. Loeser National Institute on Aging RO1 AG044034; L. Troeberg VA grants 21,776 and 22,194; C.B. Little Australian National Health and Medical Research Council (NHMRC: Project Grant APP1045890), the Hillcrest Foundation through Perpetual Philanthropies, and Arthritis Australia.

AUTHOR CONTRIBUTIONS

Individual authors independently wrote their respective sections, and all authors contributed to editing and approved the final version.

COMPETING INTERESTS

The authors have no potential or apparent conflicts of interest with regard to this work. No benefits in any form have been or will be received from a commercial party related directly or indirectly to the subject of this article.

DATA AND MATERIALS AVAILABILITY

All data associated with this study are present in the article.

PATIENT AND PUBLIC INVOLVEMENT

Although papers and studies relating to patients are cited in the article, patients/consumers were not involved in the design, conduct, or writing of this article.

DISCLOSURE

T.L. Vincent has received research funding to support the STEpUP OA Consortium from Pfizer, Galapagos, Fidia, Novartis, BioSplice. T. Alliston, M. Kapoor and L. Troeberg have nothing to disclose. R.F. Loeser has received consulting fees from Unity Biotechnology. C.B. Little has provided consulting advice for Merck Serono and Galapagos Pharmaceuticals, and has received research funding from numerous pharmaceutical companies through specific services/testing contract research agreements between and managed by The University of Sydney or the Northern Sydney Local Health District.

ACKNOWLEDGMENTS

The authors thank Dr Patrick Haubruck, Raymond Purves Research Laboratories, for producing **Fig. 2** using biorender.com.

REFERENCES

1. Global burden of 369 diseases and injuries in 204 countries and territories, 1990-2019: a systematic analysis for the Global Burden of Disease Study 2019. Lancet 2020;396(10258):1204–22.
2. Cross M, Smith E, Hoy D, et al. The global burden of hip and knee osteoarthritis: estimates from the Global Burden of Disease 2010 study. Ann Rheum Dis 2014; 73(7):1323–30.
3. Ackerman IN, Pratt C, Gorelik A, et al. Projected burden of osteoarthritis and rheumatoid arthritis in Australia: a population-level analysis. Arthritis Care Res (Hoboken) 2018;70(6):877–83.
4. Hunter DJ, Nicolson PJA, Little CB, et al. Developing strategic priorities in osteoarthritis research: proceedings and recommendations arising from the 2017 Australian Osteoarthritis Summit. BMC Musculoskelet Disord 2019;20(1):74.
5. Bedenbaugh AV, Bonafede M, Marchlewicz EH, et al. Real-world health care resource utilization and costs among US patients with knee osteoarthritis compared with controls. Clinicoecon Outcomes Res 2021;13:421–35.

6. Huizinga JL, Stanley EE, Sullivan JK, et al. Societal cost of opioid use in symptomatic knee osteoarthritis patients in the United States. Arthritis Care Res 2021.

7. Bannuru RR, Osani MC, Vaysbrot EE, et al. OARSI guidelines for the non-surgical management of knee, hip, and polyarticular osteoarthritis. Osteoarthritis Cartil 2019;27(11):1578–89.

8. Cook D, Brown D, Alexander R, et al. Lessons learned from the fate of AstraZeneca's drug pipeline: a five-dimensional framework. Nat Rev Drug Discov 2014; 13(6):419–31.

9. Little CB, Fosang AJ. Is cartilage matrix breakdown an appropriate therapeutic target in osteoarthritis: insights from studies of aggrecan and collagen proteolysis? Curr Drug Targets 2010;11(5):561–75.

10. Little CB, Hunter DJ. Post-traumatic osteoarthritis: from mouse models to clinical trials. Nat Rev Rheumatol 2013;9(8):485–97.

11. Soul J, Barter MJ, Little CB, et al. OATargets: a knowledge base of genes associated with osteoarthritis joint damage in animals. Ann Rheum Dis 2020;80(3): 376–83.

12. Hollander AP, Pidoux I, Reiner A, et al. Damage to type II collagen in aging and osteoarthritis starts at the articular surface, originates around chondrocytes, and extends into the cartilage with progressive degeneration. J Clin Invest 1995; 96(6):2859–69.

13. Lohmander LS, Atley LM, Pietka TA, et al. The release of crosslinked peptides from type II collagen into human synovial fluid is increased soon after joint injury and in osteoarthritis. Arthritis Rheum 2003;48(11):3130–9.

14. Billinghurst RC, Dahlberg L, Ionescu M, et al. Enhanced cleavage of type II collagen by collagenases in osteoarthritic articular cartilage. J Clin Invest 1997;99(7):1534–45.

15. Lim NH, Kashiwagi M, Visse R, et al. Reactive-site mutants of N-TIMP-3 that selectively inhibit ADAMTS-4 and ADAMTS-5: biological and structural implications. Biochem J 2010;431(1):113–22.

16. Neuhold LA, Killar L, Zhao W, et al. Postnatal expression in hyaline cartilage of constitutively active human collagenase-3 (MMP-13) induces osteoarthritis in mice. J Clin Invest 2001;107(1):35–44.

17. Little CB, Barai A, Burkhardt D, et al. Matrix metalloproteinase 13-deficient mice are resistant to osteoarthritic cartilage erosion but not chondrocyte hypertrophy or osteophyte development. Arthritis Rheum 2009;60(12):3723–33.

18. Coussens LM, Fingleton B, Matrisian LM. Matrix metalloproteinase inhibitors and cancer: trials and tribulations. Science 2002;295(5564):2387–92.

19. Johnson AR, Pavlovsky AG, Ortwine DF, et al. Discovery and characterization of a novel inhibitor of matrix metalloprotease-13 that reduces cartilage damage in vivo without joint fibroplasia side effects. J Biol Chem 2007;282(38):27781–91.

20. Karsdal MA, Madsen SH, Christiansen C, et al. Cartilage degradation is fully reversible in the presence of aggrecanase but not matrix metalloproteinase activity. Arthritis Res Ther 2008;10(3):R63.

21. Pratta M, Yao W, Decicco C, et al. Aggrecan protects cartilage collagen from proteolytic cleavage. J Biol Chem 2003;278:45539–45.

22. Sandy JD, Flannery CR, Neame PJ, et al. The structure of aggrecan fragments in human synovial fluid. Evidence for the involvement in osteoarthritis of a novel proteinase which cleaves the Glu 373-Ala 374 bond of the interglobular domain. J Clin Invest 1992;89:1512–6.

23. Tortorella MD, Burn TC, Pratta MA, et al. Purification and cloning of aggrecanase-1: a member of the ADAMTS family of proteins. Science 1999; 284(5420):1664–6.

24. Abbaszade I, Liu RQ, Yang F, et al. Cloning and characterization of ADAMTS11, an aggrecanase from the ADAMTS family. J Biol Chem 1999;274(33):23443–50.

25. Hurskainen TL, Hirohata S, Seldin MF, et al. ADAM-TS5, ADAM-TS6, and ADAM-TS7, novel members of a new family of zinc metalloproteases. General features and genomic distribution of the ADAM-TS family. J Biol Chem 1999;274(36): 25555–63.

26. Glasson SS, Askew R, Sheppard B, et al. Deletion of active ADAMTS5 prevents cartilage degradation in a murine model of osteoarthritis. Nature 2005; 434(7033):644–8.

27. Stanton H, Rogerson FM, East CJ, et al. ADAMTS5 is the major aggrecanase in mouse cartilage in vivo and in vitro. Nature 2005;434(7033):648–52.

28. Ismail HM, Yamamoto K, Vincent TL, et al. Interleukin-1 acts via the JNK-2 signaling pathway to induce aggrecan degradation by human chondrocytes. Arthritis Rheum 2015;67(7):1826–36.

29. Chockalingam PS, Sun W, Rivera-Bermudez MA, et al. Elevated aggrecanase activity in a rat model of joint injury is attenuated by an aggrecanase specific inhibitor. Osteoarthritis Cartil 2011;19(3):315–23.

30. Brebion F, Gosmini R, Deprez P, et al. Discovery of GLPG1972/S201086, a potent, selective, and orally bioavailable ADAMTS-5 inhibitor for the treatment of osteoarthritis. J Med Chem 2021;64(6):2937–52.

31. Clement-Lacroix P, Little CB, Smith MM, et al. Pharmacological characterization of GLPG1972/S201086, a potent and selective small molecule inhibitor of ADAMTS5. Osteoarthritis Cartilage. 2021.

32. Santamaria S, Cuffaro D, Nuti E, et al. Exosite inhibition of ADAMTS-5 by a glycoconjugated arylsulfonamide. Sci Rep 2021;11(1):949.

33. Brenneis C, Serruys B, Van Belle T, et al. Structural and symptomatic benefit of a half-live extended, systemically applied anti-ADAMTS-5 inhibitor (M6495). Osteoarthritis Cartilage. 2018;26:S299–300.

34. Larkin J, Lohr T, Elefante L, et al. The highs and lows of translational drug development: antibody-mediated inhibition of ADAMTS-5 for osteoarthritis disease modification. Osteoarthrits Cartil 2014;22:S483–4.

35. Santamaria S. ADAMTS-5: a difficult teenager turning 20. Int J Exp Pathol 2020; 101(1–2):4–20.

36. de Lange-Brokaar BJ, Ioan-Facsinay A, Yusuf E, et al. Evolution of synovitis in osteoarthritic knees and its association with clinical features. Osteoarthritis Cartilage. 2016;24(11):1867–74.

37. Wang X, Hunter DJ, Jin X, et al. The importance of synovial inflammation in osteoarthritis: current evidence from imaging assessments and clinical trials. Osteoarthritis Cartilage. 2018;26(2):165–74.

38. Benito MJ, Veale DJ, FitzGerald O, et al. Synovial tissue inflammation in early and late osteoarthritis. Ann Rheum Dis 2005;64(9):1263–7.

39. Smith MD, Triantafillou S, Parker A, et al. Synovial membrane inflammation and cytokine production in patients with early osteoarthritis. J Rheumatol 1997;24(2): 365–71.

40. Klein-Wieringa IR, de Lange-Brokaar BJ, Yusuf E, et al. Inflammatory cells in patients with endstage knee osteoarthritis: a comparison between the synovium and the infrapatellar fat pad. J Rheumatol 2016;43(4):771–8.

41. Macchi V, Stocco E, Stecco C, et al. The infrapatellar fat pad and the synovial membrane: an anatomo-functional unit. J Anat 2018;233(2):146–54.
42. Sae-Jung T, Leearamwat N, Chaiseema N, et al. The infrapatellar fat pad produces interleukin-6-secreting T cells in response to a proteoglycan aggrecan peptide and provides dominant soluble mediators different from that present in synovial fluid. Int J Rheum Dis 2021;24(6):834–46.
43. Atukorala I, Kwoh CK, Guermazi A, et al. Synovitis in knee osteoarthritis: a precursor of disease? Ann Rheum Dis 2016;75(2):390–5.
44. Ayral X, Pickering EH, Woodworth TG, et al. Synovitis: a potential predictive factor of structural progression of medial tibiofemoral knee osteoarthritis – results of a 1 year longitudinal arthroscopic study in 422 patients. Osteoarthritis Cartilage. 2005;13(5):361–7.
45. Li L, Li Z, Li Y, et al. Profiling of inflammatory mediators in the synovial fluid related to pain in knee osteoarthritis. BMC Musculoskelet Disord 2020;21(1):99.
46. Nees TA, Rosshirt N, Zhang JA, et al. Synovial cytokines significantly correlate with osteoarthritis-related knee pain and disability: inflammatory mediators of potential clinical relevance. J Clin Med 2019;8(9):1343.
47. Neogi T, Guermazi A, Roemer F, et al. Association of joint inflammation with pain sensitization in knee osteoarthritis: the multicenter osteoarthritis study. Arthritis Rheumatol 2016;68(3):654–61.
48. Lieberthal J, Sambamurthy N, Scanzello CR. Inflammation in joint injury and post-traumatic osteoarthritis. Osteoarthritis Cartilage. 2015;23(11):1825–34.
49. Rosshirt N, Trauth R, Platzer H, et al. Proinflammatory T cell polarization is already present in patients with early knee osteoarthritis. Arthritis Res Ther 2021;23(1):37.
50. Scanzello CR, Umoh E, Pessler F, et al. Local cytokine profiles in knee osteoarthritis: elevated synovial fluid interleukin-15 differentiates early from end-stage disease. Osteoarthritis Cartilage. 2009;17(8):1040–8.
51. MacFarlane LA, Yang H, Collins JE, et al. Association of changes in effusion-synovitis with progression of cartilage damage over eighteen months in patients with osteoarthritis and meniscal tear. Arthritis Rheumatol 2019;71(1):73–81.
52. Vincent TL. Mechanoinflammation in osteoarthritis pathogenesis. Semin Arthritis Rheum 2019;49:S36–8.
53. Chou CH, Jain V, Gibson J, et al. Synovial cell cross-talk with cartilage plays a major role in the pathogenesis of osteoarthritis. Sci Rep 2020;10(1):10868.
54. Griffin TM, Scanzello CR. Innate inflammation and synovial macrophages in osteoarthritis pathophysiology. Clin Exp Rheumatol. 2019;37:57–63. Suppl 120(5).
55. Menarim BC, Gillis KH, Oliver A, et al. Macrophage activation in the synovium of healthy and osteoarthritic equine joints. Front Vet Sci 2020;7:568756.
56. Chen Z, Ma Y, Li X, et al. The immune cell landscape in different anatomical structures of knee in osteoarthritis: a gene expression-based study. Biomed Res Int 2020;2020:9647072.
57. Nees TA, Rosshirt N, Zhang JA, et al. T helper cell infiltration in osteoarthritis-related knee pain and disability. J Clin Med 2020;9(8):2423.
58. Platzer H, Nees TA, Reiner T, et al. Impact of mononuclear cell infiltration on chondrodestructive MMP/ADAMTS production in osteoarthritic knee joints: an ex vivo study. J Clin Med 2020;9(5):1279.
59. Brophy RH, Tycksen ED, Sandell LJ, et al. Changes in transcriptome-wide gene expression of anterior cruciate ligament tears based on time from injury. Am J Sports Med 2016;44(8):2064–75.

60. Han D, Fang Y, Tan X, et al. The emerging role of fibroblast-like synoviocytes-mediated synovitis in osteoarthritis: an update. J Cell Mol Med 2020;24(17):9518–32.
61. Pap T, Dankbar B, Wehmeyer C, et al. Synovial fibroblasts and articular tissue remodelling: role and mechanisms. Semin Cell Dev Biol 2020;101:140–5.
62. Sandy JD, Chan DD, Trevino RL, et al. Human genome-wide expression analysis reorients the study of inflammatory mediators and biomechanics in osteoarthritis. Osteoarthritis Cartilage. 2015;23(11):1939–45.
63. de Visser HM, Mastbergen SC, Kozijn AE, et al. Metabolic dysregulation accelerates injury-induced joint degeneration, driven by local inflammation; an in vivo rat study. J Orthop Res 2018;36(3):881–90.
64. Pearson MJ, Herndler-Brandstetter D, Tariq MA, et al. IL-6 secretion in osteoarthritis patients is mediated by chondrocyte-synovial fibroblast cross-talk and is enhanced by obesity. Sci Rep 2017;7(1):3451.
65. Stannus O, Jones G, Cicuttini F, et al. Circulating levels of IL-6 and TNF-alpha are associated with knee radiographic osteoarthritis and knee cartilage loss in older adults. Osteoarthritis Cartilage. 2010;18(11):1441–7.
66. Stannus OP, Jones G, Blizzard L, et al. Associations between serum levels of inflammatory markers and change in knee pain over 5 years in older adults: a prospective cohort study. Ann Rheum Dis 2013;72(4):535–40.
67. Li Z, Wang Q, Chen G, et al. Integration of gene expression profile data to screen and verify hub genes involved in osteoarthritis. Biomed Res Int 2018;2018:9482726.
68. Persson MSM, Sarmanova A, Doherty M, et al. Conventional and biologic disease-modifying anti-rheumatic drugs for osteoarthritis: a meta-analysis of randomized controlled trials. Rheumatology (Oxford). 2018;57(10):1830–7.
69. Oo WM, Little C, Duong V, et al. The development of disease-modifying therapies for osteoarthritis (DMOADs): the evidence to date. Drug Des Devel Ther 2021;15:2921–45.
70. Glasson SS. In vivo osteoarthritis target validation utilizing genetically-modified mice. Curr Drug Targets 2007;8(2):367–76.
71. Na HS, Park JS, Cho KH, et al. Interleukin-1-interleukin-17 signaling axis induces cartilage destruction and promotes experimental osteoarthritis. Front Immunol 2020;11:730.
72. Nasi S, Ea HK, So A, et al. Revisiting the role of interleukin-1 pathway in osteoarthritis: interleukin-1α and -1β, and NLRP3 inflammasome are not involved in the pathological features of the murine menisectomy model of osteoarthritis. Front Pharmacol 2017;8:282.
73. van Dalen SC, Blom AB, Slöetjes AW, et al. Interleukin-1 is not involved in synovial inflammation and cartilage destruction in collagenase-induced osteoarthritis. Osteoarthritis Cartilage. 2017;25(3):385–96.
74. de Hooge AS, van de Loo FA, Bennink MB, et al. Male IL-6 gene knock out mice developed more advanced osteoarthritis upon aging. Osteoarthritis Cartilage. 2005;13(1):66–73.
75. Ryu JH, Yang S, Shin Y, et al. Interleukin-6 plays an essential role in hypoxia-inducible factor 2alpha-induced experimental osteoarthritic cartilage destruction in mice. Arthritis Rheum 2011;63(9):2732–43.
76. Grieshaber-Bouyer R, Kammerer T, Rosshirt N, et al. Divergent mononuclear cell participation and cytokine release profiles define hip and knee osteoarthritis. J Clin Med 2019;8(10):1631.

77. Kriegova E, Manukyan G, Mikulkova Z, et al. Gender-related differences observed among immune cells in synovial fluid in knee osteoarthritis. Osteoarthritis Cartilage. 2018;26(9):1247–56.

78. Leung YY, Huebner JL, Haaland B, et al. Synovial fluid pro-inflammatory profile differs according to the characteristics of knee pain. Osteoarthritis Cartilage. 2017;25(9):1420–7.

79. Labinsky H, Panipinto PM, Ly KA, et al. Multiparameter analysis identifies heterogeneity in knee osteoarthritis synovial responses. Arthritis Rheumatol 2020; 72(4):598–608.

80. Letarouilly JG, Salmon JH, Flipo RM. Factors affecting persistence with biologic treatments in patients with rheumatoid arthritis: a systematic literature review. Expert Opin Drug Saf 2021;20(9):1087–94.

81. Noviani M, Feletar M, Nash P, et al. Choosing the right treatment for patients with psoriatic arthritis. Ther Adv Musculoskelet Dis 2020;12. 1759720x20962623.

82. Schieker M, Conaghan PG, Mindeholm L, et al. Effects of interleukin-1β inhibition on incident hip and knee replacement: exploratory analyses from a randomized, double-blind, placebo-controlled trial. Ann Intern Med 2020;173(7): 509–15.

83. Singh JA, Arayssi T, Duray P, et al. Immunohistochemistry of normal human knee synovium: a quantitative study. Ann Rheum Dis 2004;63(7):785–90.

84. Smith MD. The normal synovium. open Rheumatol J 2011;5:100–6.

85. Oehler S, Neureiter D, Meyer-Scholten C, et al. Subtyping of osteoarthritic synoviopathy. Clin Exp Rheumatol 2002;20(5):633–40.

86. Maglaviceanu A, Wu B, Kapoor M. Fibroblast-like synoviocytes: role in synovial fibrosis associated with osteoarthritis. Wound Repair Regen 2021;29(4):642–9.

87. Estell EG, Silverstein AM, Stefani RM, et al. Cartilage wear particles induce an inflammatory response similar to cytokines in human fibroblast-like synoviocytes. J Orthop Res 2019;37(9):1979–87.

88. Kuo SJ, Liu SC, Huang YL, et al. TGF-beta1 enhances FOXO3 expression in human synovial fibroblasts by inhibiting miR-92a through AMPK and p38 pathways. Aging. 2019;11(12):4075–89.

89. Lietman C, Wu B, Lechner S, et al. Inhibition of Wnt/beta-catenin signaling ameliorates osteoarthritis in a murine model of experimental osteoarthritis. JCI Insight. 2018;3(3).

90. Remst DF, Blom AB, Vitters EL, et al. Gene expression analysis of murine and human osteoarthritis synovium reveals elevation of transforming growth factor beta-responsive genes in osteoarthritis-related fibrosis. Arthritis Rheumatol 2014;66(3):647–56.

91. Silverstein AM, Stefani RM, Sobczak E, et al. Toward understanding the role of cartilage particulates in synovial inflammation. Osteoarthritis Cartilage. 2017; 25(8):1353–61.

92. Vaamonde-Garcia C, Malaise O, Charlier E, et al. 15-Deoxy-Delta-12, 14-prostaglandin J2 acts cooperatively with prednisolone to reduce TGF-beta-induced pro-fibrotic pathways in human osteoarthritis fibroblasts. Biochem Pharmacol 2019;165:66–78.

93. Zhang L, Zhang L, Huang Z, et al. Increased HIF-1alpha in knee osteoarthritis aggravate synovial fibrosis via fibroblast-like synoviocyte pyroptosis. Oxid Med Cell Longev. 2019;2019:6326517.

94. Mattey DL, Dawes PT, Nixon NB, et al. Transforming growth factor beta 1 and interleukin 4 induced alpha smooth muscle actin expression and

myofibroblast-like differentiation in human synovial fibroblasts in vitro: modulation by basic fibroblast growth factor. Ann Rheum Dis 1997;56(7):426–31.

95. Finnson KW, Chi Y, Bou-Gharios G, et al. TGF-b signaling in cartilage homeostasis and osteoarthritis. Front Biosci 2012;4:251–68.

96. Remst DF, Blaney Davidson EN, van der Kraan PM. Unravelling osteoarthritis-related synovial fibrosis: a step closer to solving joint stiffness. Rheumatology (Oxford). 2015;54(11):1954–63.

97. Kim ES, Keating GM. Pirfenidone: a review of its use in idiopathic pulmonary fibrosis. Drugs. 2015;75(2):219–30.

98. Wei Q, Kong N, Liu X, et al. Pirfenidone attenuates synovial fibrosis and postpones the progression of osteoarthritis by anti-fibrotic and anti-inflammatory properties in vivo and in vitro. J Transl Med 2021;19(1):157.

99. Dell'Accio F, De Bari C, El Tawil NM, et al. Activation of WNT and BMP signaling in adult human articular cartilage following mechanical injury. Arthritis Res Ther 2006;8(5):R139.

100. Dell'accio F, De Bari C, Eltawil NM, et al. Identification of the molecular response of articular cartilage to injury, by microarray screening: Wnt-16 expression and signaling after injury and in osteoarthritis. Arthritis Rheum 2008;58(5):1410–21.

101. van den Bosch MH, Blom AB, Sloetjes AW, et al. Induction of canonical Wnt signaling by synovial overexpression of selected Wnts leads to protease activity and early osteoarthritis-like cartilage damage. Am J Pathol 2015;185(7):1970–80.

102. Yazici Y, McAlindon TE, Gibofsky A, et al. Lorecivivint, a novel intraarticular CDC-like kinase 2 and dual-specificity tyrosine phosphorylation-regulated kinase 1A inhibitor and Wnt pathway modulator for the treatment of knee osteoarthritis: a phase II randomized trial. Arthritis Rheumatol 2020;72(10):1694–706.

103. A study utilizing patient-reported and radiographic outcomes and evaluating the safety and efficacy of lorecivivint (SM04690) for the treatment of moderately to severely symptomatic knee osteoarthritis (STRIDES-X-ray). Updated. 2021. Available at: https://clinicaltrials.gov/ct2/show/NCT03928184. Accessed October 22, 2021.

104. Deshmukh V, O'Green AL, Bossard C, et al. Modulation of the Wnt pathway through inhibition of CLK2 and DYRK1A by lorecivivint as a novel, potentially disease-modifying approach for knee osteoarthritis treatment. Osteoarthritis Cartilage. 2019;27(9):1347–60.

105. Collins DH, Meachim G. Sulphate (35SO4) fixation by human articular cartilage compared in the knee and shoulder joints. Ann Rheum Dis 1961;20:117–22.

106. Aigner T, Fundel K, Saas J, et al. Large-scale gene expression profiling reveals major pathogenetic pathways of cartilage degeneration in osteoarthritis. Arthritis Rheum 2006;54(11):3533–44.

107. Soul J, Dunn SL, Anand S, et al. Stratification of knee osteoarthritis: two major patient subgroups identified by genome-wide expression analysis of articular cartilage. Ann Rheum Dis 2018;77(3):423.

108. Dell'Accio F, Vincent TL. Joint surface defects: clinical course and cellular response in spontaneous and experimental lesions. Eur Cells Mater. 2010;20:210–7.

109. Wiegant K, van Roermund PM, Intema F, et al. Sustained clinical and structural benefit after joint distraction in the treatment of severe knee osteoarthritis. Osteoarthritis Cartilage. 2013;21(11):1660–7.

110. Parker DA, Beatty KT, Giuffre B, et al. Articular cartilage changes in patients with osteoarthritis after osteotomy. Am J Sports Med 2011;39(5):1039–45.

111. Jansen MP, Maschek S, van Heerwaarden RJ, et al. Changes in cartilage thickness and denuded bone area after knee joint distraction and high tibial osteotomy: post-hoc analyses of two randomized controlled trials. J Clin Med 2021;10(2).
112. van der Woude J-TAD, Wiegant K, Van Roermund PM, et al. Five-year follow-up of knee joint distraction: clinical benefit and cartilaginous tissue repair in an open uncontrolled prospective study. Cartilage. 2017;8(3):263–71.
113. Ariosa-Morejon Y, Santos A, Fischer R, et al. Age-dependent changes in protein incorporation into collagen-rich tissues of mice by in vivo pulsed SILAC labelling. Elife. 2021;10:e66635.
114. Heinemeier KM, Schjerling P, Heinemeier J, et al. Radiocarbon dating reveals minimal collagen turnover in both healthy and osteoarthritic human cartilage. Sci Transl Med 2016;8(346). 346ra390.
115. Stockwell RA. Biology of cartilage cells. 1979.
116. Alsalameh S, Amin R, Gemba T, et al. Identification of mesenchymal progenitor cells in normal and osteoarthritic human articular cartilage. Arthritis Rheum 2004;50(5):1522–32.
117. Dowthwaite GP, Bishop JC, Redman SN, et al. The surface of articular cartilage contains a progenitor cell population. J Cell Sci 2004;117(Pt 6):889–97.
118. Fellows CR, Williams R, Davies IR, et al. Characterisation of a divergent progenitor cell sub-populations in human osteoarthritic cartilage: the role of telomere erosion and replicative senescence. Sci Rep 2017;7:41421.
119. De Bari C, Dell'Accio F, Tylzanowski P, et al. Multipotent mesenchymal stem cells from adult human synovial membrane. Arthritis Rheum 2001;44(8):1928–42.
120. De Bari C, Dell'Accio F, Vanlauwe J, et al. Mesenchymal multipotency of adult human periosteal cells demonstrated by single-cell lineage analysis. Arthritis Rheum 2006;54(4):1209–21.
121. Jones EA, English A, Henshaw K, et al. Enumeration and phenotypic characterization of synovial fluid multipotential mesenchymal progenitor cells in inflammatory and degenerative arthritis. Arthritis Rheum 2004;50(3):817–27.
122. Roelofs AJ, Zupan J, Riemen AHK, et al. Joint morphogenetic cells in the adult mammalian synovium. Nat Commun 2017;8:15040.
123. Poole CA, Flint MH, Beaumont BW. Chondrons in cartilage: ultrastructural analysis of the pericellular microenvironment in adult human articular cartilages. J Orthop Res 1987;5(4):509–22.
124. Tang X, Muhammad H, McLean C, et al. Connective tissue growth factor contributes to joint homeostasis and osteoarthritis severity by controlling the matrix sequestration and activation of latent TGFβ. Ann Rheum Dis 2018;77(9):1372–80.
125. Vincent T, Hermansson M, Bolton M, et al. Basic FGF mediates an immediate response of articular cartilage to mechanical injury. Proc Natl Acad Sci USA 2002;99(12):8259–64.
126. Keppie SJ, Mansfield JC, Tang X, et al. Matrix-bound growth factors are released upon cartilage compression by an aggrecan-dependent sodium flux that is lost in osteoarthritis. Function (Oxf). 2021;(5):2, zqab037.
127. Chia S-L, Sawaji Y, Burleigh A, et al. Fibroblast growth factor 2 is an intrinsic chondroprotective agent that suppresses ADAMTS-5 and delays cartilage degradation in murine osteoarthritis. Arthritis Rheum 2009;60(7):2019–27.
128. Huang L, Yi L, Zhang C, et al. Synergistic effects of FGF-18 and TGF-β3 on the chondrogenesis of human adipose-derived mesenchymal stem cells in the pellet culture. Stem Cells Int. 2018;2018. 7139485-7139410.

129. Valverde-Franco G, Binette JS, Li W, et al. Defects in articular cartilage metabolism and early arthritis in fibroblast growth factor receptor 3 deficient mice. Hum Mol Genet 2006;15(11):1783–92.
130. Moulin V. Growth factors in skin wound healing. Eur J Cell Biol 1995;68(1):1–7.
131. Styrkarsdottir U, Stefansson OA, Gunnarsdottir K, et al. GWAS of bone size yields twelve loci that also affect height, BMD, osteoarthritis or fractures. Nat Commun 2019;10(1):2054.
132. Styrkarsdottir U, Lund SH, Thorleifsson G, et al. Meta-analysis of Icelandic and UK data sets identifies missense variants in SMO, IL11, COL11A1 and 13 more new loci associated with osteoarthritis. Nat Genet 2018;50(12):1681–7.
133. Zengini E, Hatzikotoulas K, Tachmazidou I, et al. Genome-wide analyses using UK Biobank data provide insights into the genetic architecture of osteoarthritis. Nat Genet 2018;50(4):549–58.
134. Boer CG, Hatzikotoulas K, Southam L, et al. Deciphering osteoarthritis genetics across 826,690 individuals from 9 populations. Cell. 2021;184(18):4784–4818 e4717.
135. Castano-Betancourt MC, Evans DS, Ramos YF, et al. Novel genetic variants for cartilage thickness and hip osteoarthritis. Plos Genet 2016;12(10):e1006260.
136. Lohmander LS, Hellot S, Dreher D, et al. Intraarticular sprifermin (recombinant human fibroblast growth factor 18) in knee osteoarthritis: a randomized, double-blind, placebo-controlled trial. Arthritis Rheumatol 2014;66(7):1820–31.
137. Hochberg MC, Guermazi A, Guehring H, et al. Effect of intra-articular sprifermin vs placebo on femorotibial joint cartilage thickness in patients with osteoarthritis: the FORWARD randomized clinical trial. JAMA 2019;322(14):1360–70.
138. Guehring H, Moreau F, Daelken B, et al. The effects of sprifermin on symptoms and structure in a subgroup at risk of progression in the FORWARD knee osteoarthritis trial. Semin Arthritis Rheum 2021;51(2):450–6.
139. Zhu X, Chan YT, Yung PSH, et al. Subchondral bone remodeling: a therapeutic target for osteoarthritis. Front Cell Dev Biol. 2020;8:607764.
140. Chen Y, Hu Y, Yu YE, et al. Subchondral trabecular rod loss and plate thickening in the development of osteoarthritis. J Bone Miner Res 2018;33(2):316–27.
141. Goldring SR, Goldring MB. Changes in the osteochondral unit during osteoarthritis: structure, function and cartilage-bone crosstalk. Nat Rev Rheumatol 2016;12(11):632–44.
142. Kanthawang T, Bodden J, Joseph GB, et al. Obese and overweight individuals have greater knee synovial inflammation and associated structural and cartilage compositional degeneration: data from the osteoarthritis initiative. Skeletal Radiol 2021;50(1):217–29.
143. Alliston T, Hernandez CJ, Findlay DM, et al. Bone marrow lesions in osteoarthritis: what lies beneath. J Orthop Res 2018;36(7):1818–25.
144. Muratovic D, Cicuttini F, Wluka A, et al. Bone marrow lesions detected by specific combination of MRI sequences are associated with severity of osteochondral degeneration. Arthritis Res Ther 2016;18:54.
145. Muratovic D, Findlay DM, Cicuttini FM, et al. Bone matrix microdamage and vascular changes characterize bone marrow lesions in the subchondral bone of knee osteoarthritis. Bone. 2018;108:193–201.
146. Hayes KN, Giannakeas V, Wong AKO. Bisphosphonate use is protective of radiographic knee osteoarthritis progression among those with low disease severity and being non-overweight: data from the osteoarthritis initiative. J Bone Miner Res 2020;35(12):2318–26.

147. Vaysbrot EE, Osani MC, Musetti MC, et al. Are bisphosphonates efficacious in knee osteoarthritis? A meta-analysis of randomized controlled trials. Osteoarthritis Cartilage. 2018;26(2):154–64.

148. Conaghan PG, Bowes MA, Kingsbury SR, et al. Disease-modifying effects of a novel cathepsin K inhibitor in osteoarthritis: a randomized controlled trial. Ann Intern Med 2020;172(2):86–95.

149. Nakashima T, Hayashi M, Fukunaga T, et al. Evidence for osteocyte regulation of bone homeostasis through RANKL expression. Nat Med 2011;17(10):1231–4.

150. Xiong J, Onal M, Jilka RL, et al. Matrix-embedded cells control osteoclast formation. Nat Med 2011;17(10):1235–41.

151. Robling AG, Niziolek PJ, Baldridge LA, et al. Mechanical stimulation of bone in vivo reduces osteocyte expression of Sost/sclerostin. J Biol Chem 2008; 283(9):5866–75.

152. Qing H, Ardeshirpour L, Pajevic PD, et al. Demonstration of osteocytic perilacunar/canalicular remodeling in mice during lactation. J Bone Miner Res 2012; 27(5):1018–29.

153. Tang SY, Herber RP, Ho SP, et al. Matrix metalloproteinase-13 is required for osteocytic perilacunar remodeling and maintains bone fracture resistance. J Bone Miner Res 2012;27(9):1936–50.

154. Bonewald LF. The amazing osteocyte. J Bone Miner Res 2011;26(2):229–38.

155. Mazur CM, Woo JJ, Yee CS, et al. Osteocyte dysfunction promotes osteoarthritis through MMP13-dependent suppression of subchondral bone homeostasis. Bone Res 2019;7:34.

156. Bailey KN, Nguyen J, Yee CS, et al. Mechanosensitive control of articular cartilage and subchondral bone homeostasis in mice requires osteocytic transforming growth factor beta signaling. Arthritis Rheumatol 2021;73(3):414–25.

157. Youlten SE, Kemp JP, Logan JG, et al. Osteocyte transcriptome mapping identifies a molecular landscape controlling skeletal homeostasis and susceptibility to skeletal disease. Nat Commun 2021;12(1):2444.

158. Schurman CA, Verbruggen SW, Alliston T. Disrupted osteocyte connectivity and pericellular fluid flow in bone with aging and defective TGF-beta signaling. Proc Natl Acad Sci U S A 2021;118(25).

159. Anderson SA, Loeser RF. Why is osteoarthritis an age-related disease? Best Pract Res 2010;24(1):15–26.

160. Safiri S, Kolahi AA, Cross M, et al. Prevalence, deaths, and disability-adjusted life years due to musculoskeletal disorders for 195 countries and territories 1990–2017. Arthritis Rheumatol 2021;73(4):702–14.

161. Lopez-Otin C, Blasco MA, Partridge L, et al. The hallmarks of aging. Cell. 2013; 153(6):1194–217.

162. Loeser RF, Collins JA, Diekman BO. Ageing and the pathogenesis of osteoarthritis. Nat Rev Rheumatol 2016;12:412–20.

163. Gorgoulis V, Adams PD, Alimonti A, et al. Cellular senescence: defining a path forward. Cell. 2019;179(4):813–27.

164. Jeon OH, David N, Campisi J, et al. Senescent cells and osteoarthritis: a painful connection. J Clin Invest 2018;128(4):1229–37.

165. Birch J, Gil J. Senescence and the SASP: many therapeutic avenues. Genes Dev 2020;34(23–24):1565–76.

166. Copp ME, Flanders MC, Gagliardi R, et al. The combination of mitogenic stimulation and DNA damage induces chondrocyte senescence. Osteoarthritis Cartilage. 2021;29(3):402–12.

167. Chandrasekaran A, Idelchik M, Melendez JA. Redox control of senescence and age-related disease. Redox Biol 2017;11:91–102.
168. Kapoor M, Martel-Pelletier J, Lajeunesse D, et al. Role of proinflammatory cyto-kines in the pathophysiology of osteoarthritis. Nat Rev Rheumatol 2011;7(1): 33–42.
169. van den Bosch MHJ, van Lent P, van der Kraan PM. Identifying effector mole-cules, cells, and cytokines of innate immunity in OA. Osteoarthritis Cartilage. 2020;28(5):532–43.
170. Diekman BO, Sessions GA, Collins JA, et al. Expression of p16(INK)(4a) is a biomarker of chondrocyte aging but does not cause osteoarthritis. Aging Cell. 2018;e12771.
171. Liu W, Brodsky AS, Feng M, et al. Senescent tissue-resident mesenchymal stro-mal cells are an internal source of inflammation in human osteoarthritic cartilage. Front Cell Dev Biol. 2021;9:725071.
172. Xu M, Bradley EW, Weivoda MM, et al. Transplanted senescent cells induce an osteoarthritis-like condition in mice. J Gerontol A Biol Sci Med Sci 2017;72(6): 780–5.
173. Catheline SE, Bell RD, Oluoch LS, et al. IKKβ–NF-κB signaling in adult chondro-cytes promotes the onset of age-related osteoarthritis in mice. Sci Signal 2021;(701):14.
174. Hirata M, Kugimiya F, Fukai A, et al. C/EBPbeta and RUNX2 cooperate to degrade cartilage with MMP-13 as the target and HIF-2alpha as the inducer in chondrocytes. Hum Mol Genet 2012;21(5):1111–23.
175. Latourte A, Cherifi C, Maillet J, et al. Systemic inhibition of IL-6/Stat3 signalling protects against experimental osteoarthritis. Ann Rheum Dis 2016;76(4):748–55.
176. Kang D, Shin J, Cho Y, et al. Stress-activated miR-204 governs senescent phe-notypes of chondrocytes to promote osteoarthritis development. Sci Transl Med 2019;(486):11.
177. Matsuzaki T, Alvarez-Garcia O, Mokuda S, et al. FoxO transcription factors modulate autophagy and proteoglycan 4 in cartilage homeostasis and osteoar-thritis. Sci Transl Med 2018;10(428).
178. Wang C, Shen J, Ying J, et al. FoxO1 is a crucial mediator of TGF-β/TAK1 signaling and protects against osteoarthritis by maintaining articular cartilage homeostasis. Proc Natl Acad Sci U S A 2020;117(48):30488–97.
179. Jeon OH, Kim C, Laberge RM, et al. Local clearance of senescent cells attenu-ates the development of post-traumatic osteoarthritis and creates a pro-regenerative environment. Nat Med 2017;23(6):775–81.
180. Faust HJ, Zhang H, Han J, et al. IL-17 and immunologically induced senes-cence regulate response to injury in osteoarthritis. J Clin Invest 2020;130(10): 5493–507.
181. Coryell PR, Diekman BO, Loeser RF. Mechanisms and therapeutic implications of cellular senescence in osteoarthritis. Nat Rev Rheumatol 2021;17(1):47–57.
182. Felson DT. Osteoarthritis as a disease of mechanics. Osteoarthritis Cartilage. 2013;21(1):10–5.
183. Leyland KM, Hart D, Javaid MK, et al. The natural history of radiographic knee osteoarthritis: a fourteen year population-based cohort study. Arthritis Rheum 2012;64:2243–51.

The Genesis of Pain in Osteoarthritis: Inflammation as a Mediator of Osteoarthritis Pain

Matthew J. Wood, PhD[a], Rachel E. Miller, PhD[b],
Anne-Marie Malfait, MD, PhD[c],*

KEYWORDS

- Osteoarthritis • Pain • Sensitization • Inflammation • Neuroinflammation • Synovitis
- Nociceptors • Obesity

KEY POINTS

- Chronic pain is the most burdensome symptom for patients with OA, yet pain is often inadequately managed in OA.
- Nerve growth factor (NGF), inflammatory cytokines and chemokines, and DAMPs are pro-algesic through direct activation of nociceptors.
- Neuronal sprouting occurs in the synovium and subchondral bone of OA joints, and neuro-immune interactions contribute to the genesis of pain.
- Neuroinflammation in the Dorsal Root Ganglia (DRG) and the dorsal horn further amplify pain signaling and may contribute to pain chronification.
- Factors such as obesity and sex can alter systemic levels of cytokines contributing to chronic inflammation in OA, and affect sensitization and pain.

OSTEOARTHRITIS PAIN: A WORLDWIDE UNMET MEDICAL NEED

In the United States, approximately 20% of adults suffer from chronic pain, creating a substantive personal and societal burden and costing the economy up to $635 billion per year.[1,2] The musculoskeletal system is one of the leading sources of chronic pain, with osteoarthritis (OA) as the leading cause. As the most prevalent form of arthritis, OA affects over 32.5 million U.S. adults. Worldwide, 240 million individuals live with symptomatic OA,[3–6] and its prevalence is increasing as the world's population is

[a] Department of Internal Medicine, Division of Rheumatology, Rush University Medical Center, Room 340, 1735 W Harrison Street, Chicago, IL 60612, USA; [b] Department of Internal Medicine, Division of Rheumatology, Rush University Medical Center, Room 714, 1735 W Harrison Street, Chicago, IL 60612, USA; [c] Department of Internal Medicine, Division of Rheumatology, Rush University Medical Center, 1611 W Harrison Street, Suite 510, Chicago, IL 60612, USA
* Corresponding author.
E-mail address: anne-marie_malfait@rush.edu

Clin Geriatr Med 38 (2022) 221–238
https://doi.org/10.1016/j.cger.2021.11.013
0749-0690/22/© 2021 Elsevier Inc. All rights reserved.

aging.[7] It has been recognized that OA is associated with an increased risk of all-cause mortality, often because of reduced mobility.[8]

Chronic pain and disability define clinical OA, and activity-limiting pain has been shown to be the greatest burden driving patients to seek medical attention in older adults.[9] Chronic pain can have a profound negative impact on patients' physical lives as well as their mental health, and knee OA is significantly correlated with poor mental health and depressive symptoms.[10–12]

Disease-modifying and pain-alleviating therapies for OA remain elusive. Currently available analgesics are largely inadequate in addition to having adverse side effects, resulting in a major unmet medical need for patients. Therefore, furthering our understanding of the origins and mechanisms of OA pain will be critical to developing effective treatments.

PAIN IN OSTEOARTHRITIS

OA pathology is characterized by progressive joint damage, including cartilage erosion, subchondral bone sclerosis, synovitis, bone remodeling with osteophyte formation, and meniscal damage, all of which may contribute to pain. There is no simple correlation between pain and structural pathology, and in knee OA, studies have only found weak correlations between pain and radiographic findings.[13–15] In contrast, MRI studies, which image soft tissues, have uncovered that synovitis and bone marrow lesions are correlated with pain. This suggests that specific aspects of joint pathology may indeed cause OA pain, offering the prospect for targeted treatment strategies, although this has not yet led to agents that have been approved by regulatory agencies.[16] Attempts have also been made to stratify patients based on pain phenotypes, but translating this into therapeutic strategies has so far been unsuccessful.[17]

Pain in OA is complex and multi-factorial, modified by genetic, psychological, and environmental determinants. Patients struggle to self-describe pain with just "intensity," and describe numerous types of pain that vary in duration, depth, type of occurrence, impact, and rhythm.[18] Several recent reviews have thoughtfully discussed different complex aspects of the genesis of pain in OA, including peripheral mechanisms of pain and sensitization,[19,20] central pain pathways,[21] the role of innate immune responses,[22] and structural correlates of OA pain.[23] When considering the genesis of joint pain, we should bear in mind that pain is one of the cardinal signs of inflammation. While the role of low-level inflammation in the pathogenesis of OA joint damage has been extensively studied in recent years,[24] it is not at all clear how exactly inflammation contributes to the accompanying pain. Targeting inflammation in OA can provide pain relief for some patients, but the effect size for nonsteroidal antiinflammatory drugs (NSAIDs), a first-line treatment of OA, is moderate at best.[25] Likewise, intraarticular corticosteroid injections—while providing acute pain relief—have not shown long-term analgesic effects.[26,27] This illustrates that joint inflammation alone is not enough for sustaining pain in OA. Inflammatory mediators can act on many cells, including neurons, and inflammation comes in many guises, operating at many levels, including in the joint, in the nervous system ("neuro-inflammation"), and systemically. In addition, inflammation can both induce pain, as well as promote the resolution of pain. In this narrative review, we discuss recent discoveries that clarify how these different levels of inflammation may initiate, maintain, and modify pain in OA. We searched PubMed for the following terms: "osteoarthritis," "pain," "inflammation," "cytokines," "NGF," "synovium," "DRG," "obesity," and principally focused on studies published in the last 5 years.

LOCAL INFLAMMATION IN THE OSTEOARTHRITIS JOINT: CONTRIBUTIONS TO PAIN

The pain pathway can be broken down into signal detection and neuron stimulation, signal transmission to the dorsal horn via the peripheral nervous system, and transmission to the brain via the central nervous system (**Fig. 1**). A range of mechanical, thermal, and chemical stimuli—both noxious and nonnoxious—are sensed in peripheral tissues via sensory neurons. This generates action potentials that carry these signals to the dorsal horn via the dorsal root ganglia (DRG), whereby the cell bodies of sensory neurons are located. Sensory nerves are either thick, myelinated Aβ fibers which are activated by joint movement, or thinly myelinated Aδ and unmyelinated C fibers, which are activated by noxious mechanical, thermal, and chemical stimuli through specialized receptors.[28] These high-threshold pain-sensing neurons are called nociceptors (from the Latin *nocere* – to harm). For example, noxious heat is detected by the capsaicin receptor, transient receptor potential vanilloid type 1 (TRPV1),[29] generating action potentials that invade the DRG. Voltage-gated sodium channels are essential for the generation of action potentials. From the DRG, the painful signals are then transmitted to the dorsal horn in the spinal cord, whereby the first synapse occurs.[28] Second-order neurons, activated by the release of glutamate, project to supraspinal regions, and from there, the signal is relayed to higher regions of the brain, whereby pain perception occurs, and information is generated on the location and intensity of the pain, while affective aspects modify the pain experience.[30]

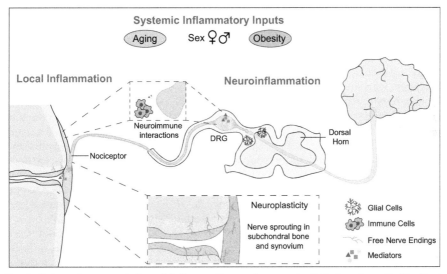

Fig. 1. Pain pathway and sites of inflammation and neuroplasticity in osteoarthritis. Nociceptors (Aδ or C- fibers) detect stimuli in joint tissues, generating action potentials that are transmitted to the dorsal horn via the dorsal root ganglia (DRG), and to the brain via the central nervous system. Inflammatory states and neuroimmune interactions can occur at multiple points along this pathway. Structural neuroplasticity occurs in the OA joint, with free nerve endings sprouting in the subchondral bone and synovium. Joint nociceptors become sensitized by mediators released in OA pathology, including nerve growth factor (NGF), inflammatory cytokines and chemokines, and damage-associated molecular patterns (DAMPs). Immune cell infiltration in synovium and DRG can include macrophages, T- and B-lymphocytes, and mast cells, which can further amplify pain mechanisms. Neuroimmune interactions also occur in the DRG and the dorsal horn. Finally, factors such as obesity, age, and sex may alter systemic inflammatory inputs and modify OA pain.

Later, we will discuss how inflammatory mediators generated in the OA joint may modify the nociceptive pathway through direct effects on sensory neurons that innervate joint tissues.

Local Inflammatory Mediators in the Joint May Affect Neuronal Activity and Neuronal Sprouting

Inflammation and tissue injury are associated with the sensitization of pain pathways, which results in augmented pain responses. For example, patients with OA are sensitized to mechanical stimuli, and quantitative sensory testing (QST) has revealed *hyperalgesia*, manifesting as lowered pain pressure thresholds when a force is applied to the joint, as well as *allodynia*, whereby nonnoxious stimuli are perceived as painful. QST measures are more closely associated with pain severity than radiographic severity and may aid in identifying people susceptible to chronic pain (reviewed in[31]). Sensitization to mechanical stimuli is also a feature of all animal models of OA.[32] Thus, it can be expected that elucidating the mechanisms underlying sensitization of joint nociceptors may be a key step in understanding the genesis of chronic OA pain.[33] Here, we will briefly discuss inflammatory mediators present in the joint that may promote pain through direct effects on joint nociceptors.

Inflammatory cytokines and chemokines

Inflammatory mediators, including cytokines, chemokines, neurotrophins, and prostaglandins can all activate nociceptors through direct binding of their cognate receptors expressed by these cells.[34] OA joint tissues and the synovial fluid contain many such pro-algesic factors, including tumor necrosis factor (TNF)-α, interleukin (IL)1-β, IL-6, and chemokine (C-C motif) ligand 2 (CCL2),[35] and *in vitro* studies have shown that OA synovial fluid induces hyperexcitability in DRG neurons.[36] In subjects with OA, synovial fluid levels of IL-7, IL-12, interferon (IFN)-γ, IL-10 and IL-13 have been correlated with knee pain.[37] Clinical trials with antibodies neutralizing traditional pro-inflammatory cytokines, including IL-1 and TNF-α, have been largely disappointing,[38] and more recent work in animal models deals with cytokines that were previously not a focus in OA research, including IL-17 and IL-33. IL-17 A causes long-lasting sensitization of joint nociceptors to mechanical stimuli when injected into the rat knee.[39] In an inflammatory model (antigen-induced arthritis), *Il17* null mice have less mechanical hyperalgesia, even though joint damage is as severe as in wild-type mice, suggesting a direct contribution of IL-17A to the genesis of pain.[40] Na *and colleagues* reported that IL-1 receptor antagonist (*IL-1Ra*) null mice have increased pain and cartilage destruction in the monosodium iodoacetate (MIA) model of OA, but the attenuation of increased IL-17 levels using IL-17/IL-1RA double-deficient mice resulted in significantly decreased pain scores.[41] Another cytokine that was recently studied in the context of OA is IL-33, a member of the IL-1 family that plays a role in innate and adaptive immunity.[42] He *and colleagues* reported increased concentrations of IL-33 in the synovial fluid of patients with OA, and increased expression of IL-33 and its receptor, suppression of tumorigenicity 2 (ST2), in OA chondrocytes.[43] IL-33 expression is also increased in mice after DMM surgery, and intraarticular administration of recombinant IL-33 caused mechanical allodynia. Neutralizing monoclonal antibodies against IL-33 and ST2 attenuated both OA progression and pain in the DMM model

There is also continued interest in the chemokine, CCL2, as a target for OA pain. CCL2 levels are increased in OA synovial fluid, and this has been correlated with symptoms.[44,45] Several laboratories have found that CCL2-CCR2 signaling is essential for the initiation and maintenance of pain-related behaviors in the DMM model (reviewed in[46]). This signaling pathway may contribute to OA pain through multiple mechanisms, including macrophage recruitment to the joint and to the DRG, as well as through direct neuronal activation.[47,48] CCR2 (the main receptor for CCL2) is expressed on intraarticular nociceptors, both in naïve mice and after the destabilization of the medial meniscus (DMM).[49] Furthermore, intraarticular injection of CCR2 receptor antagonist into the knee joint reduced knee hyperalgesia after DMM surgery, suggesting a local role for CCL2-CCR2 signaling in sensitization of joint nociceptors, and providing a possibility for therapeutic targeting of this pathway in early disease.

Finally, targeting the transcription factor, NF-κB, which is activated by both mechanical stress as well as cytokines and chemokines, remains an area of active investigation. In particular, recent work has focused on developing intraarticular therapeutic strategies that target this pathway in the context of posttraumatic OA, revealing analgesic effects.[50]

Nerve growth factor

The neurotrophin, nerve growth factor (NGF), has received much attention in the field in recent years, because clinical trials with monoclonal antibodies that neutralize NGF showed promising analgesic effects in OA of the knee.[51] However, the ill-understood risk for rapidly progressive OA in a subset of patients receiving the antibodies has prevented FDA approval of this biological therapy.[52]

During embryonic development, NGF is crucial for the growth and survival of neurons. Postnatally, NGF retains key functions, especially in inflammation, when levels are dramatically increased.[53] Pain production is a major biological effect of NGF, and local injection of NGF produces immediate and often long-lasting sensitization and pain responses in animals and humans, including when injected into the joint.[54–57] The mechanisms by which NGF exerts its pain-producing actions have been extensively reviewed, and involve both rapid effects and long-term neuroplastic changes.[58] The high-affinity receptor for NGF, tropomyosin kinase A (TrkA), is expressed by nociceptors, and NGF-TrkA signaling results in excitatory effects that lead to the functional sensitization of nociceptors, both through the transactivation of ion channels such as TRPV1, and through the retrograde transport of the NGF/TrkA complex to the cell bodies in the DRG, whereby it initiates gene expression changes that lead to the synthesis of pro-algesic peptides (substance P, CGRP) and ion channels such as $Na_V1.8$.

An important property of NGF that may contribute to its pain-promoting activity is that it can stimulate neuronal sprouting at an injured site, as has been described in models of bone fracture, bone cancer, and inflammation induced by intra-articular (i.a.) complete Freund's adjuvant, whereby anti-NGF antibodies blocked neuronal sprouting and pain.[58] This biological property may be of key importance in the context of OA, as it is becoming increasingly clear that profound neuronal plasticity of nociceptors occurs as part of OA joint pathology. Most strikingly, in human OA knees as well as in rodent models, osteochondral channels breach the tidemark between the subchondral bone and the articular cartilage, and these channels contain neurons and blood vessels.[59–62] At this time, it is not clear to which extent these newly sprouted nociceptors contribute to pain in human OA knees, but the presence of CGRP-immunoreactive nociceptors in these channels has been associated with pain.[61] Neuronal sprouting has also been reported in the medial synovium in a surgical murine model of OA.[62]

Clearly, it will be important to identify the key drivers of this neuroplasticity to enhance our understanding of the genesis of OA joint pain. Candidate molecules have been identified, such as netrin, an osteoclast-derived molecule that has been linked to neuronal sprouting in the subchondral bone in a surgical murine model.[63]

Importantly, NGF levels are elevated in the synovial fluid of OA joints,[64] and expression of NGF is increased in OA chondrocytes,[64,65] synovial fibroblasts[66] (associated with pain), and osteochondral channels[67] (also associated with pain). Therefore, it is highly likely that NGF plays a key role in the observed anatomic neuroplasticity observed in OA joints, although this has not been directly investigated.

Damage-associated molecular patterns

Products produced as part of the joint degradation process have the potential to further amplify ongoing joint damage, and innate immune mechanisms are the focus of intense research in OA pathogenesis,[68] including OA pain (recently reviewed[22]). Indeed, joint remodeling in OA generates a host of damage-associated molecular patterns (DAMPs), such as fragments of proteoglycans or inflammation-associated alarmins (eg, S100 proteins) that can bind receptors, including Toll-like receptors (TLRs) and NOD-like receptors (NLRs), which are expressed by many joint tissue cells, including nociceptors. This leads to the direct activation of nociceptors, resulting in pain. Tissue damage products can also signal to TLRs on innate immune cells, causing them to produce chemokines and cytokines that also act on pain-sensing neurons, further amplifying and maintaining pain responses.

The Role of Synovium in Osteoarthritis Pain

OA pathology involves all joint tissues, and inflammatory cytokines, chemokines, DAMPs, and NGF can exert their biological effects in all these tissues, and sensitize nociceptors. As we have discussed, neuronal sprouting has been observed in the subchondral bone of OA joints, as well as in the synovium (see **Fig. 1**). This begs the question as to how synovitis may contribute to OA pain. The synovial tissue lines the joint cavity and secretes synovial fluid, aiding in joint movement. Inflammation of the synovial tissue is observed in more than half of patients with OA throughout disease progression, including early stages of disease.[69,70] Synovitis, as detected by MRI, is associated with pain in knees with and without radiographic OA, as well as with sensitization in knee OA.[71,72] Of interest, different anatomic patterns of synovitis have been described, and a pattern including patellar sites of synovitis have been particularly associated with pain.[73] Synovitis in the OA joint is characterized by an influx of a variety of leukocytes, primarily macrophages and T-lymphocytes, but mast cells, B-lymphocytes and plasma cells can also be present.[74] The quantity of activated macrophages has been associated with OA pain severity and radiographic OA severity.[75] Correlation studies have also suggested a role for lymphocytes in OA pain; for example, Zhu and colleagues showed a positive correlation between circulating CD4+ T cells and WOMAC pain scores.[76] In the synovial tissue, proinflammatory T helper cell type 1 (Th1) infiltration has been recently reported in early patients with OA.[77] Similarly, Nees and colleagues recently investigated T cell subsets in the synovial tissue of patients with OA, with a focus on pain and disability, and found correlations between levels of both Th1 and Th2 T cells with OA-related knee pain.[78] Finally, mast cell numbers have also been found to be elevated in OA synovium,[73] and an interesting recent study in murine MIA reported that NGF-stimulated synovial mast cells produce prostaglandin D_2, which can signal to nociceptors, thus linking NGF-TrkA signaling in mast cells to OA pain.[79]

To unravel how infiltrating immune cells contribute to OA pain, it will be critical to elucidate the bidirectional cross-talk between the nervous system and the immune system. For example, targeting granulocyte macrophage colony-stimulating factor (GM-CSF) prevents pain in murine collagenase-induced osteoarthritis (CiOA).[80,81] Tewari and colleagues showed the absence of functional GM-CSF receptors on mouse nociceptors, but found that conditioned medium from GM-CSF treated macrophages could drive nociceptor transcriptional changes.[82] This exemplifies again how neuroimmune cross-talk may operate in the knee and offer avenues for targeted intervention.

Recent development of technologies such as bulk and single-cell RNA sequencing has allowed a broader approach to mapping the immune cell environment in the synovial tissue. While most studies have not yet examined a direct link of the synovial microenvironment to OA pain, they highlight that the advancement of these technologies will allow delineation of the relationship between immune cells and OA pain in the future. In particular, Chou *and colleagues* performed single-cell RNAseq on synoviocytes of 3 patients undergoing total knee replacement for medial compartment knee OA. This allowed them to identify 12 synovial cell types, including synovial fibroblasts, endothelial cells, and various types of immune cells. In addition, they were able to molecularly define the synovial cells producing particular cytokines, for example, inflammatory macrophages and dendritic cells expressing HLA-DQA1, HLA-DQA2, oxidized low-density lipoprotein receptor 1 (OLR1), or TLR2 were linked to the production of IL-1β.[83] Another study used bulk RNAseq to characterize macrophages purified from the synovial tissue of subjects with OA or with inflammatory arthritis.[84] Gene expression analyses and phenotyping revealed a heterogeneous population of macrophages within the OA samples, one of which was "inflammatory-like" macrophages that had a proliferative phenotype and aligned closely with inflammatory arthritis macrophages. While neither of these studies incorporated pain as a variable, they clearly illustrate how such approaches may aid the identification of specific cell types and their interactions with other cell types such as neurons, and how they contribute to particular aspects of the pathology, including pain. To illustrate this point, a recent single-cell RNAseq study uncovered that synovial fibroblasts from painful sites of the patellar synovium were distinct from fibroblasts from nonpainful areas, with an altered gene signature promoting fibrosis, inflammation, and growth of neurons,[85] supporting the idea that synovitis is linked to neuroplasticity, and thus pain. Finally, a bulk RNAseq study analyzed synovial biopsies collected from patients with knee OA with either low (0–3) or high (7–10) visual analog scale (VAS) pain levels at the time of surgery.[86] Interestingly, while no major differences in the cellular composition were noted between pain groups, their analysis identified neuronal genes such as *NTRK2*, encoding the receptor for the neurotrophin BDNF, as differently upregulated in the high versus low pain groups. The detailed identification and characterization of synovial tissue immune cells and molecular profiles, and their interactions with sensory neurons hold great promise for unraveling precise mechanisms of pain generation in the joint.

NEUROINFLAMMATION: AN EMERGING PLAYER IN OSTEOARTHRITIS PAIN

Inflammatory responses in the central and peripheral nervous system are considered "neuroinflammation," a process increasingly recognized to contribute to chronic pain,[87] including in OA.[88] A hallmark of neuroinflammation is the activation of glial cells, such as microglia, as well as infiltrating macrophages in the DRG and the dorsal horn, which release chemokines and other mediators, and through neuroimmune interactions, modify pain signaling. The description of neuroinflammation in OA is still in its infancy, as briefly summarized later in discussion.

DRG

Neuroinflammation has been described in several rodent models of OA. For example, in a rat CiOA model, DRG satellite glial cells become activated, alongside microglia activation in the dorsal horn—coinciding with pain development.[89] In addition to activation of resident glia, a growing body of recent research implicates immune cell infiltration of the DRG, in particular macrophages, as a contributor to pain in OA.[47,90] Raoof *and colleagues* showed in 2 rodent models of OA that M1-like macrophages accumulate in the DRG away from the injury site. Furthermore, inhibition of these M1-like macrophages in the DRG by intrathecal injection of IL-4/IL-10 fusion protein or M2-like macrophages resolved persistent pain.[90] Microarray analysis of DRGs from a murine OA model distinguished genes differentially expressed in early versus persistent OA pain, and identified genes that contribute to the initiation and maintenance of OA pain and neuroinflammation canonical pathway, including *Cx3cl1*, *Ccl2*, *Tlr1*, and *Ngf*.[91]

Dorsal Horn

Ongoing C-fiber input in the dorsal horn markedly increases second-order neuron excitability, causing activation of microglia and astrocytes, which produce a host of cytokines and chemokines that further amplify the signal.[30] In experimental models of OA, these processes are only beginning to be studied, and activated microglia have been described in the rat MIA model,[92] as well as in a surgical model of OA, whereby microgliosis was a feature of late-stage OA and was associated with persistent pain.[93] At this time, it is not clear if targeting microglia activation can modify pain. A recent study in a rat MIA model reported that the inhibition of glia with minocycline and fluorocitrate alleviated mechanical allodynia. This activation state was present alongside increased joint nociceptor innervation and DRG expression of activating transcription factor 3 (ATF3), a neuronal stress marker. The authors hypothesized that microglial activation induced proinflammatory changes that contributed to OA pain.[94]

Nuclear factor-kappa B (NF-κB) is a transcription factor with well-described roles in inflammatory responses. Previous studies have reported the association of NF-κB activity with chronic pain in the complete Freund's adjuvant (CFA) model of inflammation,[95] vincristine-induced neuropathy model,[96] and an RM-1 induced bone cancer pain model.[97] Li *and colleagues* sought to identify the mechanism NF-κB, astrocyte proliferation and pain in the rat MIA OA model. They found that both the number of astrocytes and expression of NF-κB/p65 in astrocytes in the dorsal horn increased significantly. Furthermore, on spinal inhibition of NF-κB/p65, mechanical hyperalgesia was alleviated and significant decreases were measured in the expression of inflammatory cytokines IL-1β, TNF-α, and IL-33 in the dorsal horn.[98]

While we know very little about the precise mechanisms operating in OA, neuroimmune interactions clearly modify pain pathways, not just in the joint but also in the peripheral and central nervous systems. Information on microglial and astrocyte activation in the brain is scant, but we identified one recent study that reported supraspinal astrocyte activation as a mechanism underlying anxiety-augmented pain behaviors in rat MIA.[99] Furthermore, microglia activation was recently shown in a murine model of rheumatoid arthritis, illustrating the wide impact of joint inflammation on the nervous system.[100] Hence, it can be expected that the study of neuroinflammation holds great potential for identifying specific pathways that may be targeted to attenuate pain in chronic arthritis.

SYSTEMIC INFLAMMATORY INPUTS TO PAIN

Chronic inflammation can be associated with increased systemic levels of cytokines and other mediators that may have a profound effect on the body's homeostasis, including pain. Later, we briefly discuss factors that have been associated with systemic inflammation, including obesity, and how they may affect nociception, sensitization, and chronic pain in the context of OA.

Obesity

A correlation between obesity and OA has been historically recognized, with research showing that in as many as 24% of patients with OA, disease can be attributed to being overweight or obese.[101] In addition, being overweight/obese is also associated with increased OA pain.[102] Mechanical overload of the joint may contribute to this, but obesity has also been associated with OA in nonweight bearing joints, suggesting that biomechanical loading may not be the sole cause of OA pain in obese or overweight patients and that other factors such as systemic and/or local inflammation may contribute.[103,104] In support of this, the association between metabolic syndrome and knee OA is greater for symptomatic OA than radiographic OA.[105] Links between obesity and nonmechanical painful disorders such as headaches and migraines have also been reported, suggesting a direct role for diet and intake of essential fatty acids in chronic pain, with suggested links to altered inflammatory states.[106]

Several studies in experimental models have attempted to unravel these complex relationships between obesity, adiposity, loading, inflammation, and pain. In mice with high-fat-induced OA, wheel-running is protective against joint damage rather than damaging, further suggesting that increased joint loading is not sufficient to explain OA.[107] The authors found that exercised mice had improved glucose tolerance and disrupted proinflammatory cytokine networks in the absence of weight loss. Song *and colleagues* evaluated pain behaviors in 2 strains of rats subjected to high-fat diets, one strain in which obesity is induced and one strain in which obesity is not induced. Although no changes in circulating inflammatory cytokines were measured, an infiltration of macrophages into the DRG was observed, suggesting a link between high-fat diets and the nervous system in chronic pain.[108] Finally, a recent study showed that mice with lipodystrophy were protected from joint damage and knee hyperalgesia after DMM, even under a high-fat diet. Adding back a mixture of subcutaneous and visceral adipose tissue from wild-type mice could overcome this protection.[109] This study suggests an important role for adipose tissue as a mediator of joint degeneration and associated pain in mice, independently of body weight. Although the link between obesity and OA progression may not be entirely due to overloading of joints, physical activity has long been a recommendation for the treatment of OA. The benefits of exercise for patients with OA are clear, with studies showing clear improvements in disease burden and pain scores.[110–112] Conversely, during COVID-19 lockdowns, researchers found that VAS and WOMAC scores increased significantly, correlating with a reduction in physical activity.[113] A recent study demonstrated that diet and exercise intervention in overweight and obese people suffering from knee OA resulted in an improvement of pain and function that was independent of BMI.[114] This was attributed partially to a change in serum levels of inflammatory factors, including IL-6, TNF-α, soluble IL-1 receptor, and C-reactive protein (CRP). The association of obesity and OA is clear; however, understanding the relative contribution of mechanical, inflammatory, and metabolic factors to OA pain requires further investigation.

Other Systemic Factors that can Modify the Inflammatory Aspects of Osteoarthritis Pain

Several modifiable and unmodifiable factors profoundly affect the inflammatory process. Inflammation is considered one of the mechanisms that contribute to age-related diseases, and chronic age-related stimulation of the innate immune system is termed "inflamm-aging."[115] Aging is one of the major risk factors for radiographic as well as symptomatic OA, and research is increasingly uncovering how systemic and local age-related inflammation can contribute to OA joint damage.[116] With age, levels of inflammatory mediators such as IL-6 and TNFα increase systemically and in adipose tissues, while in the joint, senescent cells accumulate and the senescence-associated secretory phenotype (SASP) creates a locally damaging environment.[117] However, the relationship of inflamm-aging and OA pain remains understudied. It has been shown that systemic levels of CRP, TNFα, and IL6 are associated with knee pain in older adults.[118] Interestingly, the authors found that when corrected for the presence of radiographic OA, these associations of inflammatory markers and knee pain remained.

Sex is a major determinant in the inflammatory process, and while differences between men and women in both the disease progression and pain burden of OA have been widely reported,[119] it is not at all yet clear how this relates to mechanisms of pain. Females have a higher symptom burden and are more likely to use health care, resulting in a higher prevalence of clinical diagnosis.[120,121] This gender discrepancy becomes particularly apparent in older adults, after 50 years of age.[120] Mun *and colleagues* hypothesized that an underlying mechanism of sex-based risk differences in developing OA might be due to exaggerated inflammatory responses to pain in women than men. The authors measured serum levels of IL-6 over time following laboratory-induced pain and found that IL-6 levels were significantly increased in women than men after painful stimulus.[122] Similarly, Perruccio *and colleagues* explored sex-based differences of systemic inflammatory markers in patients with OA scheduled for knee arthroplasty and found that IL-6 was positively correlated with knee pain in women only. Furthermore, they found positive correlations of IL-1β and IL-18 with knee pain in men, but these same cytokines were negatively correlated with knee pain in women.[123] Clearly, this will be an important area of study for the successful development of analgesics in OA.

CONCLUSIONS AND FUTURE DIRECTIONS

In summary, recent research has generated crucial novel insights into the generation of OA pain. Notably, OA joint pathology is characterized by profound neuroplasticity, with the sprouting of nociceptors in the subchondral bone and the synovium. Secondly, innate immune and inflammatory mechanisms mediate OA pathology and pain at multiple levels, and interact with sensory neurons in the joint and also in the nervous system. It can be expected that the precise molecular elucidation of these neuroimmune interactions will offer a rich substrate for targeted interventions. Several modifying systemic factors will need to be taken into account when studying these mechanisms, including sex, age, and obesity.

Finally, it should be considered that OA is strongly mechanically driven, promoted by joint overload. "Mechanoinflammation" has been suggested as a mechanical signaling pathway driving inflammatory signaling and pain in OA.[124] One potential pathway that may be of particular interest is the mechanosensitive channel, Piezo2, expressed by nociceptors. Piezo2 becomes sensitized under inflammatory conditions and plays a role in mediating mechanical allodynia.[125,126] Interestingly, a link between NGF and Piezo2 has also been proposed as a mechanism of activation of "silent nociceptors"—nociceptors that begin to sense mechanical stimuli after sensitization.[127] Therefore, the interactions between inflammatory pathways and mechanical stress on the joints may well be a unique feature of OA pathogenesis and the genesis of OA pain.

AUTHOR CONTRIBUTIONS

M.J. Wood wrote the article, R.E. Miller and A-M. Malfait edited. All three authors read and approved the final version.

ACKNOWLEDGMENTS

The authors are grateful for the support of the Rheumatology Research Foundation (M.J. Wood and A-M. Malfait funded by a Rheumatology Research Foundation 2021 Innovative Research Award) and the National Institutes of Health (National Institute of Arthritis and Musculoskeletal and Skin Diseases [NIAMS]) (R01AR060364, R01AR064251, and P30AR079206 to A.M. Malfait; R01AR077019 to R.E. Miller).

CLINICS CARE POINTS

- OA is one of the major causes of chronic pain in the world, but currently available analgesic drugs are inadequate.
- Infammatory pathways, including neuroimmune interactions, provide a rich substrate of potential targets for the development of new drugs for OA pain.
- Profound neuroplasticity is part of OA pathology. This must be taken into account when considering targeting strategies for managing pain.

DISCLOSURE

M.J. Wood and R.E. Miller: nothing to disclose; in the last 24 months, A-M. Malfait has received consulting fees from Eli Lilly, Pfizer, Vizuri, AKP, Ceva, and 23andMe.

REFERENCES

1. Dahlhamer J, Lucas J, Zelaya C, et al. Prevalence of chronic pain and high-impact chronic pain among adults — United States, 2016. MMWR Morb Mortal Wkly Rep 2018;67(36):1001–6.
2. Gaskin DJ, Richard P. The economic costs of pain in the United States. J Pain 2012;13(8):715–24.
3. Deshpande BR, Katz JN, Solomon DH, et al. Number of Persons with symptomatic knee osteoarthritis in the US: impact of Race and Ethnicity, age, sex, and obesity. Arthritis Care Res 2016;68(12):1743–50.
4. United States Bone and Joint Initiative. The burden of musculoskeletal diseases in the United States (BMUS). Fourth Edition.
5. Vos T, Lim SS, Abbafati C, et al. Global burden of 369 diseases and injuries in 204 countries and territories, 1990–2019: a systematic analysis for the Global Burden of Disease Study 2019. Lancet 2020;396(10258):1204–22. https://doi.org/10.1016/S0140-6736(20)30925-9.
6. Allen KD, Thoma LM, Golightly YM. Epidemiology of osteoarthritis. Osteoarthritis Cartilage 2021. https://doi.org/10.1016/j.joca.2021.04.020.
7. Safiri S, Kolahi A-A, Smith E, et al. Global, regional and national burden of osteoarthritis 1990-2017: a systematic analysis of the Global Burden of Disease Study 2017. Ann Rheum Dis 2020;79(6):819 LP–828.

8. Osteoarthritis: A Serious Disease. Pre Compet Consort Osteoarthr Osteoarthr Res Soc Int. Published online 2016.Available at: https://oarsi.org/education/oarsi-resources/oarsi-white-paper-oa-serious-disease (White Paper submitted to the FDA).

9. Dominick KL, Ahern FM, Gold CH, et al. Health-related quality of life and health service use among older adults with osteoarthritis. Arthritis Care Res 2004; 51(3):326–31.

10. Daniel L. Riddle, Xiangrong Kong GKF. Psychological health impact on two-year changes in pain and function in Persons with knee pain: Data from the osteoarthritis initiative. Osteoarthr Cartil 2011;19(9):1095–101.

11. Park H-M, Kim H-S, Lee Y-J. Knee osteoarthritis and its association with mental health and health-related quality of life: a nationwide cross-sectional study. Geriatr Gerontol Int 2020;20(4):379–83. https://doi.org/10.1111/ggi.13879.

12. Rathbun AM, Stuart EA, Shardell M, et al. Dynamic effects of depressive symptoms on osteoarthritis knee pain. Arthritis Care Res (Hoboken) 2018;70(1):80–8. https://doi.org/10.1002/acr.23239.

13. Neogi T, Felson D, Niu J, et al. Association between radiographic features of knee osteoarthritis and pain: results from two cohort studies. BMJ 2009; 339(7719):498–501.

14. Bacon K, Lavalley MP, Jafarzadeh SR, et al. Does cartilage loss cause pain in osteoarthritis and if so, how much? Ann Rheum Dis 2020;79(8):1105–10.

15. Wang K, Kim HA, Felson DT, et al. Radiographic knee osteoarthritis and knee pain: cross-sectional study from five different Racial/Ethnic populations. Sci Rep 2018;8(1):1–8.

16. O'Neill TW, Felson DT. Mechanisms of osteoarthritis (OA) pain. Curr Osteoporos Rep 2018;16(5):611–6.

17. Kittelson AJ, Stevens-Lapsley JE, Schmeige SJ. Determination of pain phenotypes in knee osteoarthritis: a latent class Analysis using Data from the osteoarthritis initiative. Arthritis Care Res 2017;68(5):612–20. Determination.

18. Cedraschi C, Delézay S, Marty M, et al. "Let's talk about OA pain": a qualitative analysis of the perceptions of people suffering from OA. Towards the development of a specific pain OA-related questionnaire, the Osteoarthritis Symptom Inventory Scale (OASIS). PLoS One 2013;8(11):1–10.

19. Vincent TL. Peripheral pain mechanisms in osteoarthritis. Pain 2020;161. Available at: https://journals.lww.com/pain/Fulltext/2020/09001/Peripheral_pain_mechanisms_in_osteoarthritis.15.aspx.

20. Malfait AM, Miller RE, Miller RJ. Basic mechanisms of pain in osteoarthritis: experimental Observations and new Perspectives. Rheum Dis Clin North Am 2021;47(2):165–80.

21. Clauw DJ, Hassett AL. The role of centralised pain in osteoarthritis. Clin Exp Rheumatol 2017;35(5):S79–84.

22. Miller RJ, Malfait A-M, Miller RE. The innate immune response as a mediator of osteoarthritis pain. Osteoarthr Cartil 2020;28(5):562–71.

23. Neogi T. Structural correlates of pain in osteoarthritis. Clin Exp Rheumatol 2017; 35(5):S75–8.

24. Griffin TM, Scanzello CR. Innate inflammation and synovial macrophages in osteoarthritis pathophysiology. Clin Exp Rheumatol 2019;37:57–63. Suppl 1(5). https://pubmed.ncbi.nlm.nih.gov/31621560.

25. Bannuru RR, Osani MC, Vaysbrot EE, et al. OARSI guidelines for the nonsurgical management of knee, hip, and polyarticular osteoarthritis. Osteoarthr Cartil 2019;27(11):1578–89. https://doi.org/10.1016/j.joca.2019.06.011.

26. Deyle GD, Allen CS, Allison SC, et al. Physical Therapy versus Glucocorticoid injection for osteoarthritis of the knee. N Engl J Med 2020;382(15):1420–9.

27. McAlindon TE, LaValley MP, Harvey WF, et al. Effect of intra-articular Triamcinolone vs Saline on knee cartilage Volume and pain in patients with knee osteoarthritis: a randomized clinical trial. JAMA 2017;317(19):1967–75.

28. Basbaum AI, Bautista DM, Scherrer G, et al. Cellular and molecular mechanisms of pain. Cell 2009;139(2):267–84.

29. Julius D. TRP channels and pain. Annu Rev Cell Dev Biol 2013;29(1):355–84.

30. Woller SA, Eddinger KA, Corr M, et al. An overview of pathways encoding nociception. Clin Exp Rheumatol 2017;35:40–6. Suppl 1(5). https://pubmed.ncbi.nlm.nih.gov/28967373.

31. Arant KR, Katz JN, Neogi T. Quantitative sensory testing: identifying pain characteristics in patients with osteoarthritis. Osteoarthr Cartil 2021. https://doi.org/10.1016/j.joca.2021.09.011.

32. Miller RE, Malfait A-M. Osteoarthritis pain: what are we learning from animal models? Best Pract Res Clin Rheumatol 2017;31(5):676–87.

33. Miller RE, Malfait A-M. Can we prevent chronic osteoarthritis pain? A view from the bench. *Osteoarthr Cartil* Published Online 2021. https://doi.org/10.1016/j.joca.2021.10.001.

34. Miller RJ, Jung H, Bhangoo SK, et al. Cytokine and chemokine regulation of sensory neuron function. Handb Exp Pharmacol 2009;194:417–49.

35. Scanzello CR. Chemokines and inflammation in osteoarthritis: insights from patients and animal models. J Orthop Res 2017;35(4):735–9. https://doi.org/10.1002/jor.23471.

36. Chakrabarti S, Jadon DR, Bulmer DC, et al. Human osteoarthritic synovial fluid increases excitability of mouse dorsal root ganglion sensory neurons: an in-vitro translational model to study arthritic pain. Rheumatology 2020;59(3):662–7.

37. Nees TA, Rosshirt N, Zhang JA, et al. Synovial cytokines significantly correlate with osteoarthritis-related knee pain and disability: inflammatory mediators of potential clinical Relevance. J Clin Med 2019;8(9). https://doi.org/10.3390/jcm8091343.

38. Persson MSM, Sarmanova A, Doherty M, et al. Conventional and biologic disease-modifying anti-rheumatic drugs for osteoarthritis: a meta-analysis of randomized controlled trials. Rheumatology 2018;57(10):1830–7.

39. Richter F, Natura G, Ebbinghaus M, et al. Interleukin-17 sensitizes joint nociceptors to mechanical stimuli and contributes to arthritic pain through neuronal interleukin-17 receptors in rodents. Arthritis Rheum 2012;64(12):4125–34. https://doi.org/10.1002/art.37695.

40. Ebbinghaus M, Natura G, Segond von Banchet G, et al. Interleukin-17A is involved in mechanical hyperalgesia but not in the severity of murine antigen-induced arthritis. Sci Rep 2017;7(1):10334.

41. Na HS, Park J-S, Cho K-H, et al. Interleukin-1-Interleukin-17 signaling Axis induces cartilage Destruction and promotes experimental osteoarthritis. Front Immunol 2020;11:730. https://www.frontiersin.org/article/10.3389/fimmu.2020.00730.

42. Liew FY, Girard J-P, Turnquist HR. Interleukin-33 in health and disease. Nat Rev Immunol 2016;16(11):676–89.

43. He Z, Song Y, Yi Y, et al. Blockade of IL-33 signalling attenuates osteoarthritis. Clin Transl Immunol 2020;9(10):e1185. https://doi.org/10.1002/cti2.1187.

44. Haraden CA, Huebner JL, Hsueh M-F, et al. Synovial fluid biomarkers associated with osteoarthritis severity reflect macrophage and neutrophil related inflammation. Arthritis Res Ther 2019;21(1):146.

45. Li L, Jiang B-E. Serum and synovial fluid chemokine ligand 2/monocyte chemoattractant protein 1 concentrations correlates with symptomatic severity in patients with knee osteoarthritis. Ann Clin Biochem 2014;52(2):276–82.

46. Miller RE, Malfait A-M. Can we target CCR2 to treat osteoarthritis? The trick is in the timing. Osteoarthr Cartil 2017;25(6):799–801.

47. Miller RE, Tran PB, Das R, et al. CCR2 chemokine receptor signaling mediates pain in experimental osteoarthritis. Proc Natl Acad Sci U S A 2012;109(50):20602–7.

48. Miotla Zarebska J, Chanalaris A, Driscoll C, et al. CCL2 and CCR2 regulate pain-related behaviour and early gene expression in post-traumatic murine osteoarthritis but contribute little to chondropathy. Osteoarthr Cartil 2017;25(3):406–12.

49. Ishihara S, Obeidat AM, Wokosin DL, et al. The role of intra-articular neuronal CCR2 receptors in knee joint pain associated with experimental osteoarthritis in mice. Arthritis Res Ther 2021;23(1):103.

50. Berke IM, Jain E, Yavuz B, et al. NF-κB-mediated effects on behavior and cartilage pathology in a non-invasive loading model of post-traumatic osteoarthritis. Osteoarthr Cartil 2021;29(2):248–56.

51. Dietz BW, Nakamura MC, Bell MT, et al. Targeting nerve growth factor for pain management in osteoarthritis—clinical Efficacy and Safety. Rheum Dis Clin North Am 2021;47(2):181–95.

52. Wise BL, Seidel MF, Lane NE. The evolution of nerve growth factor inhibition in clinical medicine. Nat Rev Rheumatol 2021;17(1):34–46.

53. Hefti FF, Rosenthal A, Walicke PA, et al. Novel class of pain drugs based on antagonism of NGF. Trends Pharmacol Sci 2006;27(2):85–91.

54. Rukwied R, Mayer A, Kluschina O, et al. NGF induces non-inflammatory localized and lasting mechanical and thermal hypersensitivity in human skin. Pain 2010;148(3). Available at: https://journals.lww.com/pain/Fulltext/2010/03000/NGF_induces_non_inflammatory_localized_and_lasting.11.aspx.

55. Weinkauf B, Obreja O, Schmelz M, et al. Differential time course of NGF-induced hyperalgesia to heat versus mechanical and electrical stimulation in human skin. Eur J Pain (United Kingdom) 2015;19(6):789–96.

56. Andresen T, Nilsson M, Nielsen AK, et al. Intradermal injection with nerve growth factor: a Reproducible model to induce experimental allodynia and hyperalgesia. Pain Pract 2016;16(1):12–23.

57. Ashraf S, Mapp PI, Burston J, et al. Augmented pain behavioural responses to intra-articular injection of nerve growth factor in two animal models of osteoarthritis. Ann Rheum Dis 2014;73(9):1710 LP–1718.

58. Denk F, Bennett DL, McMahon SB. Nerve growth factor and pain mechanisms. Annu Rev Neurosci 2017;40(1):307–25.

59. Suri S, Gill SE, Massena de Camin S, et al. Neurovascular invasion at the osteochondral junction and in osteophytes in osteoarthritis. Ann Rheum Dis 2007;66(11):1423–8.

60. Mapp PI, Sagar DR, Ashraf S, et al. Differences in structural and pain phenotypes in the sodium monoiodoacetate and meniscal transection models of osteoarthritis. Osteoarthr Cartil 2013;21(9):1336–45.

61. Aso K, Shahtaheri SM, Hill R, et al. Contribution of nerves within osteochondral channels to osteoarthritis knee pain in humans and rats. Osteoarthr Cartil 2020; 28(9):1245–54. https://doi.org/10.1016/j.joca.2020.05.010.

62. Obeidat AM, Miller RE, Miller RJ, et al. The nociceptive innervation of the normal and osteoarthritic mouse knee. Osteoarthr Cartil 2019;27(11):1669–79.

63. Zhu S, Zhu J, Zhen G, et al. Subchondral bone osteoclasts induce sensory innervation and osteoarthritis pain. J Clin Invest 2019;129(3):1076–93.

64. Iannone F, De Bari C, Dell'Accio F, et al. Increased expression of nerve growth factor (NGF) and high affinity NGF receptor (p140 TrkA) in human osteoarthritic chondrocytes. Rheumatology 2002;41(12):1413–8.

65. Driscoll C, Chanalaris A, Knights C, et al. Nociceptive Sensitizers are regulated in damaged joint tissues, including articular cartilage, when osteoarthritic mice Display pain behavior. Arthritis Rheumatol (Hoboken, Nj) 2016;68(4):857–67.

66. Stoppiello LA, Mapp PI, Wilson D, et al. Structural associations of symptomatic knee osteoarthritis. Arthritis Rheumatol (Hoboken, Nj) 2014;66(11):3018–27.

67. Aso K, Shahtaheri SM, Hill R, et al. Associations of symptomatic knee osteoarthritis with Histopathologic features in subchondral bone. Arthritis Rheumatol 2019;71(6):916–24.

68. van den Bosch MHJ, van Lent PLEM, van der Kraan PM. Identifying effector molecules, cells, and cytokines of innate immunity in OA. Osteoarthr Cartil 2020;28(5):532–43.

69. Roemer FW, Guermazi A, Felson DT, et al. Presence of MRI-detected joint effusion and synovitis increases the risk of cartilage loss in knees without osteoarthritis at 30-month follow-up: the MOST study. Ann Rheum Dis 2011;70(10): 1804 LP–1809.

70. Benito MJ, Veale DJ, FitzGerald O, et al. Synovial tissue inflammation in early and late osteoarthritis. Ann Rheum Dis 2005;64(9):1263 LP–1267.

71. Baker K, Grainger A, Niu J, et al. Relation of synovitis to knee pain using contrast-enhanced MRIs. Ann Rheum Dis 2010;69(10):1779–83.

72. Neogi T, Guermazi A, Roemer F, et al. Association of joint inflammation with pain sensitization in knee osteoarthritis: the Multicenter osteoarthritis study. Arthritis Rheumatol (Hoboken, Nj) 2016;68(3):654–61.

73. de Lange-Brokaar BJE, Ioan-Facsinay A, Yusuf E, et al. Association of pain in knee osteoarthritis with distinct patterns of synovitis. Arthritis Rheumatol 2015; 67(3):733–40. https://doi.org/10.1002/art.38965.

74. Mathiessen A, Conaghan PG. Synovitis in osteoarthritis: current understanding with therapeutic implications. Arthritis Res Ther 2017;19(1):18.

75. Kraus VB, McDaniel G, Huebner JL, et al. Direct in vivo evidence of activated macrophages in human osteoarthritis. Osteoarthr Cartil 2016;24(9):1613–21.

76. Zhu W, Zhang X, Jiang Y, et al. Alterations in peripheral T cell and B cell subsets in patients with osteoarthritis. Clin Rheumatol 2020;39(2):523–32.

77. Rosshirt N, Trauth R, Platzer H, et al. Proinflammatory T cell polarization is already present in patients with early knee osteoarthritis. Arthritis Res Ther 2021;23(1):37.

78. Nees TA, Rosshirt N, Zhang JA, et al. T helper cell infiltration in osteoarthritis-related knee pain and disability. J Clin Med 2020;9(8):2423.

79. Sousa-Valente J, Calvo L, Vacca V, et al. Role of TrkA signalling and mast cells in the initiation of osteoarthritis pain in the monoiodoacetate model. Osteoarthr Cartil 2018;26(1):84–94.

80. Cook AD, Pobjoy J, Steidl S, et al. Granulocyte-macrophage colony-stimulating factor is a key mediator in experimental osteoarthritis pain and disease development. Arthritis Res Ther 2012;14(5):R199.

81. Lee KM-C, Prasad V, Achuthan A, et al. Targeting GM-CSF for collagenase-induced osteoarthritis pain and disease in mice. Osteoarthr Cartil 2020;28(4): 486–91.

82. Tewari D, Cook AD, Lee M-C, et al. Granulocyte-macrophage colony stimulating factor As an Indirect mediator of nociceptor activation and pain. J Neurosci 2020;40(11):2189–99.

83. Chou C-H, Jain V, Gibson J, et al. Synovial cell cross-talk with cartilage plays a major role in the pathogenesis of osteoarthritis. Sci Rep 2020;10(1):10868.

84. Wood MJ, Leckenby A, Reynolds G, et al. Macrophage proliferation distinguishes 2 subgroups of knee osteoarthritis patients. JCI insight 2019;4(2): e125325.

85. Nanus DE, Badoume A, Wijesinghe SN, et al. Synovial tissue from sites of joint pain in knee osteoarthritis patients exhibits a differential phenotype with distinct fibroblast subsets. EBioMedicine 2021;72:103618.

86. Bratus-Neuenschwander A, Castro-Giner F, Frank-Bertoncelj M, et al. Pain-associated transcriptome changes in synovium of knee osteoarthritis patients. Genes (Basel) 2018;9(7):338.

87. Matsuda M, Huh Y, Ji R-R. Roles of inflammation, neurogenic inflammation, and neuroinflammation in pain. J Anesth 2019;33(1):131–9.

88. Geraghty T, Winter DR, Miller RJ, et al. Neuroimmune interactions and osteoarthritis pain: focus on macrophages. Pain Rep 2021;6(1):e892.

89. Adães S, Almeida L, Potes CS, et al. Glial activation in the collagenase model of nociception associated with osteoarthritis. Mol Pain 2017;13. 1744806916688219-1744806916688219.

90. Raoof R, Martin Gil C, Lafeber FPJG, et al. Dorsal root ganglia macrophages maintain osteoarthritis pain. J Neurosci 2021. JN-RM-1787-20.

91. Miller RE, Tran PB, Ishihara S, et al. Microarray analyses of the dorsal root ganglia support a role for innate neuro-immune pathways in persistent pain in experimental osteoarthritis. Osteoarthr Cartil 2020;28(5):581–92.

92. Ogbonna AC, Clark AK, Malcangio M. Development of monosodium acetate-induced osteoarthritis and inflammatory pain in ageing mice. Age (Omaha) 2015;37(3):54.

93. Tran PB, Miller RE, Ishihara S, et al. Spinal microglial activation in a murine surgical model of knee osteoarthritis. Osteoarthr Cartil 2017;25(5):718–26.

94. Bourassa V, Deamond H, Yousefpour N, et al. Pain-related behavior is associated with increased joint innervation, ipsilateral dorsal horn gliosis, and dorsal root ganglia activating transcription factor 3 expression in a rat ankle joint model of osteoarthritis. PAIN Rep 2020;5(5). Available at: https://journals.lww.com/painrpts/Fulltext/2020/10000/Pain_related_behavior_is_associated_with_increased.4.aspx.

95. Hartung JE, Eskew O, Wong T, et al. Nuclear factor-kappa B regulates pain and COMT expression in a rodent model of inflammation. Brain Behav Immun 2015; 50:196–202.

96. Zhou L, Hu Y, Li C, et al. Levo-corydalmine alleviates vincristine-induced neuropathic pain in mice by inhibiting an NF-kappa B-dependent CXCL1/CXCR2 signaling pathway. Neuropharmacology 2018;135:34–47. https://doi.org/10.1016/j.neuropharm.2018.03.004.

97. Xu J, Zhu M-D, Zhang X, et al. NFκB-mediated CXCL1 production in spinal cord astrocytes contributes to the maintenance of bone cancer pain in mice. J Neuroinflammation 2014;11:38.
98. Li Y, Yang Y, Guo J, et al. Spinal NF-kB upregulation contributes to hyperalgesia in a rat model of advanced osteoarthritis. Mol Pain 2020;16. 1744806920905691.
99. Burston JJ, Valdes AM, Woodhams SG, et al. The impact of anxiety on chronic musculoskeletal pain and the role of astrocyte activation. Pain 2019;160(3). Available at: https://journals.lww.com/pain/Fulltext/2019/03000/The_impact_of_anxiety_on_chronic_musculoskeletal.13.aspx.
100. Matsushita T, Otani K, Oto Y, et al. Sustained microglial activation in the area postrema of collagen-induced arthritis mice. Arthritis Res Ther 2021;23(1):273.
101. Silverwood V, Blagojevic-Bucknall M, Jinks C, et al. Current evidence on risk factors for knee osteoarthritis in older adults: a systematic review and meta-analysis. Osteoarthr Cartil 2015;23(4):507–15.
102. Whittaker JL, Runhaar J, Bierma-Zeinstra S, et al. A lifespan approach to osteoarthritis prevention. Osteoarthr Cartil 2021. https://doi.org/10.1016/j.joca.2021.06.015.
103. Grotle M, Hagen KB, Natvig B, et al. Obesity and osteoarthritis in knee, hip and/or hand: an epidemiological study in the general population with 10 years follow-up. BMC Musculoskelet Disord 2008;9:1–5.
104. Kluzek S, Newton JL, Arden NK. Is osteoarthritis a metabolic disorder? Br Med Bull 2015;115(1):111–21.
105. Berenbaum F, Griffin TM, Liu-Bryan R. Review: metabolic regulation of inflammation in osteoarthritis. Arthritis Rheumatol 2017;69(1):9–21. https://doi.org/10.1002/art.39842.
106. Razeghi Jahromi S, Ghorbani Z, Martelletti P, et al. Association of diet and headache. J Headache Pain 2019;20(1):1–11.
107. Griffin TM, Huebner JL, Kraus VB, et al. Induction of osteoarthritis and metabolic inflammation by a very high-fat diet in mice: effects of short-term exercise. Arthritis Rheum 2012;64(2):443–53. https://doi.org/10.1002/art.33332.
108. Song Z, Xie W, Chen S, et al. High-fat diet increases pain behaviors in rats with or without obesity. Sci Rep 2017;7(1):10350.
109. Collins KH, Lenz KL, Pollitt EN, et al. Adipose tissue is a critical regulator of osteoarthritis. Proc Natl Acad Sci U S A 2021;118(1). e2021096118.
110. Anwer S, Alghadir A, Brismeé JM. Effect of Home exercise Program in patients with knee osteoarthritis: a systematic review and meta-analysis. J Geriatr Phys Ther 2016;39(1):38–48.
111. Kraus VB, Sprow K, Powell KE, et al. Effects of physical activity in knee and hip osteoarthritis: a systematic Umbrella review. Med Sci Sports Exerc 2019;51(6):1324–39.
112. Messier SP, Mihalko SL, Legault C, et al. Effects of intensive diet and exercise on knee joint loads, inflammation, and clinical outcomes among overweight and obese adults with knee osteoarthritis: the IDEA randomized clinical trial. JAMA 2013;310(12):1263–73.
113. Endstrasser F, Braito M, Linser M, et al. The negative impact of the COVID-19 lockdown on pain and physical function in patients with end-stage hip or knee osteoarthritis. Knee Surgery, Sport Traumatol Arthrosc 2020;28(8):2435–43.
114. Runhaar J, Beavers DP, Miller GD, et al. Inflammatory cytokines mediate the effects of diet and exercise on pain and function in knee osteoarthritis independent of BMI. Osteoarthr Cartil 2019;27(8):1118–23.

115. Franceschi C, Garagnani P, Parini P, et al. Inflammaging: a new immune–metabolic viewpoint for age-related diseases. Nat Rev Endocrinol 2018; 14(10):576–90.
116. Greene MA, Loeser RF. Aging-related inflammation in osteoarthritis. Osteoarthr Cartil 2015;23(11):1966–71.
117. Coryell PR, Diekman BO, Loeser RF. Mechanisms and therapeutic implications of cellular senescence in osteoarthritis. Nat Rev Rheumatol 2021;17(1):47–57.
118. Stannus OP, Jones G, Blizzard L, et al. Associations between serum levels of inflammatory markers and change in knee pain over 5 years in older adults: a prospective cohort study. Ann Rheum Dis 2013;72(4):535 LP–540.
119. Srikanth VK, Fryer JL, Zhai G, et al. A meta-analysis of sex differences prevalence, incidence and severity of osteoarthritis. Osteoarthr Cartil 2005;13(9): 769–81.
120. Laitner MH, Erickson LC, Ortman E. Understanding the impact of sex and gender in osteoarthritis: Assessing research Gaps and unmet needs. J Women's Heal 2021;30(5):634–41.
121. Tschon M, Contartese D, Pagani S, et al. Gender and sex are key determinants in osteoarthritis not only Confounding variables. A systematic review of clinical Data. J Clin Med 2021;10(14). https://doi.org/10.3390/jcm10143178.
122. Mun CJ, Letzen JE, Nance S, et al. Sex differences in interleukin-6 responses over time following laboratory pain testing among patients with knee osteoarthritis. J Pain 2020;21(5):731–41.
123. Perruccio AV, Badley EM, Power JD, et al. Sex differences in the relationship between individual systemic markers of inflammation and pain in knee osteoarthritis. Osteoarthr Cartil Open 2019;1(1):100004.
124. Vincent TL. Mechanoflammation in osteoarthritis pathogenesis. Semin Arthritis Rheum 2019;49(3, Supplement):S36–8.
125. Murthy SE, Loud MC, Daou I, et al. The mechanosensitive ion channel Piezo2 mediates sensitivity to mechanical pain in mice. Sci Transl Med 2018;10(462): eaat9897.
126. Szczot M, Liljencrantz J, Ghitani N, et al. PIEZO2 mediates injury-induced tactile pain in mice and humans. Sci Transl Med 2018;10(462):eaat9892.
127. Prato V, Taberner FJ, Hockley JRF, et al. Functional and molecular characterization of Mechanoinsensitive "silent" nociceptors. Cell Rep 2017;21(11):3102–15.

Osteoarthritis Flares

Martin J. Thomas, PhD[a,b,*], Francis Guillemin, MD, PhD[c],
Tuhina Neogi, MD, PhD[d]

KEYWORDS

- Osteoarthritis • Flare • Pain • Acute • Exacerbation • Symptom variability
- Management

KEY POINTS

- Osteoarthritis (OA) flares are episodic sudden-onset increases in signs and symptoms that can be distressing and disabling.
- The triggers and impact of OA flares vary between people and within people across the disease course.
- All health care professionals can help patients recognize and understand their own flare behaviors.
- Viewing and managing OA as an "acute-on-chronic" condition, with a practical distinction between short-term "fast" flare management strategies and long-term "slower" management strategies may be beneficial.

INTRODUCTION

Osteoarthritis (OA) is a leading cause of long-term disability worldwide[1] and places a significant burden on individuals, health care providers, and the wider economy.[2] Multifactorial in onset[3] and heterogeneous in course (eg, Ref.[4]), the OA disease process can affect the whole joint complex.[5] Clinical interventions for OA prioritize personalized symptom management, with a range of strategies designed to minimize distress and disability.[6]

OA-related pain is best understood through a biopsychosocial perspective[7] and patients' active engagement with available treatments and interventions is central to their efficacy. For example, the known benefits of exercise and weight control for prevention and management are largely achieved and maintained by motivated lifestyle adherence, with the support of health care professionals.

The inherent variability in OA prognosis is mirrored in daily life, which is commonly experienced as periods of relative comfort punctuated by episodic flares

[a] Primary Care Centre Versus Arthritis, School of Medicine, Keele University, Staffordshire ST5 5BG, UK; [b] Haywood Academic Rheumatology Centre, Midlands Partnership NHS Foundation Trust, Haywood Hospital, Burslem, Staffordshire ST6 7AG, UK; [c] APEMAC, Université de Lorraine, Nancy, France; [d] Department of Medicine, Section of Rheumatology, Boston University School of Medicine, 650 Albany Street, Suite X-200, Boston, MA 02118, USA
* Corresponding author. Primary Care Centre Versus Arthritis, School of Medicine, Keele University, Staffordshire ST5 5BG, United Kingdom.
E-mail address: m.thomas@keele.ac.uk

Clin Geriatr Med 38 (2022) 239–257
https://doi.org/10.1016/j.cger.2021.11.001
0749-0690/22/© 2021 Elsevier Inc. All rights reserved.

(exacerbations) often of unpredictable frequency, intensity, and duration. These can be physically and psychologically distressing and disrupt self-management routines.[8] In the community, between 23% and 32% of people with knee OA experience significant pain variability,[9] and average flare episode frequency of 2.4 per year among people with hip, knee, or hand OA,[10] illustrating the scale of the problem, which can also impact work productivity.[11]

Historically, physical, behavioral, and mind-body flare management has only received sporadic research attention compared with pharmacologic management. Previously, there has been a longstanding focus on flare-design trials, whereby flare episodes are induced by suspending current treatment before testing new pharmacologic treatment effectiveness (eg, nonsteroidal anti-inflammatory drugs [NSAIDs]). These studies appear to produce comparable findings to nonflare trial designs,[12] but cannot be presumed to characterize "naturally occurring" flares.[13] More recently, empirical studies are emerging internationally, as are coordinated efforts to address key issues in the area of "naturally occurring" flares with an emphasis on improving patient care.

In this article, we undertake a critical narrative synthesis of evidence on recognizing and defining OA flares, present conceptual ideas for exploring their behavior in clinical practice, provide an overview of best-practice treatment approaches, and offer suggestions on the timing of self-management strategies.

RECOGNIZING AND DEFINING OA FLARES

A challenge for both patient education and the research endeavor is recognizing and defining what is meant by a flare. From the patient perspective, flares are recognized as discrete episodes of increased pain, often with rapid onset, that can impact daily activities.[14] Despite researcher efforts to develop diagnostic criteria[15] and formal flare assessment,[16] a wide variety of flare definitions exist within the literature.[13,17] Spontaneous or "naturally occurring" flares should be considered distinct from induced flares in drug withdrawal trials,[13] and the cardinal defining feature of flares has been pain.[17]

Recent observational studies have predominantly defined flares as a 0 to 10 numerical rating scale change score of ≥ 2 from baseline "usual" pain[18–21] versus participant self-report.[22] Flares have been perceived as transient events that can occur multiple times a day[23] or viewed as distinct episodes, or changes in state, that must endure for prespecified periods beyond usual within-day/between-day pain fluctuations (eg, ≥ 8 hours,[18,20] ≥ 24 hours,[22] 48 hours[19]). The distinction between a flare versus worsening of symptoms into a persistent, progressive state can be unclear. Clinically, flares are discrete sudden-onset episodes that resolve. Worsening that persists (ie, deteriorating state as opposed to a short-term fluctuation in disease activity) would therefore not be considered a flare, but this may be difficult to distinguish in the early stages.

A growing consensus that flares are more than just pain is reflected in a position statement reached by an international community of clinicians and patients recently proposing and further endorsing 5 key domains, that represent worsening from peoples "usual" state, and endure for a few days[24,25]:

- Pain
- Swelling
- Stiffness
- Psychological aspects (eg, low mood, irritation)
- Impact of symptoms (eg, sleep/activity changes, function)

Flare experiences themselves are heterogeneous and likely to exist on a continuum. For example, there may be circumstances where people experiencing flares have no swelling[15] or no perceived distress. Despite this, there is some evidence that patient and physician flare recognition correlates well[15], and imposing a dichotomized definition of flare informed by available evidence follows the convention across many conditions. Clinical definitions (diagnoses) are most helpful if they have prognostic significance or inform treatment selection.[26]

Capturing flares as they occur often presents a significant challenge, and a valid patient-reported outcome measure has recently been developed (Traore Y, Epstein J, Spitz E, et al. Development and validation of the Flare-OA questionnaire for measuring flare in knee and hip osteoarthritis. Submitted (undergoing revision).). The Flare-OA questionnaire will offer the ability to adopt a more standardized approach for identifying flare occurrence and reoccurrence to better inform planned interventions.

Furthermore, people often consult health services with flares not just because they are disruptive but because of concerns about what they mean and whether they might signal something serious in underlying pathologic change. These may or may not relate to OA. A challenge when recognizing and defining flares is judging and excluding rare but serious underlying causes[27] (eg, insufficiency fracture, malignancy, or infection).

TRIGGERS FOR OA FLARES

The underlying susceptibility to flares is likely to include distal causes (eg, possibly obesity) and proximal triggers (eg, unaccustomed activity). Bracken's "Cone of causation" simultaneously acknowledges causal contributors, induction periods between risk factors in a causal chain, and time.[28] The cone shape reflects greater number of earlier distal factors than proximal factors in causation.[28] Although little is known about distal causes that increase susceptibility to flares, they might reasonably look similar to those associated with OA incidence and progression. **Fig. 1** outlines a conceptual model of causality recognizing the potential role of both distal and proximal causes of OA flares. Although the relative contribution, number, and timing of distal and proximal causes are unknown, this may represent a useful framework to

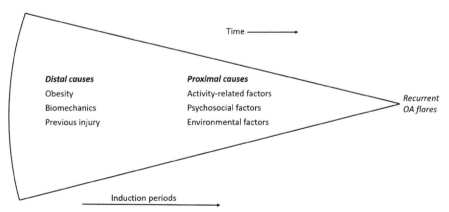

Fig. 1. Conceptual model of causality for OA flares acknowledging the contribution of potential distal and proximal causes. Illustration based on the "Cone of causation." (*Adapted from* Bracken MB. Risk, chance, and causation: Investigating the origins and treatment of disease. New Haven: Yale University press; 2013; with permission.)

conceptualize OA flares. The remainder of this section focuses on synthesizing evidence from studies on proximal triggers.

The episodic nature of flares means that exposures (triggers) are commonly time-varying events with short induction times. Investigating flare triggers in daily life is challenging. Self-controlled case-crossover study methodology[29] combined with mechanisms for "real-time" data capture, such as Web-based platforms, have facilitated empirical observation of flare triggers in community settings. This design enables study participants to provide data at the time of a flare and the days leading up to it, and compares these observations with equivalent data collected during non-flare periods. Questions in this context are not concerned with why people experience flares ("Why me?"), but aim to examine what might trigger flares ("Why now?").[30]

Table 1 summarizes potential trigger exposures examined for hip/knee OA,[31] knee OA,[19,21,22,32–34] and hip OA.[20,35–38] Broadly, positive proximate trigger exposures for flare onset fall into categories of activity-related, psychosocial, and environmental factors. However, the exact mechanisms by which exposures precipitate flares and their relationship to each other remain unclear. Collectively across hip and knee studies, triggers with supportive evidence from one or more other studies are activity-related factors, including moderate physical activity,[21,22] squatting or kneeling, lifting or moving heavy objects, climbing ladders,[19,22] joint buckling/giving way[20,22,33]; psychosocial factors, including worse mental health,[31] higher negative effect and passive coping strategies,[32] low mood/depression, feeling angry, irritable or hostile,[22] and poor sleep[22,35]; and environmental factors, including weather temperature changes.[22,38] Contrasting observations across studies in terms of direction and magnitude of associations might be explained by differences in OA and flare definition, sample size, exposure measurement, and observed induction times.

A strength of within-person case-crossover methodology is that person-level and slow-varying potential confounders are controlled by design. A potential weakness of how most OA case-crossover studies have typically been designed is with retrospective exposure measurement. Consequently, there may be differential recall between hazard and control periods leading to some inherent bias. With the exception of objective weather analyses,[34,38] only one previous case-crossover analysis used prospective self-reported daily measurement,[19] and the advantages of intensive 3-month daily diary study over periodic measurement must be considered in terms of acceptable participant burden.

A common patient belief is that weather changes can trigger flares. A 15-month prospective study of 2658 UK-based participants with several long-term pain conditions observed that relative humidity, pressure, and wind speed had a modest significant relationship with pain.[44] Furthermore, in a subgroup analysis limited to those with OA, OA pain remained positively associated with relative humidity. This observation contrasts 3 OA flare studies.[22,34,38] However, these study samples were smaller and Thomas and colleagues'[22] retrospective exposure measurements were vulnerable to recall bias. Dixon and colleagues[44] also found a positive association between pain events and low mood, but not high physical activity. Contrasting physical activity associations with those in **Table 1** may be explained by recall bias, smaller sample sizes, and differences in exposure measurement.

Currently, the literature appears to indicate that flare triggering effects of weather are likely modest. In general, activity-related and psychosocial triggers have been observed more consistently and are likely to be more amenable to modification. Further investigation to understand flare triggers and their relationship with OA pathophysiology is warranted.

Table 1
Potential trigger exposures and association with osteoarthritis flares

Study	Design	Mode of Data Collection	OA Definition	Flare Definition	Sample Size	Sample Age (years), Mean (SD); Sex	Exposure-Flare Onset Induction Time	Potential Trigger Exposure and Association with Flare Onset
Hip/knee								
Wise et al.[31] United States	12 week telephone-based case-crossover study	Retrospective, self-reported	Physician clinically diagnosed hip or knee OA	WOMAC score in highest 30% of all WOMAC scores (yes/no)	91	65 (8.8); 79% female	1 week prior	*Positive risk factor* Worse mental health
Knee								
Efrani et al.[32] Australia	90 day Web-based case-crossover study	Retrospective, self-reported	Meet ≥1 ACR criteria for knee OA[39] and ≥2 KL[40] tibiofemoral OA or patellofemoral OA[41] on plain radiography	NRS (0-10) change score of ≥2 from baseline mildest knee pain, lasting >8 hours	149 & 54	62.1 (8.1); 66% female & 62.7 (9.0); 65% female	Affect measures 10 days prior; pain coping/perceived stress 30 days prior	*Positive risk factors* Higher negative affect; passive coping strategies. *Protective factor* Higher active coping strategies *None* Positive affect; all coping strategies; problem-focused coping; emotion-focused coping; pain catastrophizing; control over pain; ability to decrease pain; overall coping strategies effectiveness, perceived stress

(continued on next page)

Table 1
(continued)

Study	Design	Mode of Data Collection	OA Definition	Flare Definition	Sample Size	Sample Age (years), Mean (SD); Sex	Exposure-Flare Onset Induction Time	Potential Trigger Exposure and Association with Flare Onset
Zobel et al.[33] Australia	90 day Web-based case-crossover study	Retrospective, self-reported	Meet ≥1 ACR criteria for knee OA[39] and ≥2 KL[40] tibiofemoral OA or patellofemoral OA[41] on plain radiography	NRS (0-10) change score of ≥2 from baseline mildest knee pain, lasting >8 hours	157	61.8 (8.4) years; 66% female	Knee injury 7 days prior; knee buckling 2 days prior	*Positive risk factors* Knee injury; knee buckling
Ferriera et al.[34] Australia	90 day Web-based case-crossover study	Prospective, objective	Meet ≥1 ACR criteria for knee OA[39] and ≥2 KL[40] tibiofemoral OA or patellofemoral OA[41] on plain radiography	NRS (0-10) change score of ≥2 from baseline mildest knee pain, lasting >8 hours	171 (404 hazards, 1021 control)	61.7 (8.7); 64% female	72 hours prior	*None* Temperature; relative humidity; barometric pressure; precipitation
Parry et al.[19] England, UK	3 month pen-paper daily diary study	Prospective, self-reported	GP defined & self-reported knee symptoms on ≥1 day in last 12 months	NRS (0-10) change score of ≥2 from baseline in last 24 hours, last ≥2 days	67	62 (10.6); 55% female	48 hours prior	*Positive risk factors* ≥1 selected physical activity (prolonged kneeling, lifting/ moving heavy objects, climbing stairs, prolonged squatting, climbing ladders)
Atukorala et al.[21] Sri Lanka	3 month telephone-based case-crossover study	Retrospective, self-reported	Meet ACR criteria for knee OA[39]	NRS (0-10) change score of ≥2 from baseline usual knee	120	59.9 (7.3); 90% female	Footwear use/being barefoot 2 days prior;	*Positive risk factors* Moderate physical activity 1,2 and 3-7

						Physical activity 7 days prior; pain, lasting ≥4 hours; days prior; using footwear 1 and 2 days before
Thomas et al.[22] England, UK	13 week Web-based case-crossover study	Retrospective, self-reported	GP defined/ self-reported	Self-reported sudden onset of worsening signs and symptoms sustained for ≥24 hours (568 hazards, 867 controls) 376	61.8 (10.1); 68% female	24 hours prior

Protective factor
Increased duration barefoot (>8 hours) 1 and 2 days prior

Positive risk factors
Squatting or kneeling; standing for long periods without rest; lifting or moving heavy objects; going up and down ladders, moderate-to-vigorous physical activity; knee buckling; slip trip or fall; taking extra analgesia in anticipation of increased physical activity; poor night's sleep; low mood/depression; feeling angry, irritable or hostile; cold/damp weather

Protective factors
Sitting for long periods without a break; missing or reducing planned medication; cough, cold or minor infection

None

(continued on next page)

Table 1
(continued)

Study	Design	Mode of Data Collection	OA Definition	Flare Definition	Sample Size	Sample Age (years), Mean (SD); Sex	Exposure-Flare Onset Induction Time	Potential Trigger Exposure and Association with Flare Onset
								Going up/down stairs; driving; stressful events at home, work and family-related stress
Hip								
Fu et al.[20] Australia	90 day Web-based case-crossover study	Retrospective, self-reported	Meet ACR criteria for hip OA[42] and ≥2 KL[43] hip OA	NRS (0-10) change score of ≥2 from baseline mildest hip pain, lasting >8 hours	133	62.5 (8.3); 85% female	Hip injury 7 days prior; hip giving way 2 days prior	*Positive risk factors* Hip injury; hip giving way
Fu et al.[35] Australia	90 day Web-based case-crossover study	Retrospective, self-reported	Meet ACR criteria for hip OA[42] and ≥2 KL[43] hip OA	NRS (0-10) change score of ≥2 from baseline mildest hip pain, lasting >8 hours	130	62.5 (8,1); 85% female	7 days prior	*Positive risk factors* Poor sleep; increased fatigue
Fu et al.[36] Australia	90 day Web-based case-crossover study	Retrospective, Self-reported	Meet ACR criteria for hip OA[42] and ≥2 KL[43] hip OA	NRS (0-10) change score of ≥2 from baseline mildest hip pain, lasting >8 hours	137	62.6 (9.8); 83% female	24 hours prior	*Protective factors* Shoes with heel height ≥2.5 cm; longer duration of heel height ≥2.5 cm
Fu et al.[37] Australia	90 day Web-based case-crossover study	Retrospective, self-reported	Meet ACR criteria for hip OA[42] and ≥2 KL[43] hip OA	NRS (0-10) change score of ≥2 from baseline mildest hip pain, lasting >8 hours	131	62.5 (8,1); 86% female	7 days prior	*Positive risk factors* Pain catastrophizing; pain self-efficacy beliefs *None* Depression; anxiety; stress; positive effect; negative affect

Fu et al.[38] Australia	90 day Web-based case-crossover study	Prospective, objective	Meet ACR criteria for hip OA[42] and ≥2 KL[43] hip OA	NRS (0-10) change score of ≥2 from baseline mildest hip pain, lasting >8 hours	129	62.9 (8.0); 86% female	72 hours prior	*Positive risk factors* Temperature variation
								None Maximum/minimum temperature; relative humidity; precipitation; barometric pressure

Abbreviations: ACR, American College of Rheumatology; KL, Kellgren and Lawrence; NRS, Numerical Rating Scale; OA, Osteoarthritis; SD, Standard Deviation; WOMAC, Western Ontario and McMaster Universities Osteoarthritis Index.

OA FLARE PATTERNS AND SYMPTOM VARIABILITY

Flares appear to occur from the earliest phases of OA[45] but the predictability of episodic pain appears to diminish in later phases, when their impact can also become more distressing[45] and unacceptable.[46]

In terms of predicting flares in people with knee OA, Atukorala and colleagues[47] suggested that baseline risk factors, including increasing age, years lived with OA, body mass index, background/worse levels of pain, knee injury, buckling, intermittent and constant pain score, and footwear type/heel height, predicted a pain flare within 30 days. In adults with, or at risk of, knee OA, Thomas and colleagues[22] reported that flares appeared to be slightly more common among adults of working age, women, and people with more frequent pain.

Preventing or reducing flares by understanding and anticipating daily life circumstances that might trigger onset, and modifying these if possible, provides an opportunity for people to develop personalized flare prevention strategies. Focused consultation support to help patients understand their own flare patterns and recognize potential triggers would appear beneficial, particularly as a recent study found that in adults with, or at risk of, knee OA, 70% of reported flares were unexpected.[22]

Studies that capture flare episode duration are broadly comparable, with flares typically lasting around 3 to 8 days.[19,22,48] For patients, flares of unfamiliar impact (eg, resulting in time off work) or that last longer than usual should perhaps signal a need to seek additional health care. Potential relationships between different triggers and flare duration are unknown and likely to vary across the disease course.

In the short term, flares can be distressing and disrupt daily life. Whether flares have implications for long-term prognosis remains unclear. It has previously been proposed that the theoretical natural history could chart a course where intermittent and benign flare episodes may cumulate over time and occur with increased frequency, duration, and intensity, eventually leading to consequences that culminate in joint failure[49] (**Fig. 2**). Future empirical demonstration of the relationship between potential flare triggers, episode duration, and flare frequency may help to establish the potential longer-term consequences of flares and identify people most at risk of poor outcomes earlier in the disease course. This could potentially help steer people onto more favorable trajectories.[48] Flare patterns are likely to be heterogeneous, both between-people and within-people over time.

Symptom variability (within-day and between-day) may also be an important related yet distinct phenomenon. For example, in other conditions such as cardiovascular disease, blood pressure variability is a strong predictor of stroke.[50] Although prospective studies examining short-term symptom variability exist within the OA literature (eg, Refs. 23,51–53), extending the application of intensive longitudinal designs[54] to studies of OA symptom fluctuations may offer new perspectives on clinically relevant short-term changes and their impact on longer-term outcomes. Furthermore, attempting to reduce symptom variability itself may be a worthy treatment target[55] that might also have utility as part of self-monitoring or behavior change strategies in clinical settings.[56]

ACUTE FLARE MANAGEMENT AND LONG-TERM OA MANAGEMENT
Access to Care

OA is predominantly managed in primary care settings by general practitioners/physicians and more recently other health professionals, such as physiotherapists.[57,58] Flare episodes and consultations do not always align well, but when they do, they represent opportunistic encounters to share key messages and advice[59] at times when people may be most receptive to change behavior. Although access to care varies,[60] adequate knowledge and understanding of OA as a condition, that gives rise to appropriate acute flare and long-term condition management, are skills that all first contact clinicians should equip themselves with to positively frame patient care and provide consistent messages. A recent qualitative literature synthesis promotes the notion of participatory discourse where positive communication focuses on what patients can, rather than cannot, do to facilitate physical activity engagement.[61]

Consequences of poor flare management, particularly early in the disease course, may be escalating treatment and unnecessary health care utilization. For example, the prescription of stronger opioid-based medication, MRI, or referral for surgical opinion may occur earlier than desirable in response to poorly managed flares. This could be detrimental to patient self-management behaviors and self-efficacy, leading to poor outcomes. The potential role of pharmacists to support timely flare management advice and education in community settings could also be better utilized.

Physical, Behavioral, and Lifestyle Interventions for Acute OA Flare Management

In terms of evidence-based practice, a recent scoping review concluded that robust evidence for a range of OA flare management strategies (behavioral, lifestyle, and adjunctive treatments) is lacking.[62] Although 2 studies examining retrowalking[63] (walking backward) and modified "rescue" exercise[64] during a flare of knee OA found tentative evidence of safety and pain improvement, the clinical meaningfulness of these physical activities/exercise outcomes was unclear.[62] Furthermore, the predominant focus on knee pain means broader inclusion of other joint sites (eg, hip or hand) and other flare symptoms (eg, stiffness, swelling, or psychological distress) are

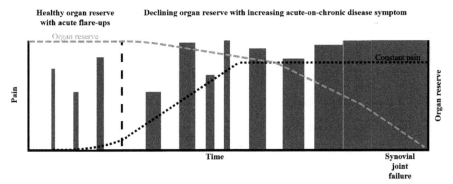

Fig. 2. Theoretical natural history of symptomatic OA progression. The impact of intermittent discrete (potentially benign) flare-up episodes (red bars) progress in frequency, intensity (height of bars), and duration (width of bars), with reducing periods of remission and capacity for complete symptom resolution. These acute symptom events drive the underlying disease process, eventually resulting in constant pain, complete loss of organ reserve (capacity to restore homeostasis), and synovial joint failure. Each red bar representing a flare-up is preceded by potential exposure flare-up triggers. The black vertical dashed line represents a period of time after which flare-ups may no longer be potentially benign. The black dotted line represents the course of pain over time. The blue dotted line represents the organ reserve over time, which theoretically may diminish whth repeated and/or frequent flare-ups. (*From* Thomas MJ, Neogi T. Flare-ups of osteoarthritis: what do they mean in the short-term and the long-term?. Osteoarthritis Cartilage. 2020;28(7):870-873. doi:10. 1016/j.joca.2020.01.005; with permission.)

lacking.[62] Although flares often co-occur with increased or unaccustomed physical activity, and appear to relate to movement mechanics,[65,66] exercise-induced flares are likely to decrease with graded exposure to exercise[67] and patient-focused physical activity promotion. For example, a recent study concluded that knee pain flares were associated with recent knee injury, more severe radiographic OA, and lower quadriceps strength.[68] Factoring such presentations into treatment planning may provide more targeted care.[68]

Pharmacologic Management of Acute OA Flares

Pharmacologic management options for OA broadly involve topical NSAIDs applied directly to affected joints, oral medications (eg, paracetamol, NSAIDs), and intra-articular steroid injections for moderate-to-severe pain (eg, Refs.[69–72]). Pharmacologic efficacy is often complicated by a lack of data relating to patient usage habits.[69] Data observing oral NSAIDs use for acute knee pain flares identified favorable recovery trajectories within 3 to 5 days, with pain levels, activity interference, stiffness, and swelling following a similar course.[48] Recent meta-analyzed data from knee OA clinical trials concluded pain and function improvements from NSAIDs use peaking at 2 weeks.[73] Owing to the heterogeneity of pharmacologic efficacy and side-effect profiles, the lowest effective dose for the shortest possible duration is advocated[69–72] and patients should be encouraged to regularly rationalize medication use in the context of comorbidities via shared decision-making with health care professionals.[69–72]

Managing OA as an "Acute-on-Chronic" Condition

Lack of evidence to underpin flare management recommendations, alongside chronic disease management, in current international clinical guidelines highlights further research opportunities. Better understanding flare mechanisms,[74] their potential role in OA etiopathogenesis, and their response to treatment could lead to new insights for clinical intervention. The notion that complementary chronic disease and acute pain care models could help OA management is not new.[75] However, the increased emphasis of OA as an "acute-on-chronic"[76] condition could support strategies designed to manage (i) the underlying (chronic) disease course, (ii) (acute) flare episodes, and (iii) behavior modification to potentially avoid or minimize exposure to flare triggers.[49] Patient management in the context of these 3 inter-related components could guide personalized care.

Short-Term and Long-Term OA Management Strategies

One proposed way to frame currently recommended self-management strategies is by recognizing 2 sets of actions: short-term "fast" strategies and long-term "slower" strategies. The goal of short-term management strategies is to act "fast" to reduce acute flare episode duration, minimize their impact, and empower patients to feel more in control of their symptoms, with a focus on short-term outcomes. Although empirical evidence underpinning short-term "fast" management strategies would be needed, examples of fast-action response models for flare interventions include NSAIDs use for the shortest possible period[75] and short-term decrease in usual activities/exercise.[64]

The goal of long-term "slower" management strategies is to optimize chronic condition management and reduce acute flare episode frequency. These can include core best-practice elements; education, support with weight loss (as required), and physical activity/exercise participation.[69–71] An overall goal is to support people to develop and maintain physically active lifestyles. Avoidance of flare-provoking triggers may be advisable in some contexts but for others may not always be practical, for example, if frequent kneeling is a feature of occupation. Periods of decreased activity or avoid-ance, if needed, should be followed by a return to usual activities as much as possible on flare resolution. This will prevent negative emotions due to increased sedentary time and inactivity[77] and prevent deconditioning, which themselves may lead to more flare episodes. Patients should be educated to try to avoid catastrophizing activity-related pain increases[78] and flares, and be supported to expect and manage their periodic occurrence. Partner support[79] and social interactions[80] can also posi-tively affect the OA pain experience.

Adopting short-term "fast" management strategies has implications for the speed of access to health care. As discussed earlier, patient flares and health care consulta-tions rarely coincide and patients' ability to establish fast-response strategies as required may need to be developed through self-management education (**Fig. 3**, eg). More responsive health care, for example, through digital platforms, may also facilitate quicker supportive action. Furthermore, integrated "fast" and "slower" man-agement strategies could reduce the disruption to chronic condition management caused by flares.

There remain several research knowledge gaps around OA condition management and timing of treatment responses. Viewing and managing OA as an "acute-on-chronic" condition with current core and adjunctive interventions contributing to short-term "fast" management and long-term "slower" management strategies could translate into improvements in patient care.

OA Flare Management and Joint Deterioration

Currently, there is no evidence to suggest that flares signify deterioration of joint struc-tures. However, the extent to which painful inflammatory flare responses in OA are necessary processes for the joint to restore homeostasis versus reactions within the joint that should be minimized to preserve joint health remains unclear.[48] This poten-tially has implications for how NSAIDs are prescribed. For example, in the theoretic context of **Fig. 2**, whether NSAIDs might be more or less effective early or late in the disease course is unknown. In consultation with patients, health care professionals should focus on managing the cumulative daily disability caused by flares, rather than structural joint changes.

SUMMARY

OA is a chronic long-term condition, and yet the lived experience is often familiar day-to-day pain punctuated by distinct episodic flares that likely vary in predictability, fre-quency, duration, and intensity across the disease course. By emphasizing OA as an "acute-on-chronic" condition, patient education and self-management advice can proactively support patients to formulate bespoke sets of strategies for acute flare episode management and chronic condition management to facilitate the primary goal of maintaining an active lifestyle.

CLINICS CARE POINTS

- Recognizing, defining, and exploring OA flares in clinical practice should include consideration of joint pain, swelling and stiffness, psychological distress, and the impact of symptoms on functioning and activities, whilst excluding serious underlying causes.

- A broad range of activity-related, psychosocial, and environmental factors can trigger OA flares, many of which are potentially modifiable if patients are supported to understand their symptoms and gain more control over them.

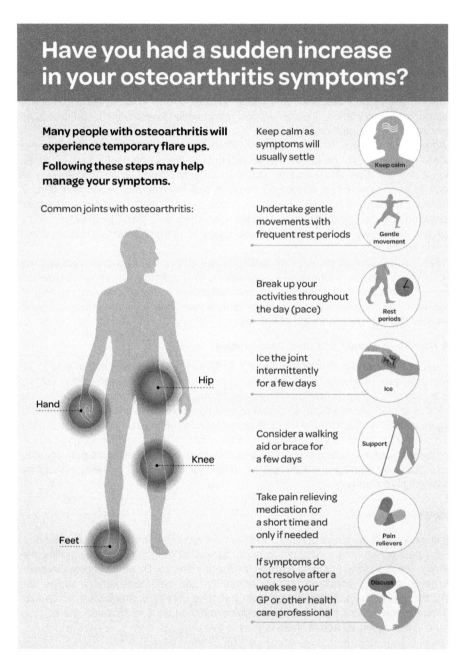

Fig. 3. Examples of currently recommended self-management strategies and advice for OA[69,71] that may serve well as short-term "fast" flare management strategies. Patients could be taught how to implement these alongside long-term "slower" management strategies such as condition education, weight loss (as required), and physical activity/exercise participation.[69–71] (*Courtesy of* J Bowden, PhD and J Eyles, PhD, Institute of Bone and Joint Research, Sydney, NSW, Australia.)

- Flare patterns are often unique to each individual and likely to change over time, therefore flare management strategies may need to evolve within patients over the course of the condition and continual monitoring may be beneficial.
- In addition to acute flare episode prevention and management, aiming to reduce overall symptom variability may also be beneficial for optimizing self-care and prognosis.
- All health care professionals involved in the provision of patient care should provide consistent messages about OA, flares, and management options, which may reduce unnecessary health care utilization and treatment escalation.
- Framing current OA best-practice guidance as short-term "fast" management and long-term "slower" management strategy interventions may help to optimize patient self-management and better conceptualize OA as an "acute-on-chronic" condition.
- Helping patients better explore and understand their own flare behaviors and triggers should be discussed in the context of maintaining an active lifestyle and not catastrophizing their occurrence.

DISCLOSURE

Dr. Neogi is supported by grant number NIH K24 AR070892.

ACKNOWLEDGMENTS

The authors would like to thank Professor George Peat for his comments during the drafting of this article.

REFERENCES

1. GBD 2019 Diseases and Injury Collaborators. Global burden of 369 diseases and injuries in 204 countries and territories, 1990-2019: a systematic analysis for the Global Burden of Disease Study 2019. Lancet 2020;396(10258):1204–22.
2. Hunter DJ, Schofield D, Callander E. The individual and socioeconomic impact of osteoarthritis. Nat Rev Rheumatol 2014;10(7):437–41.
3. Brandt KD, Dieppe P, Radin EL. Etiopathogenesis of osteoarthritis. Rheum Dis Clin North Am 2008;34(3):531–59.
4. Wieczorek M, Rotonda C, Coste J, et al. Trajectory analysis combining pain and physical function in individuals with knee and hip osteoarthritis: results from the French KHOALA cohort. Rheumatology (Oxford) 2020;59(11):3488–98.
5. Brandt KD, Radin EL, Dieppe PA, et al. Yet more evidence that osteoarthritis is not a cartilage disease. Ann Rheum Dis 2006;65(10):1261–4.
6. Hunter DJ, Bierma-Zeinstra S. Osteoarthritis. Lancet 2019;393(10182):1745–59.
7. Neogi T. The epidemiology and impact of pain in osteoarthritis. Osteoarthr Cartil 2013;21(9):1145–53.
8. Peat G, Thomas E. When knee pain becomes severe: a nested case-control analysis in community-dwelling older adults. J Pain 2009;10(8):798–808.
9. Parry E, Ogollah R, Peat G. Significant pain variability in persons with, or at high risk of, knee osteoarthritis: preliminary investigation based on secondary analysis of cohort data. BMC Musculoskelet Disord 2017;18(1):80.
10. Fautrel B, Hilliquin P, Rozenberg S, et al. Impact of osteoarthritis: results of a nationwide survey of 10,000 patients consulting for OA. Joint Bone Spine 2005;72(3):235–40.
11. Ricci JA, Stewart WF, Chee E, et al. Pain exacerbation as a major source of lost productive time in US workers with arthritis. Arthritis Rheum 2005;53(5):673–81.

12. Smith TO, Zou K, Adbullah N, et al. Does flare trial design affect the effect size of non-steroidal anti-inflammatory drugs in symptomatic osteoarthritis? A systematic review and meta-analysis. Ann Rheum Dis 2016;75(11):1971–8.

13. Parry EL, Thomas MJ, Peat G. Defining acute flares in knee osteoarthritis: a systematic review. BMJ Open 2018;8(7):019804.

14. Parry E. Acute flares in knee osteoarthritis. Doctor of Philosophy. Staffordshire: Keele University; 2019.

15. Marty M, Hilliquin P, Rozenberg S, et al. Validation of the KOFUS (Knee Osteoarthritis Flare-Ups Score). Joint Bone Spine 2009;76(3):268–72.

16. Scott-Lennox JA, McLaughlin-Miley C, Lennox RD, et al. Stratification of flare intensity identifies placebo responders in a treatment efficacy trial of patients with osteoarthritis. Arthritis Rheum 2001;44(7):1599–607.

17. Cross M, Dubouis L, Mangin M, et al. Defining flare in osteoarthritis of the hip and knee: a systematic literature review – OMERACT virtual special interest group. J Rheumatol 2017;44(12):1920–7.

18. Makovey J, Metcalf B, Zhang Y, et al. Web-based study of risk factors for pain exacerbation in osteoarthritis of the knee (SPARK-Web): design and rationale. JMIR Res Protoc 2015;4(3):e80.

19. Parry E, Ogollah R, Peat G. 'Acute flare-ups' in patients with, or at high risk of, knee osteoarthritis: a daily diary study with case-crossover analysis. Osteoarthr Cartil 2019;27(8):1124–8.

20. Fu K, Makovey J, Metcalf B, et al. Role of hip injury and giving way in pain exacerbation in hip osteoarthritis: an internet-based case-crossover study. Arthritis Care Res (Hoboken) 2019;71(6):742–7.

21. Atukorala I, Pathmeswaran A, Batuwita N, et al. Is being barefoot, wearing shoes and physical activity associated with knee osteoarthritis pain flares? Data from a usually barefoot Sri Lankan cohort. Int J Rheum Dis 2021;24(1):96–105.

22. Thomas MJ, Rathod-Mistry T, Parry EL, et al. Triggers for acute flare in adults with, or at risk of, knee osteoarthritis: a web-based case-crossover study in community-dwelling adults. Osteoarthr Cartil 2021;29(7):956–64.

23. Murphy SL, Lyden AK, Kratz AL, et al. Characterizing pain flares from the perspective of individuals with symptomatic knee osteoarthritis. Arthritis Care Res (Hoboken) 2015;67(8):1103–11.

24. Guillemin F, Ricatte C, Barcenilla-Wong A, et al. Developing a preliminary definition and domains of flare in knee and hip osteoarthritis (OA): consensus building of the flare-in-OA OMERACT Group. J Rheumatol 2019;46(9):1188–91.

25. King LK, Epstein J, Cross M, et al. Endorsement of the domains of knee and hip osteoarthritis (OA) flare: a report from the OMERACT 2020 inaugural virtual consensus vote from the flares in OA working group. Semin Arthritis Rheum 2021;51(3):618–22.

26. Hemingway H, Croft P, Perel P, et al. Prognosis research strategy (PROGRESS) 1: a framework for researching clinical outcomes. BMJ 2013;346:e5595.

27. Kompel AJ, Roemer FW, Murakami AM, et al. Intra-articular corticosteroid injections in the hip and knee: perhaps not as safe as we thought? Radiology 2019; 293(3):656–63.

28. Braken MB. Risk, chance, and causation: Investigating the origins and treatment of disease. New Haven: Yale University press; 2013.

29. Maclure M. The case-crossover design: a method for studying transient effects on the risk of acute events. Am J Epidemiol 1991;133(2):144–53.

30. Maclure M. 'Why me?' versus 'why now?' – differences between operational hypotheses in case-control versus case-crossover studies. Pharmacoepidemiol Drug Saf 2007;16(8):850–3.
31. Wise BL, Niu J, Zhang Y, et al. Psychological factors and their relation to osteoarthritis pain. Osteoarthr Cartil 2010;18(7):883–7.
32. Efrani T, Keefe F, Bennell K, et al. Psychological factors and pain exacerbation in knee osteoarthritis: a web-based case-crossover study. Rheumatol (Sunnyvale) 2015;S6:005.
33. Zobel I, Erfani T, Bennell KL, et al. Relationship of buckling and knee injury to pain exacerbation in knee osteoarthritis: a web-based case-crossover study. Interact J Med Res 2016;5(2):e17.
34. Ferreira ML, Zhang Y, Metcalf B, et al. The influence of weather on the risk of pain exacerbation in patients with knee osteoarthritis – a case-crossover study. Osteoarthr Cartil 2016;24(12):2042–7.
35. Fu K, Makovey J, Metcalf B, et al. Sleep quality and fatigue are associated with pain exacerbations of hip osteoarthritis: an internet-based case-crossover study. J Rheumatol 2019;46(11):1524–30.
36. Fu K, Metcalf BR, Bennell KL, et al. Is heel height associated with pain exacerbations in hip osteoarthritis patients?-Results from a case-crossover study. J Clin Med 2020;9(6):1872.
37. Fu K, Metcalf B, Bennell KL, et al. The association between psychological factors and pain exacerbations in hip osteoarthritis. Rheumatology (Oxford) 2021;60(3): 1291–9.
38. Fu K, Metcalf B, Bennell KL, et al. Association of weather factors with the risk of pain exacerbations in people with hip osteoarthritis. Scand J Rheumatol 2021; 50(1):68–73.
39. Altman R, Asch E, Bloch D, et al. Development of criteria for the classification and reporting of osteoarthritis. Classification of osteoarthritis of the knee. Diagnostic and Therapeutic Criteria Committee of the American Rheumatism Association. Arthritis Rheum 1986;29(8):1039–49.
40. Kellgren J, Lawrence JS. Atlas of standard radiographs. Oxford: Blackwell Scientific; 1963.
41. Felson DT, McAlindon TE, Anderson JJ, et al. Defining radiographic osteoarthritis for the whole knee. Osteoarthr Cartil 1997;5(4):241–50.
42. Altman R, Alarcón G, Appelrouth D, et al. The American College of Rheumatology criteria for the classification and reporting of osteoarthritis of the hip. Arthritis Rheum 1991;34(5):505–14.
43. Kellgren JH, Lawrence JS. Radiological assessment of osteo-arthrosis. Ann Rheum Dis 1957;16(4):494–502.
44. Dixon WG, Beukenhorst AL, Yimer BB, et al. How the weather affects the pain of citizen scientists using a smartphone app. NPJ Digit Med 2019;2:105.
45. Hawker GA, Stewart L, French MR, et al. Understanding the pain experience in hip and knee osteoarthritis-an OARSI/OMERACT initiative. Osteoarthr Cartil 2008;16(4):415–22.
46. Liu A, Kendzerska T, Stanaitis I, et al. The relationship between knee pain characteristics and symptom state acceptability in people with knee osteoarthritis. Osteoarthr Cartil 2014;22(2):178–83.
47. Atukorala I, Pathmeswaran A, Makovey J, et al. Can pain flares in knee osteoarthritis be predicted? Scand J Rheumatol 2021;50(3):198–205.

48. Thomas MJ, Yu D, Nicholls E, et al. Short-term recovery trajectories of acute flares in knee pain: a UK-Netherlands multicenter prospective cohort analysis. Arthritis Care Res (Hoboken) 2020;72(12):1687–92.
49. Thomas MJ, Neogi T. Flare-ups of osteoarthritis: what do they mean in the short-term and the long-term? Osteoarthr Cartil 2020;28(7):870–3.
50. Rothwell PM, Howard SC, Dolan E, et al. Prognostic significance of visit-to-visit variability, maximum systolic blood pressure, and episodic hypertension. Lancet 2010;375(9718):895–905.
51. Hutchings A, Calloway M, Choy E, et al. The Longitudinal Examination of Arthritis Pain (LEAP) study: relationships between weekly fluctuations in patient-rated joint pain and other health outcomes. J Rheumatol 2007;34(11):2291–300.
52. Allen KD, Coffman CJ, Golightly YM, et al. Daily pain variations among patients with hand, hip, and knee osteoarthritis. Osteoarthr Cartil 2009;17(10):1275–82.
53. Trouvin A-P, Marty M, Goupille P, et al. Determinants of daily pain trajectories and relationship with pain acceptability in hip and knee osteoarthritis. A national prospective cohort study on 886 patients. Joint Bone Spine 2019;86(2):245–50.
54. Mun CJ, Suk HW, Davis MC, et al. Investigating intraindividual pain variability: methods, applications, issues, and directions. Pain 2019;160(11):2415–29.
55. Schneider S, Junghaenel DU, Keefe FJ, et al. Individual differences in the day-to-day variability of pain, fatigue, and well-being in patients with rheumatic disease: associations with psychological variables. Pain 2012;153(4):813–22.
56. Allen KD. The value of measuring variability in osteoarthritis pain. J Rheumatol 2007;34(11):2132–3.
57. Décary S, Fallaha M, Pelletier B, et al. Diagnostic validity and triage concordance of a physiotherapist compared to physicians' diagnoses for common knee disorders. BMC Musculoskelet Disord 2017;18(1):445.
58. Walker A, Williams R, Sibley F, et al. Improving access to better care for people with knee and/or hip pain: service evaluation of allied health professional-led primary care. Musculoskeletal Care 2018;16(1):222–32.
59. Canerio JP, O'Sullivan PB, Roos EM, et al. Three steps to changing the narrative about knee osteoarthritis care: a call to action. Br J Sports Med 2020;54(5):256–8.
60. Desai RJ, Jin Y, Franklin PD, et al. Association of geography and access to health care providers with long-term prescription opioid use in medicare patients with severe osteoarthritis: a cohort study. Arthritis Rheumatol 2019;71(5):712–21.
61. Bunzli S, Taylor N, O'Brien P, et al. How do people communicate about knee osteoarthritis? A discourse analysis. Pain Med 2021;22(5):1127–48.
62. Bowden JL, Kobayashi S, Hunter DJ, et al. Best-practice clinical management of flares in people with osteoarthritis: a scoping review of behavioural, lifestyle and adjunctive treatments. Semin Arthritis Rheum 2021;51(4):749–60.
63. Gondhalekar GA, Deo MV. Retrowalking as an adjunct to conventional treatment versus conventional treatment alone on pain and disability in patients with acute exacerbation of chronic knee osteoarthritis: a randomized clinical trial. N Am J Med Sci 2013;5(2):108–12.
64. Bartholdy C, Klokker L, Bandak E, et al. A standardized "rescue" exercise program for symptomatic flare-up of knee osteoarthritis: description and safety considerations. J Orthop Sports Phys Ther 2016;46(11):942–6.
65. Boyer KA, Hafer JF. Gait mechanics contribute to exercise induced pain flares in knee osteoarthritis. BMC Musculoskelet Disord 2019;20(1):107.
66. Skou ST, Grønne DT, Roos EM. Prevalence, severity, and correlates of pain flares in response to a repeated sit-to-stand activity: a cross-sectional study of 14902

patients with knee and hip osteoarthritis in primary care. J Orthop Sports Phys Ther 2020;50(6):309–18.

67. Sandal LF, Roos EM, Bøgesvang SJ, et al. Pain trajectory and exercise-induced pain flares during 8 weeks of neuromuscular exercise in individuals with knee and hip pain. Osteoarthr Cartil 2016;24(4):589–92.

68.. Liu Q, Li Z, Ferreira M, et al. Recent injury, severe radiographic change, and lower quadriceps strength increase risk of knee pain exacerbation during walking: a within-person knee-matched study. J Orthop Sports Phys Ther 2021;51(6):298–304.

69. National Institute for Health and Care Excellence. Osteoarthritis: care and management in adults. Clinical guidance 177. London: NICE; 2014.

70. Bannuru RR, Osani MC, Vaysbrot EE, et al. OARSI guidelines for the non-surgical management of knee, hip, and polyarticular osteoarthritis. Osteoarthr Cartil 2019; 27(11):1578–89.

71. Kolasinski SL, Neogi T, Hochberg MC, et al. 2019 American College of Rheumatology/Arthritis Foundation guideline for the management of osteoarthritis of the hand, hip and knee. Arthritis Care Res (Hoboken) 2020;72(2):149–62.

72. Sellam J, Courties A, Eymard F, et al. Recommendations of the French Society of Rheumatology on pharmacological treatment of knee osteoarthritis. Joint Bone Spine 2020;87(6):548–55.

73. Osani MC, Vaysbrot EE, Zhou M, et al. Duration of symptom relief and early trajectory of adverse events for oral nonsteroidal anti-inflammatory drugs in knee osteoarthritis: a systematic review and meta-analysis. Arthritis Care Res (Hoboken) 2020;72(5):641–51.

74. Dan J, Izumi M, Habuchi H, et al. A novel mice model of acute flares in osteoarthritis elicited by intra-articular injection of cultured mast cells. J Exp Orthop 2021; 8(1):75.

75. Moskowitz RW, Sunshine A, Hooper M, et al. An analgesic model for assessment of acute pain response in osteoarthritis of the knee. Osteoarthr Cartil 2006;14(11): 1111–8.

76. Tsai CL, Camergo CA Jr. Methodological considerations, such as directed acyclic graphs, for studying "acute on chronic" disease epidemiology: chronic obstructive pulmonary disease example. J Clin Epidemiol 2009;62(9):982–90.

77. Zhaoyang R, Martire LM. Daily sedentary behavior predicts pain and affect in knee arthritis. Ann Behav Med 2019;53(7):642–51.

78. Lazaridou A, Martel MO, Cornelius M, et al. The association between daily physical activity and pain among patients with knee osteoarthritis: the moderating role of pain catastrophizing. Pain Med 2019;20(5):916–24.

79. Carriere JS, Lazaridou A, Martel MO, et al. The moderating role of pain catastrophizing on the relationship between partner support and pain intensity: a daily diary study in patients with knee osteoarthritis. J Behav Med 2020;43(5):807–16.

80. Rivera NV, Parmelee PA, Smith DM. The impact of social interactions and pain on daily positive and negative affect in adults with osteoarthritis of the knee. Aging Ment Health 2020;24(1):8–14.

The Challenges in the Primary Prevention of Osteoarthritis

Jos Runhaar, PhD[a],*, Sita M.A. Bierma-Zeinstra, PhD[b]

KEYWORDS

• Primary prevention • Osteoarthritis • Illness • Disease • Risk factors

KEY POINTS

• Many experts call for a focus on the primary prevention of osteoarthritis.
• Preventing the development of osteoarthritis is not as straightforward as it may seem.
• Osteoarthritis prevention research should be deemed highly important to oppose the predicted increase in osteoarthritis development and associated costs to health care and society in the near future.

INTRODUCTION
The Need for Primary Osteoarthritis Prevention

For years, osteoarthritis (OA) has been ranked among the diseases with the largest impact on patients and society.[1] In the absence of disease-modifying drugs and small to moderate efficacy of symptom relieving therapies, the urge for primary prevention increases.[2–4]

The theoretic basis of primary prevention of OA might sound simple, appealing, and feasible: preventing the onset of OA among subjects without but at high risk for OA. Nevertheless, there are many pitfalls in different aspects related to the initiation of preventive measures in both clinical and research settings. To name a few: how and where can we identify the appropriate target groups? What interventions have an acceptable risk-benefit profile in the absence of symptoms in the ones we treat? How do we establish adherence to the intervention when patients cannot experience any benefits of the intervention? How do we evaluate the preventive effectiveness of the intervention in a slowly developing disease such as OA? The current review addresses some of these key challenges in preventing OA, provides insights into our current knowledge, and highlights some essential knowledge gaps in OA prevention. For

[a] Department of General Practice, Erasmus MC University Medical Center Rotterdam, PO-Box 2040, Rotterdam 3000 CA, the Netherlands; [b] Department of General Practice and Orthopedics & Sports Medicine, Erasmus MC University Medical Center Rotterdam, PO-box 2040, Rotterdam 3000 CA, the Netherlands
* Corresponding author.
E-mail address: j.runhaar@erasmusmc.nl

Clin Geriatr Med 38 (2022) 259–271
https://doi.org/10.1016/j.cger.2021.11.012
geriatric.theclinics.com

this, we use a slightly modified version of the well-known PICO approach; in the absence of OA at the initiation of any primary preventive therapy, the P for "patient" in the traditional PICO should be replaced by either "population" or "target group." As trivial as this might seem, this has important implications, mainly for the choice and uptake of a preventive intervention. Given the high prevalence, we will focus on knee, hip, and hand OA.

IDENTIFYING THE TARGET GROUP
Risk Factors for Osteoarthritis Illness and Disease

The traditional approach to identify a target population for preventive measures for any condition is through identifying its risk factors. For OA, many risk factors have been identified over the years. Some of the most studied and well-known risk factors for knee OA development include older age, female sex, overweight/obesity, joint trauma, genetic predisposition, and occupational loading.[5–8] Although less strong, over-weight/obesity has also been established as a risk factor for hip OA development.[9,10] Other risk factors for hip OA development include altered joint shape, high-impact sports, occupational loading, and genetic predisposition.[7,8,11–13] Female sex, older age, overweight/obesity, occupational loading, local muscle weakness, and genetic predisposition are all known to increase the risk for incident hand OA.[8,14–16]

A very important point to consider here is the fact that most studies on risk factors for OA development have focused on the development of OA disease, that is, pathologic changes in joint tissues. In the available systematic reviews on risk factors for OA development, very little evidence is available for risk factors for OA illness, that is, symptoms and complaints of OA.[17] Nevertheless, it is the actual OA illness that drives the large burden for patients and causes major direct and indirect costs for society and health care. Moreover, radiographic OA (OA disease) in the absence of pain was not associated with mortality, whereas OA pain (illness) in the presence and absence of radiographic OA was associated with a 35% to 37% increased risk for mortality in the general population.[18] Given the general importance of OA illness over OA disease, the focus of OA prevention should be on OA illness, and better insights into risk factors for the onset of OA illness are required.

After selecting established risk factors for OA development in the joint of interest, taking the OA illness versus disease concept into account, the identification of a target group for the prevention of OA could focus either on those at risk for a certain risk factor (eg, those at risk for knee joint trauma or at risk for overweight/obesity) or on those with a certain risk factor (eg, those with a recent knee joint trauma or those with over-weight/obesity). The list of risk factors described here is far from exhaustive but is rather meant to illustrate that a strong risk factor for OA development does not always easily translate into the identification of a feasible target population. Both modifiable and nonmodifiable risk factors will be addressed; modifiable risk factors (eg, lifestyle, body weight, occupational loading) are amenable to interventions and therefore help to shape the preventive interventions, whereas nonmodifiable risk factors (eg, age, sex, genetic predisposition) are not amenable to interventions but can be used to identify the right target population.

Identification of Individuals at Risk for Osteoarthritis Risk Factors

For one of the strongest risk factors for knee OA development, joint trauma,[5,6,19] identification of individuals at risk seems relatively straight forward; sports that put players at increased risk for joint trauma include soccer and rugby for meniscal injuries and American football, soccer, and gymnastics for anterior cruciate ligament (ACL) injuries.[20,21] Selecting individuals participating in these "high-risk sports" could be a very feasible approach to identify a potential target population for preventive measures. Nevertheless, the incidence of ACL injuries per 1000 hours of athlete exposure ranges between 0.10 and 0.17 only, which leads to very high "numbers needed to treat."[20] Also, for other risk factors for OA development in the knee, hip, or hand, for example, overweight/obesity or high occupational loading, different groups of individuals at risk for these risk factors can fairly easily be identified, for instance, low socioeconomic status girls/women who have an increased risk for overweight/obesity[22] and students in training for occupations with a known risk for OA development.[7,14] For other OA risk factors, the identification of the right target group to prevent these risk factors might be more challenging. Local muscle weakness is a known risk factor for both knee and hand OA development.[14,23] Being highly modifiable, local muscle weakness could be seen as a great target for preventive interventions. However, with an average of only 1% decline in muscle mass (a proxy for muscle strength) per year from a peak between the age of 20 and 30 years,[24] identifying those at risk for local muscle weakness is challenging, as there is no threshold to define the presence of muscle weakness. Indications for a stronger decline after the age of 50 years and the strong link to physical inactivity could help to identify those at risk for local muscle weakness. One has to keep in mind that local muscle weakness could also be an early sign of OA disease and therefore not causally related to OA development. If so, targeting local muscle weakness in order to prevent OA development will be ineffective.

Identification of Individuals with Osteoarthritis Risk Factors

Focusing on risk factors for OA illness, identifying individuals with overweight/obesity (for knee and hip OA illness), participating in high-impact sports (for hip OA illness), or having physically demanding jobs (for hip OA illness) seems doable.[17] Although the presence of other OA illness risk factors such as hip shape morphology, (mild) hip dysplasia, and local muscle strength can be determined accurately and reliably, the feasibility of screening for the presence of these risk factors among subjects free of OA symptoms can be questioned. Besides the low prevalence of these risk factors in the open population, for example, 0% to 13% for cam impingement among nonselective populations,[25] the exposure to radiation required for the determination of the presence of some of these risk factors should be carefully considered.

Given the aging population, many studies highlight the importance of older age as a risk factor for OA development.[2,5] From a prevention perspective, the importance of the association between aging and OA incidence is somewhat questionable. Not only is age itself nonmodifiable, the impact on the number of years lived in good health will be less substantial when preventing OA among elderly individuals (eg, 80+ years) than among middle-aged individuals. Next to that, the exposure to/development of many risk factors for OA incidence occurs during adolescence and early adulthood (eg, joint injuries, overweight/obesity, and occupational overload). When using these risk factors to define potential target populations for preventive interventions, the optimal "window of opportunity" likely has passed at an older age. That is why experts in the field call for a lifespan approach to OA prevention (**Fig. 1**): prevention and treatment of risk factors for OA development at those stages of life where these risk factors are developing or amendable to treatment.[17]

Looking Beyond the Single-Risk Factors Approach

Despite the fact that there are multiple known strong risk factors for OA development,[6,7,11,14] it is the actual combination of the prevalence of the risk factor and the

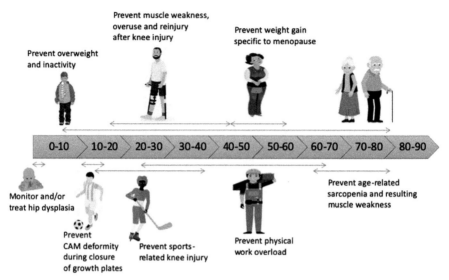

Fig. 1. Opportunities for preventing OA across the lifespan.

strength of its association to OA development that will determine the importance of that risk factor, in the light of OA prevention. For example, knee joint injuries are one of the strongest risk factors for future knee OA development.[6,19] By calculating the population attributable fraction, an estimation of the proportion of new cases in the population that could be avoided if the risk factor was removed, Silverwood and colleagues showed that the number of new cases of knee OA/pain in a 3-year follow-up study of 3907 middle-aged men and women (aged 50 years and older) that could be attributed to knee injuries was only 5.1%.[5] Hence, preventing all knee injuries among these 3907 individuals would only have led to a 5.1% lower incidence of knee OA. Despite the fact that the association between overweight/obesity and knee OA development is less strong than that for knee injuries, the higher prevalence of overweight/obesity resulted in a population attributable fraction of 24.6%.[5] These results might look very promising for a preventive trial on weight loss among overweight/obese subjects free of knee OA/pain. Nevertheless, with a total incidence of knee pain of only 24% in 3 years,[26] the actual effect of preventing all cases of overweight/obesity in the given population would result in a reduction of the total incidence of 24.6% × 24% = 6% in the first 3 years. A quick sample size calculation for a trial with 24.6% incidence in the control group and 18.6% in the intervention group would require 2 groups of 735 individuals followed-up for 3 years ($\alpha = 95\%$, $\beta = 80\%$).[27]

The aforementioned examples illustrate the importance of the selection of target populations based on the interaction of multiple risk factors for future preventive interventions. Risk factors such as female sex/gender or genetic predisposition might not be relevant on their own for the selection of a target population for OA prevention, as these factors are nonmodifiable. However, given the known interaction between female sex/gender, knee joint injuries, and adiposity on knee OA development,[28] focusing on the prevention of weight gain among female athletes who suffered from a knee injury might provide a more feasible treatment target. Unfortunately, little is known about the interaction of risk factors for OA development and should therefore be a focus of future research initiatives.[17] To better communicate individuals' risk for OA development and to visualize the potential of certain interventions, risk stratification tools, such as those for cardiovascular events in which multiple risk factors are incorporated, might improve the understanding among high-risk individuals and could also help to motivate them to adhere to any preventive intervention.

DESIGNING THE INTERVENTION

So, for the selection of OA risk factors, either to prevent the occurrence of the risk factor or to intervene once the risk factor is present, both the prevalence of the risk factor and the strength of its association with OA development are of great importance for the relevance of the selected target population. Obviously, the next step to consider is if and when the selected risk factor is modifiable (ie, amenable to any intervention).

Challenges in Preventing Osteoarthritis Risk Factors

As indicated earlier, overweight/obesity is one of the major drivers for the development of OA.[5,6] The main cause for the high prevalence of overweight/obesity worldwide is the overconsumption of processed, energy-dense food.[29] The purchase and consumption of food are influenced by the interaction of pricing, palatability, and cultural and ethnic habits.[30] Given these complex interactions, designing interventions that prevent overweight/obesity is very challenging. Despite the multidisciplinary nature of primary care, which is generally seen as the optimal setting for targeting the prevention of overweight/obesity, there is little to no evidence for effective interventions.[31] Given the potential of population-based approaches and effective examples from these kinds of approaches on, for example, smoking and alcohol usage,[32] already in 2007, there was a call from the World Health Organization for more upstream interventions by countries to "develop its own needs-driven portfolio of appropriate and realistic interventions, and involve many stakeholders from all relevant sectors in a transparent and explicit process."[33] Unfortunately, nowadays implementation of such strategies is limited.[34]

The initiatives for the prevention of joint injuries illustrate another major challenge when designing a preventive intervention, namely adherence/uptake. There is sufficient high-quality evidence available showing that injury prevention programs (ie, plyometrics, strengthening, and agility exercises) are effective in the prevention of anterior cruciate ligament injuries.[35] Nevertheless, implementation of these programs into real-world settings is a major challenge, as adherence to these programs in the real world is generally very low.[36] This observation closely relates to a broader challenge for preventive therapies, as "there is no glory in prevention." To further OA prevention, we need to align our efforts and knowledge with experts from behavioral research. How can we motivate individuals at risk for OA risk factors to modify their lifestyle, if there is no positive feedback from that actual intervention? After all, these individuals do not have any joint symptoms, so they cannot experience any relief of symptoms to keep them motivated to adhere to an intervention. Are individuals at risk for OA risk factors willing to consider medical interventions or should we aim for nonpharmacologic interventions only? How should we educate these individuals regarding their future risk of OA in order to motivate them to get into action, rather than demoralizing them by presenting a future with a chronic condition? These questions highlight some of the current knowledge gaps in OA prevention.

Challenges in Treating Osteoarthritis Risk Factors

When designing a preventive intervention, the presence of a (modifiable) risk factor for OA might help to overcome the lack of motivation for preventive measures among the target population. For instance, among those with overweight/obesity, tracking the body weight over time to illustrate their weight loss will provide participants with a measure of their progress during the intervention. Still, we know that achieving sustainable lifestyle changes among subjects with overweight/obesity is very hard, and adherence to these interventions remains a challenge.[37–39] Similarly, targeting individuals with a history of joint trauma might facilitate the willingness for preventive interventions, as these individuals have a strong preference to keep physically active but also often fear for a reinjury.[40] Unfortunately, little is known about the mechanisms through which joint injuries lead to the early onset of OA.[41,42] A recently developed framework for an intervention for managing knee OA risk factors after ACL injuries does show that the first steps toward OA prevention after knee joint injuries are currently being taken.[43]

The presence of an OA risk factor does not always facilitate the process of OA prevention. Participating in high-impact sports puts individuals at risk for hip OA development, and high occupational loading is known to increase the risk for hand and hip OA. Nevertheless, targeting these risk factors to prevent the subsequent onset of OA will be challenging. How to motivate athletes to change the sport they participate in toward one with less/no risk for OA development? Also, most employees with high occupational loadings will require retraining in order to take on new jobs, are likely to have a preference for their current job, and might lack a track-record to be competitive when applying for another and less burdensome job. Given the lack of preventive trials in OA research, the selection of effective interventions for the prevention of OA is very hard.[3,17] Next to that, there are other aspects that challenge the design of future preventive interventions, as described in the earlier section. Again, the list of examples is far from exhaustive, but rather an impetus for an in-depth discussion on what interventions will be effective and feasible in a preventive setting.

MEASURING THE EFFECT

Every trial or intervention requires predefined primary outcome and/or treatment goal. In a preventive intervention aimed to prevent the onset of OA, obviously, the development of OA should be evaluated primarily. As easy as this may seem, defining the actual outcome for a preventive trial in OA has some challenges and implications.

Measuring the Incidence of Osteoarthritis Illness

As indicated earlier, it is the illness of OA (ie, symptoms and complaints of OA) that seems the most important outcome for OA prevention. Pain is often defined as the most important complaint by patients with OA.[2] Nevertheless, how we measure pain or define the presence of pain in OA is very variable. Current clinical guidelines use the presence of "activity-related joint pain" (irrespective of frequency or severity) to define the presence of pain in hip and knee OA.[44,45] Scientific reports using the American College of Rheumatology (ACR) classification criteria to evaluate clinical hip/knee OA define the presence of pain as "pain on most days of the month," without specifying whether this is during any specific activity.[46–48] Others specifically measure pain during an activity, such as walking, stair descending/ascending, or rising from a chair, using specific questions from validated OA questionnaires such as WOMAC and KOOS/HOOS[49,50] or a cut-off in the overall pain subscales.[51] Another way of defining a clinically relevant outcome in OA is the patient-acceptable symptom state (PASS)[52–54]; before an intervention, each patient defines his/her "acceptable state," and the percentage of patients reaching that state is used in the comparison of the intervention arm. Up to now, the clinical relevance and feasibility of PASS have never been tested in a preventive setting.

An important aspect to consider when choosing a potential outcome of symptomatic OA is the fact that in early stage OA, pain can be absent for prolonged periods of time, with short and very sudden short flare-ups.[55,56] For patients with early-stage OA, it is this intermittent pain that is extremely burdensome.[57] When pain is highly fluctuating, one can question the clinical relevance of a single measure in time of something like "pain during walking" or the PASS. To illustrate this fluctuation problem, although 52% of first-time presenters in primary care with knee and/or hip pain fulfilled the ACR-criteria for clinical knee/hip OA at baseline, only 17.5% fulfilled these criteria at each of the 5 follow-up measures over a 10-year period and only 14% never fulfilled these criteria during follow-up.[46]

Most likely, measuring symptomatic outcomes more often (eg, daily) over a longer period (eg, several weeks or months) will provide a better insight into the symptoms of patients with early stage OA. With the use of mobile applications for data capture, this will be feasible[58] but will require advanced statistical methods to properly evaluate intervention effects in these highly correlated repeated measures. Measuring multiple domains of pain is highly recommended in the field of chronic pain research/management.[59] Given the challenges in measuring OA *illness* in a preventive setting, state-of-the-art knowledge from related fields (eg, chronic pain and pain assessment) needs to find its way into OA prevention.

Measuring the Incidence of Osteoarthritis Disease

Whether defined using traditional radiography and Kellgren and Lawrence criteria,[60] or using more sensitive measures of OA features on MRI to define the incidence of OA,[61] the clinical relevance of preventing OA disease (ie, structural features of OA) is questionable.[17] Structural features of OA do matter when considering total joint arthroplasty, as patients with only mild structural OA are significantly more dissatisfied after an arthroplasty than those with more severe structural OA.[62] Moreover, in the light of cost savings, preventing arthroplasties due to OA will save on health care costs, as these are primarily attributable to these joint arthroplasties. However, when targeting subjects without disease for preventive intervention and evaluating the effects on joint arthroplasties, one will need to have multiple decades of follow-up to reach sufficient numbers of cases that underwent surgery; this scenario seems very unrealistic.

The Need for Surrogate Outcomes

Both OA illness and OA disease develop very slowly. Therefore, when evaluating potential outcomes for preventive trials in OA, the annual incidence rate of the outcome is an important feature for the feasibility of such a trial. Annual incidence rates of OA (either hands, knees or hips) within subjects at high risk are only ±2% to 5% for OA illness and disease.[38,46,63–67]

To overcome this challenge, OA prevention urgently needs validated surrogate outcomes. These surrogate outcomes can lead to a "reduction in sample size and trial duration when a [...] distant disease is replaced by a more frequent or proximal endpoint," and this could "reduce costs and enhance the feasibility" of preventive clinical trials.[68–70] Because of the success of surrogate outcomes in many other chronic diseases, treatment effects of certain medications are no longer evaluated using primary outcomes that have direct impact on patients (eg, cardiovascular events or mortality). For instance, in 436 registered randomized controlled trials on diabetes drugs, most trials (82%) used glycosylated hemoglobin as the primary outcome rather than patient-oriented outcomes.[71] One of the few existing examples of the evaluation of surrogate outcomes for OA development showed that a measure of cartilage integrity on MRI was significantly affected by weight loss and that its change was related to long-term knee OA development.[72] Unfortunately, in another study, none of the changes in structural MRI features were related to long-term pain progression among patients with knee pain and a meniscal tear that were randomized over after meniscal surgery and physical therapy.[73] Exploring and validating more potential surrogate outcomes for different target groups and different potential preventive interventions is deemed a top priority for the field of OA prevention research.

CONCLUSIONS AND RECOMMENDATIONS

With the aforementioned examples, we have tried to illustrate some of the key challenges in OA prevention (**Table 1**). Despite the call for shifting the focus of OA research toward the early disease stage and OA prevention, there is a clear lack of knowledge for many aspects of the early phase of OA.[2–4,17]

Given the association with OA incidence in several joints, combined with the increasing prevalence of overweight/obesity worldwide, lifestyle interventions to prevent weight gain or to treat the presence of overweight are of great importance for the prevention of OA. Of course, OA prevention is not the only reason to strife for a healthy lifestyle in the population; positive health effects of a healthy lifestyle and a healthy body weight are known for, for example, diabetes, coronary heart disease, hypertension, cancer, and early death.[39] From a research perspective, it would be naïve to not align initiatives to gain knowledge on OA prevention with ongoing and future efforts with these other medical fields. From a societal perspective, perhaps focusing efforts on preventing overweight/obesity would be more appealing and therefore more feasible, than narrowing the scope down to OA prevention only. Given the important effect of OA pain on mortality[18] and the huge burden on health care costs,[2,74] OA outcomes should then be considered a major concern for the overall population that should be taken into account when evaluating the societal effects of interventions focusing on preventing overweight/obesity.[75]

Table 1
Summary of key challenges in osteoarthritis prevention

Target group	• Prevention of OA risk factors
	  ○ Targeting risk factors for OA *disease* or OA *illness*?
	  ○ Is the risk (factor) modifiable?
	    ■ If so, in which stage of life?
	  ○ Focus on a single or a combination of risk factors?
	  ○ How to identify the target population?
	• Prevention among those with OA risk factors
	  ○ Targeting risk factors for OA *disease* or OA *illness*?
	  ○ Are the risk factors modifiable?
	    ■ If so, in which stage of life?
	  ○ Focus on a single or a combination of risk factors?
	  ○ How to identify the target population?

Intervention	• Adherence/uptake to the intervention • Motivation of participants • Education of participants
Outcome	• How to capture OA *illness* in the early disease stage? • Is it relevant to measure OA *disease*? • How to overcome the slow-developing nature of OA? • Validation of potential surrogate outcomes

Two essential aspects of OA prevention clearly lack solid high-quality scientific evidence: risk factors for OA illness and surrogate outcomes. Inevitably, the signs of OA illness (ie, joint pain, functional limitations, health-related quality of life) form the burden to patients, drive patients to seek health care, and lead to early retirement.[17] Therefore, the selection of target populations and potential interventions should be informed by knowledge on risk factors for the development of OA illness. To facilitate future studies on OA prevention, also the evaluation and validation of surrogate outcomes for long-term OA development are urgently needed. Surrogate outcomes have the potential to shorten future trials on OA prevention and with that reduce costs and enhance the feasibility. As many studies in the field of OA have measured both short-term (ie, 1–2 years) changes in OA-related features (eg, patient-reported outcomes, objective physical functional test, and imaging) and have evaluated the long-term (ie, >5 years) development of OA, there is a huge potential for the identification and validation of surrogate markers already. Based on a stepwise approach, not only data from RCTs can be used for the validation of surrogate outcomes but also data from observational studies can help to build the evidence around potential surrogate outcomes for OA development.[68] In the absence of validated surrogate outcomes, and in line with the narrative of the societal approach to OA prevention, an alternative approach to enhance the feasibility of preventive trials could be to set strong OA risk factors as primary outcome for preventive trials (eg, ACL injuries) and estimate the subsequent preventive effect on OA development, rather than following all patients long enough for OA to develop.

In conclusion, despite the urge for a more proactive rather than a reactive approach to OA treatment, there are still many challenges in OA prevention. All aspects of OA prevention, selecting the proper target population, designing an optimal intervention, and measuring the intervention effects, still hold many challenges and have important knowledge gaps. Nevertheless, given the enormous burden of OA for patients and society, and the expected increase in OA prevalence, OA prevention is a very important field that deserves our attention and dedication.

CLINICS CARE POINTS

- To prevent osteoarthritis development, the onset and interaction of multiple osteoarthritis risk factors should direct preventive strategies, for example, weight gain after menopause and muscle strength loss after joint trauma.
- Behavioral strategies, such as Motivational Interviewing, should be applied to explore the internal motivation for lifestyle changes in individuals at risk for osteoarthritis development.

DISCLOSURE

All authors declare no conflicts of interest related to the content of this article.

REFERENCES

1. Diseases GBD, Injuries C. Global burden of 369 diseases and injuries in 204 countries and territories, 1990-2019: a systematic analysis for the Global Burden of Disease Study 2019. Lancet 2020;396(10258):1204–22.
2. Hunter DJ, Bierma-Zeinstra S. Osteoarthritis. Lancet 2019;393(10182):1745–59.
3. Runhaar J, Zhang Y. Can we prevent OA? Epidemiology and public health insights and implications. Rheumatology (Oxford) 2018;57(suppl_4):iv3–9.

4. Roos EM, Arden NK. Strategies for the prevention of knee osteoarthritis. Nat Rev Rheumatol 2016;12(2):92–101.

5. Silverwood V, Blagojevic-Bucknall M, Jinks C, et al. Current evidence on risk factors for knee osteoarthritis in older adults: a systematic review and meta-analysis. Osteoarthritis Cartilage 2015;23(4):507–15.

6. Blagojevic M, Jinks C, Jeffery A, et al. Risk factors for onset of osteoarthritis of the knee in older adults: a systematic review and meta-analysis. Osteoarthritis Cartilage 2010;18(1):24–33.

7. Canetti EFD, Schram B, Orr RM, et al. Risk factors for development of lower limb osteoarthritis in physically demanding occupations: a systematic review and meta-analysis. Appl Ergon 2020;86:103097.

8. Spector TD, MacGregor AJ. Risk factors for osteoarthritis: genetics. Osteoarthritis Cartilage 2004;12(Suppl A):S39–44.

9. Jiang L, Rong J, Wang Y, et al. The relationship between body mass index and hip osteoarthritis: a systematic review and meta-analysis. Joint Bone Spine 2011;78(2):150–5.

10. Lievense AM, Bierma-Zeinstra SM, Verhagen AP, et al. Influence of obesity on the development of osteoarthritis of the hip: a systematic review. Rheumatology (Oxford) 2002;41(10):1155–62.

11. van Buuren MMA, Arden NK, Bierma-Zeinstra SMA, et al. Statistical shape modeling of the hip and the association with hip osteoarthritis: a systematic review. Osteoarthritis Cartilage 2021;29(5):607–18.

12. Lievense AM, Bierma-Zeinstra SM, Verhagen AP, et al. Influence of sporting activities on the development of osteoarthritis of the hip: a systematic review. Arthritis Rheum 2003;49(2):228–36.

13. Lievense A, Bierma-Zeinstra S, Verhagen A, et al. Influence of work on the development of osteoarthritis of the hip: a systematic review. J Rheumatol 2001;28(11):2520–8.

14. Kalichman L, Hernandez-Molina G. Hand osteoarthritis: an epidemiological perspective. Semin Arthritis Rheum 2010;39(6):465–76.

15. Jiang L, Xie X, Wang Y, et al. Body mass index and hand osteoarthritis susceptibility: an updated meta-analysis. Int J Rheum Dis 2016;19(12):1244–54.

16. Leung GJ, Rainsford KD, Kean WF. Osteoarthritis of the hand I: aetiology and pathogenesis, risk factors, investigation and diagnosis. J Pharm Pharmacol 2014;66(3):339–46.

17. Whittaker JL, Runhaar J, Bierma-Zeinstra MA, et al., A lifespan approach to osteoarthritis prevention. Osteoarthritis Cartilage, 2021. (in press).

18. Leyland KM, Gates LS, Sanchez-Santos MT, et al. Knee osteoarthritis and time-to all-cause mortality in six community-based cohorts: an international meta-analysis of individual participant-level data. Aging Clin Exp Res 2021;33(3):529–45.

19. Poulsen E, Goncalves GH, Bricca A, et al. Knee osteoarthritis risk is increased 4-6 fold after knee injury - a systematic review and meta-analysis. Br J Sports Med 2019;53(23):1454–63.

20. Bram JT, Magee LC, Mehta NN, et al. Anterior cruciate ligament injury incidence in adolescent athletes; A systematic review and meta-analysis. Am J Sports Med 2021;49(7):1962–72.

21. Snoeker BA, Bakker EW, Kegel CA, et al. Risk factors for meniscal tears: a systematic review including meta-analysis. J Orthop Sports Phys Ther 2013;43(6):352–67.

22. Newton S, Braithwaite D, Akinyemiju TF. Socio-economic status over the life course and obesity: systematic review and meta-analysis. PLoS One 2017; 12(5):e0177151.
23. Oiestad BE, Juhl CB, Eitzen I, et al. Knee extensor muscle weakness is a risk factor for development of knee osteoarthritis. A systematic review and meta-analysis. Osteoarthritis Cartilage 2015;23(2):171–7.
24. Montero-Fernandez N, Serra-Rexach JA. Role of exercise on sarcopenia in the elderly. Eur J Phys Rehabil Med 2013;49(1):131–43.
25. van Klij P, Heerey J, Waarsing JH, et al. The prevalence of Cam and Pincer morphology and its association with development of hip osteoarthritis. J Orthop Sports Phys Ther 2018;48(4):230–8.
26. Jinks C, Jordan KP, Blagojevic M, et al. Predictors of onset and progression of knee pain in adults living in the community. A prospective study. Rheumatology (Oxford) 2008;47(3):368–74.
27. Tibrewala R, et al. Principal Component analysis of Simultaneous PET-MRI Reveals patterns of Bone-cartilage interactions in osteoarthritis. J Magn Reson Imaging 2020;52(5):1462–74.
28. Toomey CM, Whittaker JL, Nettel-Aguirre A, et al. Higher Fat mass is associated with a history of knee injury in Youth sport. J Orthop Sports Phys Ther 2017; 47(2):80–7.
29. Swinburn BA, Sacks G, Hall KD, et al. The global obesity pandemic: shaped by global drivers and local environments. Lancet 2011;378(9793):804–14.
30. Seidell JC, Halberstadt J. The global burden of obesity and the challenges of prevention. Ann Nutr Metab 2015;66(Suppl 2):7–12.
31. Peirson L, Douketis J, Ciliska D, et al. Prevention of overweight and obesity in adult populations: a systematic review. CMAJ Open 2014;2(4):E268–72.
32. Capewell S, Dowrick C. Healthful Diet and physical activity for cardiovascular disease prevention in adults without known risk factors: is behavioral Counselling Necessary? JAMA Intern Med 2017;177(9):1254–5.
33. Organisation, W.H., The challenge of obesity in the WHO European Region and the strategies for response, F. Branca, H. Nikogosian, and T. Lobstein, Editors. 2007.
34. Seidell JC, Halberstadt J, Noordam H, et al. An integrated health care standard for the management and prevention of obesity in The Netherlands. Fam Pract 2012;29(Suppl 1):i153–6.
35. Huang YL, Jung J, Mulligan CMS, et al. A Majority of anterior cruciate ligament injuries can Be prevented by injury prevention programs: a systematic review of randomized controlled trials and Cluster-randomized controlled trials with meta-analysis. Am J Sports Med 2020;48(6):1505–15.
36. Owoeye OBA, McKay CD, Verhagen E, et al. Advancing adherence research in sport injury prevention. Br J Sports Med 2018;52(17):1078–9.
37. Runhaar J, de Vos BC, van Middelkoop M, et al. Prevention of incident knee osteoarthritis by moderate weight loss in overweight and obese females. Arthritis Care Res (Hoboken) 2016;68(10):1428–33.
38. Runhaar J, van Middelkoop M, Reijman M, et al. Prevention of knee osteoarthritis in overweight females: the first preventive randomized controlled trial in osteoarthritis. Am J Med 2015;128(8):888–895 e4.
39. Kohl HW 3rd, Craig CL, Lambert EV, et al. The pandemic of physical inactivity: global action for public health. Lancet 2012;380(9838):294–305.
40. Filbay SR, Crossley KM, Ackerman IN. Activity preferences, lifestyle modifications and re-injury fears influence longer-term quality of life in people with knee

symptoms following anterior cruciate ligament reconstruction: a qualitative study. J Phys 2016;62(2):103–10.

41. Whittaker JL, Roos EM. A pragmatic approach to prevent post-traumatic osteoarthritis after sport or exercise-related joint injury. Best Pract Res Clin Rheumatol 2019;33(1):158–71.

42. Kramer WC, Hendricks KJ, Wang J. Pathogenetic mechanisms of posttraumatic osteoarthritis: opportunities for early intervention. Int J Clin Exp Med 2011;4(4): 285–98.

43. Davies AM, Wong R, Steinhart K, et al., Development of an Intervention to Manage Knee Osteoarthritis Risk and Symptoms Following Anterior Cruciate Ligament Injury. Osteoarthritis Cartilage, 2021. (in press).

44. Excellence, N.I.o.H.C., Osteoarthritis: Care and Management in Adults. 2014: London.

45. Zhang W, Doherty M, Peat G, et al. EULAR evidence-based recommendations for the diagnosis of knee osteoarthritis. Ann Rheum Dis 2010;69(3):483–9.

46. Schiphof D, Runhaar J, Waarsing JH, et al. The clinical and radiographic course of early knee and hip osteoarthritis over 10 years in CHECK (Cohort Hip and Cohort Knee). Osteoarthritis Cartilage 2019;27(10):1491–500.

47. Fernandes GS, Bhattacharya A, McWilliams DF, et al. Risk prediction model for knee pain in the Nottingham community: a Bayesian modelling approach. Arthritis Res Ther 2017;19(1):59.

48. Skou ST, Koes BW, Gronne DT, et al. Comparison of three sets of clinical classification criteria for knee osteoarthritis: a cross-sectional study of 13,459 patients treated in primary care. Osteoarthritis Cartilage 2020;28(2):167–72.

49. Liu Q, Li Z, Ferreira M, et al. Recent injury, severe radiographic change, and lower Quadriceps strength increase risk of knee pain Exacerbation during walking: a within-person knee-matched study. J Orthop Sports Phys Ther 2021; 51(6):298–304.

50. Liu Q, Lane NE, Hunter D, et al. Co-existing patterns of MRI lesions were differentially associated with knee pain at rest and on joint loading: a within-person knee-matched case-controls study. BMC Musculoskelet Disord 2020;21(1):650.

51. Wang Y, Teichtahl AJ, Abram F, et al. Knee pain as a predictor of structural progression over 4 years: data from the Osteoarthritis Initiative, a prospective cohort study. Arthritis Res Ther 2018;20(1):250.

52. Mahler EAM, Boers N, Bijlsma JWJ, et al. Patient Acceptable symptom state in knee osteoarthritis patients Succeeds across different patient-reported outcome measures assessing physical function, but Fails across other Dimensions and Rheumatic diseases. J Rheumatol 2018;45(1):122–7.

53. Bijsterbosch J, Watt I, Meulenbelt I, et al. Clinical and radiographic disease course of hand osteoarthritis and determinants of outcome after 6 years. Ann Rheum Dis 2011;70(1):68–73.

54. Tubach F, Ravaud P, Martin-Mola E, et al. Minimum clinically important improvement and patient acceptable symptom state in pain and function in rheumatoid arthritis, ankylosing spondylitis, chronic back pain, hand osteoarthritis, and hip and knee osteoarthritis: results from a prospective multinational study. Arthritis Care Res (Hoboken) 2012;64(11):1699–707.

55. Carlesso LC, Hawker GA, Torner J, et al. Association of intermittent and constant knee pain patterns with knee pain severity, radiographic knee osteoarthritis duration and severity. Arthritis Care Res (Hoboken) 2020.

56. Thomas MJ, Neogi T. Flare-ups of osteoarthritis: what do they mean in the short-term and the long-term? Osteoarthritis Cartilage 2020;28(7):870–3.

57. Liu A, Kendzerska T, Stanaitis I, et al. The relationship between knee pain characteristics and symptom state acceptability in people with knee osteoarthritis. Osteoarthritis Cartilage 2014;22(2):178–83.
58. Bedson J, Hill J, White D, et al. Development and validation of a pain monitoring app for patients with musculoskeletal conditions (The Keele pain recorder feasibility study). BMC Med Inform Decis Mak 2019;19(1):24.
59. Fillingim RB, Loeser JD, Baron R, et al. Assessment of chronic pain: domains, methods, and mechanisms. J Pain 2016;17(9 Suppl):T10–20.
60. Kellgren JH, Lawrence JS. Radiological assessment of osteo-arthrosis. Ann Rheum Dis 1957;16(4):494–502.
61. Hunter DJ, Guermazi A, Lo GH, et al. Evolution of semi-quantitative whole joint assessment of knee OA: MOAKS (MRI Osteoarthritis Knee Score). Osteoarthritis Cartilage 2011;19(8):990–1002.
62. Leppanen S, Niemelainen M, Huhtala H, et al. Mild knee osteoarthritis predicts dissatisfaction after total knee arthroplasty: a prospective study of 186 patients aged 65 years or less with 2-year follow-up. BMC Musculoskelet Disord 2021; 22(1):657.
63. de Vos BC, Landsmeer MLA, van Middelkoop M, et al. Long-term effects of a lifestyle intervention and oral glucosamine sulphate in primary care on incident knee OA in overweight women. Rheumatology (Oxford) 2017;56(8):1326–34.
64. Lo GH, Strayhorn MT, Driban JB, et al. Subjective Crepitus as a risk factor for incident symptomatic knee osteoarthritis: data from the osteoarthritis initiative. Arthritis Care Res (Hoboken) 2018;70(1):53–60.
65. Lohmander LS, Englund PM, Dahl LL, et al. The long-term consequence of anterior cruciate ligament and meniscus injuries: osteoarthritis. Am J Sports Med 2007;35(10):1756–69.
66. Snyder EA, Alvarez C, Golightly YM, et al. Incidence and progression of hand osteoarthritis in a large community-based cohort: the Johnston County Osteoarthritis Project. Osteoarthritis Cartilage 2020;28(4):446–52.
67. Yu D, Jordan KP, Bedson J, et al. Population trends in the incidence and initial management of osteoarthritis: age-period-cohort analysis of the Clinical Practice Research Datalink, 1992-2013. Rheumatology (Oxford) 2017;56(11):1902–17.
68. Ciani O, Buyse M, Drummond M, et al. Time to review the Role of surrogate End points in health Policy: state of the art and the way forward. Value Health 2017; 20(3):487–95.
69. Prentice RL. Surrogate endpoints in clinical trials: definition and operational criteria. Stat Med 1989;8(4):431–40.
70. Vanderweele TJ. Surrogate measures and consistent surrogates. Biometrics 2013;69(3):561–9.
71. Gandhi GY, Murad MH, Fujiyoshi A, et al. Patient-important outcomes in registered diabetes trials. JAMA 2008;299(21):2543–9.
72. Runhaar J, Dam EB, Oei EHG, et al. Medial cartilage Surface integrity as a surrogate measure for incident radiographic knee osteoarthritis following weight changes. Cartilage 2019. 1947603519892305.
73. Katz JN, Collins JE, Jones M, et al. Association between structural change over 18 months and subsequent symptom change in middle-aged persons treated for meniscal tear. Arthritis Care Res (Hoboken) 2021.
74. White AG, Birnbaum HG, Janagap C, et al. Direct and indirect costs of pain therapy for osteoarthritis in an insured population in the United States. J Occup Environ Med 2008;50(9):998–1005.
75. (OARSI), O.R.S.I., Osteoarthritis: A Serious Disease, Submitted to the. 2016.

Phenotypes in Osteoarthritis
Why Do We Need Them and Where Are We At?

Murillo Dório, MD, PhD[a],*, Leticia A. Deveza, MD, PhD[b]

KEYWORDS

• Osteoarthritis • Phenotypes • Endotypes • Machine learning

KEY POINTS

• The multifactorial pathogenesis of osteoarthritis (OA), the heterogeneity of clinical manifestations, and the mixed population have contributed to the failure of multiple drugs in trials.
• Dividing OA patients into subgroups (phenotypes) with common characteristics may guide therapy and improve management.
• Phenotypes can be categorized based on mechanisms of disease (endotypes), prognosis, and treatment response.
• Machine learning (an application of artificial intelligence) is being increasingly applied to large data sets in OA, including imaging, biochemical biomarker, and genetic information, for the purpose of identifying OA phenotypes.

INTRODUCTION

Osteoarthritis (OA) is a common and serious disease that affects predominantly older adults.[1] It has been defined as "the disease which manifests first as a molecular derangement (abnormal joint tissue metabolism) followed by anatomic, and/or physiologic derangements, characterized by cartilage degradation, bone remodeling, osteophyte formation, joint inflammation, and loss of normal joint function".[2] OA can affect one or multiple joints in a person, most often the knees, finger joints, hips, and spine. It is a major and growing contributor to disability worldwide and is associated with increased comorbidity and mortality.[1]

[a] Division of Rheumatology, Hospital das Clínicas da Faculdade de Medicina da Universidade de São Paulo, Avendia Dr. Arnaldo 455, sala 3142, Cerqueira César, São Paulo, SP CEP 01246-903, Brazil; [b] Rheumatology Department, Royal North Shore Hospital and Institute of Bone and Joint Research, Kolling Institute, University of Sydney, Reserve Road, Sydney, New South Wales 2065, Australia
* Corresponding author:
E-mail address: murillodorio@gmail.com

Clin Geriatr Med 38 (2022) 273–286
https://doi.org/10.1016/j.cger.2021.11.002
geriatric.theclinics.com
0749-0690/22/© 2021 Elsevier Inc. All rights reserved.

Current guidelines recommend as core treatments for OA both nondrug (such as exercise) and drug therapies (such as anti-inflammatory agents).[3,4] However, most have only short-term to medium-term benefits, and effect sizes are small to moderate at best.[5,6] Furthermore, the use of drugs is restricted in patients with comorbidities due to the risk of adverse events.[3] Having failed these options, knee/hip arthroplasty is usually an effective definitive treatment, but it is expensive and there is the risk of medical and postsurgical complications.[1]

Although many clinical trials have been conducted, there are still no approved disease-modifying therapies, although some drugs have shown positive results in trials more recently.[7,8] This is at least in part due to the heterogeneity of this complex disease.[9] Most trials for OA treatment have defined OA for inclusion criteria as the presence of symptoms and definite radiographic changes (eg, osteophytes or joint space narrowing). This does not account for the different mechanisms leading to joint damage, which can be due to mechanical dysfunction, inflammation, metabolic factors, prior injury, and so forth, or even a combination of these. Nor does it take into account the diversity of clinical manifestations (ie, number of involved joints, presence of pain sensitization, etc.), chronicity, comorbidities, or other aspects of the disease in individuals that may affect their response to the studied therapy.[10] The complexity of OA and the difficulties to identify a single treatment modality for all patients are associated with the heterogeneity of the disease.[11]

To address the heterogeneity of OA to improve practice and clinical research, a new model of understanding OA based on a phenotype-guided approach is needed and has gained attention in OA research over the past 10 years. This review covers the main aspects of OA phenotyping research, including the concepts and rationale, the current approaches to OA phenotyping, recent advances in this area, and future directions.

WHAT ARE OA PHENOTYPES?

Mobasheri and colleagues[12] defined phenotypes, in medicine, as "any observable characteristic or trait of a disease, such as morphology, development, biochemical or physiologic properties, or behavior, without any implication of a molecular mechanism or pathway." In clinical medicine, patients with common characteristics are often grouped together to guide therapy and improve management. In contrast, an endotype is "a subtype of a disease or condition, which is defined by a distinct functional or pathobiological mechanism."[12] Endotype implies the presence of a well-defined molecular mechanism.[12]

Phenotyping is very useful for studying, diagnosing, and treating diseases, particularly those that are multifactorial and chronic. OA phenotyping research has the purpose of better identifying individuals at higher risk of progression and better delineating subgroups with distinct risk factors and disease mechanisms that would be suitable for prevention strategies and targeted treatment.[9] Such classifications are only relevant and clinically useful if they can inform on differences in underlying pathophysiology, clinical outcomes, or management. At present, clinical phenotypes are the most common method of subgrouping OA, although this strategy has a few drawbacks. First, there is no consensus definition for specific OA subgroups as yet. Second, there may be no specific tests or biomarkers that identify a particular phenotype compared with another. For this reason, poorly understood subgroups may go undiagnosed and untreated and put together with others.[12] The importance of identifying endotypes for targeted treatment has gained much attention, particularly from the point of view of drug discovery, where identifying the right target is key for success.[12] How to best subset OA into phenotypes and endotypes is an important issue that has not yet been fully addressed. Identifying phenotypes of OA is an important research priority because it allows us to gain a better understanding of the pathways and mechanisms that may be involved in each distinct phenotype and target them more effectively using a variety of preventive and treatment strategies.[13]

HISTORICAL BACKGROUND—HOW HAS OA PHENOTYPING RESEARCH STARTED?

Brandt and colleagues,[14] in 2009, suggested that dividing OA into classical primary and secondary subsets is not useful since "all OA is secondary" and that any attempt to subset OA had to take into account the fact that OA is largely a condition driven by the response to mechanical stress on the joint. They suggested that subsetting OA should be done based on the mechanical abnormalities responsible for OA in a group of individuals, which could include joint trauma, neuromuscular factors that affect the ability to absorb loading, congenital or developmental anatomic abnormalities causing joint incongruities or postinfectious. Research on potential OA phenotypes has gained recent attention in the medical literature, although the heterogeneity of OA has been known for many decades.[15]

In a review of this literature in 2016, there was evidence for 6 potential clinical phenotypes that may be linked to different disease mechanisms: chronic pain with central sensitization, inflammatory, metabolic syndrome, bone and cartilage metabolism, mechanical overload, and minimal joint disease (an outcome-based phenotype).[16] In a subsequent paper by the same group, Dell'Isola and colleagues used data from the osteoarthritis initiative (OAI; n = 599), a large population-based knee OA cohort, to classify individuals into these predefined groups, comparing them for demographic and OA outcomes.[17] Participants who fell into more than one phenotype were assigned a separate "complex knee OA" group. The authors were able to allocate phenotypes for 84% of cases with an overlap of 20%. Disease duration was shorter in the minimum joint disease, while they found that the chronic pain phenotype included more women (81%). This study demonstrated the feasibility of using a classification system for knee OA individuals and placing them in distinct phenotypes based on subgroup-specific characteristics.[17]

Several classifications were subsequently proposed, which motivated a recent effort to standardize the conduct and reporting of OA phenotyping studies.[18] In this consensus-based international collaboration, phenotypes were defined as "subtypes of OA that share distinct underlying pathobiological and pain mechanisms and their structural and functional consequences," that should differ from others in disease-driving factors and/or outcomes.

APPROACHES FOR OA PHENOTYPING

There is a critical need to accurately define the factors that could contribute to OA phenotyping from a large number of potentially relevant variables. However, simply defining OA phenotypes based on risk factors is insufficient. Many individuals have more than one risk factor, and, as already noted in the case of mechanics, there are shared mechanisms among risk factors likely contributing to OA.[9] For phenotyping to be successful, data sets with a diverse set of variables and well-defined outcomes are needed (**Fig. 1**). This may include various sociodemographic factors and clinical, imaging, and biochemical marker measurements in addition to mechanical measures. Considering the best evidence to date, we describe below 3 main categories for OA phenotyping, which has previously been discussed in other articles[9,19] (**Fig. 2**). In this review, we focus on knee OA phenotypes where there is more research evidence,

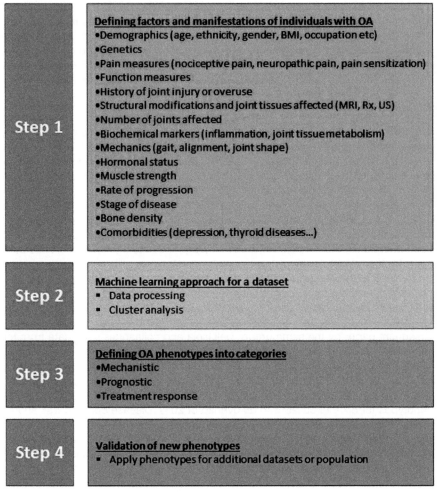

Fig. 1. Workflow for OA phenotyping.

although heterogeneity in disease mechanisms and response to treatment is also well known for hip and hand OA.

Mechanistic Phenotypes

Established by endotypes and pathophysiologic mechanisms of disease, this is a sub-type of disease defined functionally and pathologically by a molecular mechanism. It is important to note that a given OA manifestation (eg, medial tibiofemoral OA) may be common to multiple endotypes (ie, different mechanisms leading to the same manifestation). Example:

- IL-1β is a critical proinflammatory cytokine in OA, resulting in elevated levels of matrix metalloproteinases and cartilage matrix protein degradation.[20] This might indicate that IL-1β is one of the drivers of OA pathogenesis. However, some trials of anti–IL-1α/β showed poor results in improving OA outcomes.[21] Some factors such as differences in disease stage among included participants might have hindered the identification of an effect of the drug in specific subgroups. Yet,

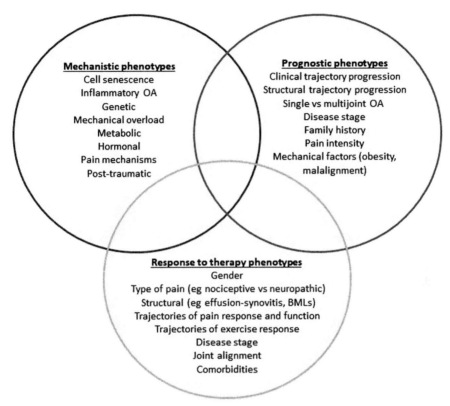

Fig. 2. Examples of subgroups in the 3 main classification categories for OA phenotyping.

selecting particular molecular endotypes rather than clinical phenotypes may still help identify patient subgroups that could benefit from targeted anti-inflammatory strategies such as IL-1β blockade.

Prognostic Phenotypes

This approach refers to subgroups that are more likely, within a specified period, to reach a specific outcome of interest (eg, disease progression defined by deterioration in joint structural features and worsening pain). Treatment stratification and decision to treat could be supported by this phenotyping approach.[9] Example:

- A latent class analysis used to cluster clinical and imaging data from the OAI database identified 4 clusters that represented mild OA, "classical" OA with minor areas of denuded bone (defined as areas where cartilage has been eroded completely so the underlying bone becomes visible or intrachondral osteophytes protruding to the joint surface), and 2 severe groups of "aggressive OA" with larger areas of denuded bone. Prognostic groups were differentiated based on the extent of denuded bone, with more severe subgroups showing a higher prevalence of progression.[22]

Treatment Response Phenotypes

Subgroups are more likely to respond to a specific intervention with an outcome of interest (eg, improved pain or function), also named prescriptive phenotypes. They could also help to identify patients more likely to experience side effects.[9] Example:

- A study of predictors of response to corticosteroids injections in OA knees has shown that the presence of effusion, withdrawal of fluid from the knee, severity of disease, and greater symptoms at baseline may improve the likelihood of response to intra-articular corticosteroids.[23] A subsequent meta-analysis using individual patient data supported that patients with more severe pain at baseline were more likely to improve following an intra-articular corticosteroid injection compared with placebo but has not found differences in response in patients with or without signs of inflammation.[24]

CURRENT STATUS OF OA PHENOTYPING—WHERE ARE WE AT?
Progress on Mechanistic Phenotypes

Preclinical studies are key to understanding endotypes and how different etiologies such as age-related and post-traumatic OA may be associated with differences in disease pathophysiology and expression.

An endotype related to aging or cell senescence has been suggested by a few studies.[25,26] Recent research on the senescence-associated secretory phenotype in chondrocytes from OA cartilage has revealed phenotypic alterations at the cellular level, including chondrosenescence,[27,28] metabolic alterations at the mitochondrial and glycolytic levels, and molecular changes in the secretome and cartilage. Research in this field has looked at developing therapeutics (namely, senolytics and senomorphics) that eliminate or alter senescent cells to stop disease progression and pathogenesis, potentially providing relief for patients with OA.[29]

A collaborative study between 7 expert OA laboratories raised the challenge to identify common gene signatures in 6 murine models of OA representative of clinical phenotypes in OA patients using standard operating procedures and centralized analyses.[30] As TGF-β is a key player in cartilage homeostasis and OA pathology, the study analyzed the TGF-β pathway by transcriptomic analysis in 6 mouse models of OA mimicking clinical phenotypes. The analysis revealed specific gene signatures in each of the 6 models; however, no gene was deregulated in all 6 OA models, highlighting the OA animal model heterogeneity and the need for caution when extrapolating results from one model to another.[30]

Another recent preclinical study has identified model-specific (medial-meniscal-destabilization or antigen-induced-arthritis) associations between articular cartilage, synovium, and bone, providing further evidence that pathologic interaction between joint tissues in OA is dependent on the disease phenotype.[31] Although no causal relationships can be established from the data presented in this study, the different associations between joint pathologies may have implications when considering the potential for therapeutic interventions targeting one tissue to treat global OA-joint pathology.[31]

Another potential phenotype that has attracted great research attention is the inflammatory endotype that would have a shared mechanism related to a specific cytokine that could be targeted for therapy. In this way, some members of the tyrosine kinase family, including FGFR-1, DDR1, DDR2, EGFR, VEGFR, TrkA, ROR2, FAK, and Fyn, have been found to induce chondrocyte hypertrophy in articular cartilage, an initial phenomenon in OA pathogenesis.[32] Thus, the use of inhibitors that impair the activity of these tyrosine kinases could be considered as a potential treatment for OA. For example, Nintedanib is an oral tyrosine kinase inhibitor approved for clinical use for pulmonary fibrosis with specificity against VEGFRs, FGFRs, and PDGFRs, which might be interesting for drug repurposing as a disease-modifying osteoarthritic drug.[32]

Pain endotypes have also been investigated. Individuals with or at risk of knee OA who displayed greater features of sensitization, such as pressure pain sensitivity and temporal summation, experienced worse clinical outcomes in cross-sectional studies[33,34] and were more likely to develop incident persistent pain after 2 years in a longitudinal analysis.[35] The presence of psychological characteristics, such as pain catastrophizing, has additionally been shown to negatively influence pain outcomes.[36] Identifying individuals with those characteristics and tailoring pain therapies to each patient's needs may be vital to achieving better clinical outcomes.

Progress on Prognostic Subgroups

Trajectory analysis is a statistical methodology that uses a data-driven approach to identify clusters of individuals following different trajectories in a given outcome over time. Prediction models use characteristics that can be obtained through the clinical history, physical examination, or radiographic assessment to facilitate their use in research or clinical practice. Recent studies have applied these techniques to study OA outcomes heterogeneity over time. Similar to studies using radiographs for outcome assessment,[37,38] a study using MRI has shown that a minority of knee OA individuals (approximately 10%) experience medial cartilage thickness loss over 2 years.[39] This subgroup had greater odds of experiencing concurrent pain progression and requiring total knee replacement (TKR).

Other studies have also defined prediction models to identify knee OA progression[40–42] and incident knee OA with fast progression,[43] although there were different definitions of progression in these studies, such as reduction in medial joint space on radiographs[41] and increase in Kellgren-Lawrence grade.[42] Roemer and colleagues[44] recently studied the association of knee OA structural phenotypes to risk for progression over 48 months. Knees were stratified into subchondral bone, cartilage/meniscus, and inflammatory phenotypes based on MRI semiquantitative assessment. The bone phenotype was associated with an increased risk of having both radiographic and pain progression. The same group has recently published a simplified MRI scoring instrument for knee OA (ROAMES), which allows stratification of potential candidates to be included in disease-modifying OA drugs (DMOAD) trials into 5 different structural phenotypes (inflammatory, subchondral bone, meniscus/cartilage, atrophic, or hypertrophic).[45] Potentially, the suggested phenotypic stratification may result in more targeted populations in DMOAD trials considering the potential specific mode of action of a given pharmacologic compound.[45]

Trajectories of clinical progression have also been used to define OA subgroups.[46–48] Most individuals follow a stable course over several years with mild to moderate symptoms, whereas others experience a more severe disease course with persistent intense pain and disability or significant decline over a few years, highlighting differences in prognosis. Baseline characteristics that more frequently predicted worse trajectory outcomes include high body mass index, lower education, more severe symptoms and worse radiographic disease at baseline, psychological factors (eg, depression), and presence of concomitant hip pain.[49]

Progress on Treatment Response Subgroups

Personalizing care according to clinically relevant characteristics may optimize the effects of OA treatments.[9] To date, most analyses investigating subgroup effects of interventions in OA have been post hoc and exploratory.

Heterogeneous response after exposure to interventions has also been investigated by trajectory analysis. Lee and colleagues[50] found 4 patterns of response to exercise over 12 weeks among knee OA patients, with over 70% of patients displaying early improvement, whereas a minority experienced delayed improvement (15%) or no improvement (10%). An unfavorable trajectory was associated with poorer physical and psychosocial status at baseline. These findings evidence that early treatment is important to reduce pain and disability and suggest that appropriate stratification may be needed to triage patients according to their probability of improvement with different interventions. As another example, OA models of care, characterized by a multidisciplinary approach to personalize the treatment plan, have been implemented in several countries.[51] However, a decision support tool to identify who would be best targeted by specific interventions and who would benefit the most from those programs is still lacking.

Knoop and colleagues[52,53] described and found mixed results regarding the construct validity of a model of stratified exercise therapy, consisting of (i) a stratification algorithm allocating patients with knee OA into 1 of the 3 subgroups ("high muscle strength subgroup" representing a post-traumatic phenotype, "low muscle strength subgroup" representing an age-induced phenotype, and "obesity subgroup" representing a metabolic phenotype) and (ii) subgroup-specific exercise therapy. It is a valid instrument to consistently allocate patients into subgroups, although subgroups did not differ substantially in the effects of usual exercise therapy.

Lentz and colleagues[54] recently found that almost 50% of Medicare beneficiaries in the United States with knee OA had a phenotype characterized by one or more concordant conditions, suggesting that perpetuation of existing management models that rely on single (or dominant) specialty providers are insufficient for a large proportion of older adults with knee OA. Key comorbidity differences among older adults with knee OA compared with those without OA included a higher frequency of other musculoskeletal conditions, rheumatic diseases, and chronic pain, which were especially prevalent in hypothyroid/osteoporosis and high comorbidity phenotypes. Results of this study could potentially help to guide health care systems in the development of specific integrated comorbidity care pathways.[54]

A phenotype classification of varus osteoarthritic knees was also recently proposed: type 1 "neutral," type 2 "intra-articular varus," type 3 "extra-articular varus," and type 4 "valgoid type." This classification may be potentially relevant for treatment response evaluation because it can help planning and performance of corrective osteotomies, unicompartmental, and TKR.[55]

Treatment response phenotypes can be defined for pain outcomes. Among other previous proposals, a recent study[56] found 4 OA phenotypes using a large population from the OAI cohort and a clinical trial testing the effect of vitamin D in knee OA[57]: low-fluctuating, mild-increasing, moderate-treatment-sensitive, and severe-treatment-insensitive pain. Over time, functional knee limitation followed the same trajectory as pain with almost complete concordance (94.3%) between pain and functional limitation trajectory groups. Notably, the study identified a phenotype with severe pain that did not benefit from available treatments, and another one most likely to benefit from knee replacement.[56]

Treatment response phenotyping can also be used to identify individuals more likely to experience serious side effects from interventions. A subgroup of patients receiving anti–nerve growth factor (NGF) experience more rapid progression of their structural changes, which is a serious concern that could limit its use. A recent trial was designed to mitigate the risk of this adverse event before treatment was initiated, and it has shown that tanezumab (an anti-NGF drug) still resulted in more joint safety events than nonsteroidal anti-inflammatory drugs (NSAIDs) in patients previously on a stable dose of NSAIDs.[58]

USE OF BIG DATA AND MACHINE LEARNING FOR OA PHENOTYPING

Data sets in medicine are becoming larger, and to use these vast amounts of data, researchers are increasingly using artificial intelligence (AI) methodologies. In machine learning, a computer learns from a variety of examples, eventually "learning" to classify new information based on these inputs.[59] There are many machine learning methodologies, including artificial neural networks, deep learning, support vector machines, decision trees, and so forth. A variety of these methodologies, used primarily for image analysis in OA,[60,61] are being applied to large data sets, often including biochemical biomarkers, genetic information, and detailed imaging for the purpose of identifying OA phenotypes.[62–64] Linking confirmatory analysis with the scientific discovery process, while considering expert opinion, is relevant as data sets become larger and incorporate more complex objects.

Advantages of machine learning methodologies include the ability to treat all available data together, even when there are thousands of them, reducing bias related to variable selection, and the need to adjust for multiple comparisons. Several variables or contributors to outcomes of interest can be identified using one method of analysis. Limitations include the inherent limitations of a big data set (eg, missing data), generalizability, which requires both internal and external validation, and the need for additional analyses to determine the importance of the associated variables.[9]

To date, the use of AI in OA research has been predominantly in the area of image analysis. These studies have used various AI methods for analyzing radiographic or MRI, in some cases to increase efficiency (as reading these images is currently time-consuming and reader-dependent) and in others to identify novel features that may define phenotypes.[10]

To exemplify the application of machine learning in OA phenotyping research, a recent study has used multiple clinical, laboratory, and imaging features to identify groups that did and did not progress by pain and radiographic measures.[63] MRI variables were important features to differentiate progressors from nonprogressors, whereas demographic/clinical and biochemical biomarkers were not as useful. Features with the greatest contribution to the identified differences (bone marrow lesions, osteophytes, medial meniscal extrusion, and urine C-terminal crosslinked telopeptide type II collagen [CTX-II]) were identified.[63]

Recently, Namiri and colleagues[65] built a convolutional neural network, a type of deep learning tool, to stratify knees into morphologic phenotypes and examined associations of structural phenotypes according to ROAMES[45] with odds of concurrent and incident OA, and incidence of TKR within 96 months from baseline. All phenotypes, particularly the meniscus/cartilage and hypertrophic phenotypes, were associated with concurrent structural OA. In addition, all phenotypes increased the odds of concurrent symptomatic OA. Among knees with no baseline OA, the bone phenotype and hypertrophic phenotype each, respectively, increased odds of incident structural OA and symptomatic OA over 48 months. All phenotypes except meniscus/cartilage increased odds of TKR within 96 months after adjustment for potential confounders. They concluded that AI can rapidly stratify knees into structural phenotypes associated with incident OA and TKR, which may aid in stratifying patients for clinical trials of targeted therapeutics.[65]

FUTURE DIRECTIONS

There are probably multiple molecular and clinical OA phenotypes that are important to take into account in preclinical and clinical research. A major goal in this field is to identify the clinical phenotypes and define their related molecular endotypes. This is a difficult task because many of these phenotypes are interconnected and mechanistically related, but it would allow the development of biomarker panels that might predict disease progression and determine which patients have a better potential for joint repair. We may even be able to distinguish between patients who will respond better to nonpharmacologic or pharmacologic interventions and those who will benefit from earlier joint replacement surgery. This will enhance clinical trials design, favor more effective OA drug development pipelines, and lead to significant savings in health care management.[12] OA phenotyping research should also focus on identifying individuals at higher risk of progression and those more likely to benefit from a given already existing treatment. Ultimately, all approaches aim to achieve improved clinical outcomes for individual OA patients.

AI methodologies are just beginning to be used in this area. The potential of these approaches to define higher risk groups and direct potential targeted therapies in future clinical trials is promising. It is likely that further progress in the areas of OA phenotyping, endotyping, and precision medicine, using various aspects of AI, will dramatically impact the design and implementation of clinical studies in the near future.[10]

CLINICS CARE POINTS

- Osteoarthritis (OA) is a common and serious disease of older adults and can affect one or multiple joints in a person, most often the knees, finger joints, hips, and spine. It is a major and growing contributor to disability worldwide and is associated with increased comorbidity and excess mortality.

- The multifactorial pathogenesis of OA, the heterogeneity in clinical manifestations, and the mixed population included have contributed to the failure of multiple drugs in trials.

- A significant research effort has emerged aimed to define a classification of OA phenotypes (subgroups) for the purpose of better identifying individuals at higher risk of progression and to better delineate OA subpopulations with distinct risk factors and disease mechanisms that would be suitable for targeted treatment and prevention strategies.

- Phenotypes can be categorized according to mechanisms of disease (endotypes), prognosis, and response to treatment.

- Mechanistic phenotypes or endotypes are a subtype of disease defined functionally and pathologically by a molecular mechanism. The importance of identifying endotypes comes from drug discovery, where identifying the right target is key for success.

- Prognostic phenotypes are subgroups that are more likely, within a specified period, to reach a specific outcome of interest. The decision to treat with disease-modifying OA drugs, when available, could be supported by this phenotyping approach.

- Treatment response phenotypes are subgroups more likely to respond to a specific intervention with an outcome of interest. They could also help to identify patients more likely to experience side effects of treatments.

- Machine learning (an application of artificial intelligence) is being increasingly applied to large data sets in OA, including imaging, biochemical biomarker, and genetic information, for the purpose of identifying OA phenotypes. This methodology has a rising potential to impact the design and implementation of clinical studies and OA treatment in the near future.

DISCLOSURE

The authors have nothing to disclose.

REFERENCES

1. Hunter DJ, Bierma-Zeinstra S. Osteoarthritis. Lancet 2019;393(10182):1745–59.
2. Kraus VB, Blanco FJ, Englund M, et al. Call for standardized definitions of osteoarthritis and risk stratification for clinical trials and clinical use. Osteoarthritis Cartilage 2015;23(8):1233–41.
3. Bannuru RR, Osani MC, Vaysbrot EE, et al. OARSI guidelines for the non-surgical management of knee, hip, and polyarticular osteoarthritis. Osteoarthritis Cartilage 2019;27(11):1578–89.
4. Bruyère O, Honvo G, Veronese N, et al. An updated algorithm recommendation for the management of knee osteoarthritis from the European society for clinical and economic aspects of osteoporosis, osteoarthritis and musculoskeletal diseases (ESCEO). Semin Arthritis Rheum 2019;49(3):337–50.
5. Machado GC, Maher CG, Ferreira PH, et al. Efficacy and safety of paracetamol for spinal pain and osteoarthritis: systematic review and meta-analysis of randomised placebo controlled trials. BMJ 2015;350:h1225.
6. Fransen M, McConnell S, Harmer AR, et al. Exercise for osteoarthritis of the knee. Cochrane Database Syst Rev 2015;(1):CD004376.
7. Hochberg MC, Guermazi A, Guehring H, et al. Effect of intra-articular sprifermin vs placebo on femorotibial joint cartilage thickness in patients with osteoarthritis: the FORWARD randomized clinical trial. JAMA 2019;322(14):1360–70.
8. Conaghan PG, Bowes MA, Kingsbury SR, et al. Disease-modifying effects of a novel cathepsin K inhibitor in osteoarthritis: a randomized controlled trial. Ann Intern Med 2020;172(2):86–95.
9. Deveza LA, Nelson AE, Loeser RF. Phenotypes of osteoarthritis: current state and future implications. Clin Exp Rheumatol 2019;37(Suppl 120):64–72.
10. Nelson AE. How feasible is the stratification of osteoarthritis phenotypes by means of artificial intelligence? Expert Rev Precis Med Drug Dev 2021;6(2):83–5.
11. Bierma-Zeinstra SM, Verhagen AP. Osteoarthritis subpopulations and implications for clinical trial design. Arthritis Res Ther 2011;13(2):213.
12. Mobasheri A, Saarakkala S, Finnilä M, et al. Recent advances in understanding the phenotypes of osteoarthritis. F1000Res 2019;8.
13. Bierma-Zeinstra SM, van Middelkoop M. Osteoarthritis: in search of phenotypes. Nat Rev Rheumatol 2017;13(12):705–6.
14. Brandt KD, Dieppe P, Radin EL. Commentary: is it useful to subset "primary" osteoarthritis? A critique based on evidence regarding the etiopathogenesis of osteoarthritis. Semin Arthritis Rheum 2009;39(2):81–95.
15. Bjelle A. On the heterogeneity of osteoarthritis. Clin Rheumatol 1983;2(2):111–3.
16. Dell'Isola A, Allan R, Smith SL, et al. Identification of clinical phenotypes in knee osteoarthritis: a systematic review of the literature. BMC Musculoskelet Disord 2016;17(1):425.
17. Dell'Isola A, Steultjens M. Classification of patients with knee osteoarthritis in clinical phenotypes: data from the osteoarthritis initiative. PLoS One 2018;13(1): e0191045.
18. van Spil WE, Bierma-Zeinstra SMA, Deveza LA, et al. A consensus-based framework for conducting and reporting osteoarthritis phenotype research. Arthritis Res Ther 2020;22(1):54.
19. Deveza LA, Loeser RF. Is osteoarthritis one disease or a collection of many? Rheumatology (Oxford) 2018;57(suppl_4):iv34–42.
20. Goldring SR, Goldring MB. The role of cytokines in cartilage matrix degeneration in osteoarthritis. Clin Orthop Relat Res 2004;(427 Suppl):S27–36.

21. Kloppenburg M, Peterfy C, Haugen IK, et al. Phase IIa, placebo-controlled, randomised study of lutikizumab, an anti-interleukin-1α and anti-interleukin-1β dual variable domain immunoglobulin, in patients with erosive hand osteoarthritis. Ann Rheum Dis 2019;78(3):413–20.

22. Waarsing JH, Bierma-Zeinstra SM, Weinans H. Distinct subtypes of knee osteoarthritis: data from the Osteoarthritis Initiative. Rheumatology (Oxford) 2015; 54(9):1650–8.

23. Maricar N, Callaghan MJ, Felson DT, et al. Predictors of response to intra-articular steroid injections in knee osteoarthritis–a systematic review. Rheumatology (Oxford) 2013;52(6):1022–32.

24. van Middelkoop M, Arden NK, Atchia I, et al. The OA Trial Bank: meta-analysis of individual patient data from knee and hip osteoarthritis trials show that patients with severe pain exhibit greater benefit from intra-articular glucocorticoids. Osteoarthritis Cartilage 2016;24(7):1143–52.

25. Collins JA, Diekman BO, Loeser RF. Targeting aging for disease modification in osteoarthritis. Curr Opin Rheumatol 2018;30(1):101–7.

26. Jeon OH, Kim C, Laberge RM, et al. Local clearance of senescent cells attenuates the development of post-traumatic osteoarthritis and creates a pro-regenerative environment. Nat Med 2017;23(6):775–81.

27. Mobasheri A, Matta C, Zákány R, et al. Chondrosenescence: definition, hallmarks and potential role in the pathogenesis of osteoarthritis. Maturitas 2015;80(3): 237–44.

28. van der Kraan P, Matta C, Mobasheri A. Age-related alterations in signaling pathways in articular chondrocytes: implications for the pathogenesis and progression of osteoarthritis - a mini-review. Gerontology 2017;63(1):29–35.

29. Xie J, Wang Y, Lu L, et al. Cellular senescence in knee osteoarthritis: molecular mechanisms and therapeutic implications. Ageing Res Rev 2021;70:101413.

30. Maumus M, Noël D, Ea HK, et al. Identification of TGFβ signatures in six murine models mimicking different osteoarthritis clinical phenotypes. Osteoarthritis Cartilage 2020;28(10):1373–84.

31. Zaki S, Smith MM, Smith SM, et al. Differential patterns of pathology in and interaction between joint tissues in long-term osteoarthritis with different initiating causes: phenotype matters. Osteoarthritis Cartilage 2020;28(7):953–65.

32. Ferrao Blanco MN, Domenech Garcia H, Legeai-Mallet L, et al. Tyrosine kinases regulate chondrocyte hypertrophy: promising drug targets for Osteoarthritis. Osteoarthritis Cartilage 2021;29(10):1389–98.

33. Cardoso JS, Riley JL, Glover T, et al. Experimental pain phenotyping in community-dwelling individuals with knee osteoarthritis. Pain 2016;157(9): 2104–14.

34. Frey-Law LA, Bohr NL, Sluka KA, et al. Pain sensitivity profiles in patients with advanced knee osteoarthritis. Pain 2016;157(9):1988–99.

35. Carlesso LC, Segal NA, Frey-Law L, et al. Pain susceptibility phenotypes in those free of knee pain with or at risk of knee osteoarthritis: the multicenter osteoarthritis study. Arthritis Rheumatol 2019;71(4):542–9.

36. Egsgaard LL, Eskehave TN, Bay-Jensen AC, et al. Identifying specific profiles in patients with different degrees of painful knee osteoarthritis based on serological biochemical and mechanistic pain biomarkers: a diagnostic approach based on cluster analysis. Pain 2015;156(1):96–107.

37. Bartlett SJ, Ling SM, Mayo NE, et al. Identifying common trajectories of joint space narrowing over two years in knee osteoarthritis. Arthritis Care Res (Hoboken) 2011;63(12):1722–8.

38. Collins JE, Neogi T, Losina E. Trajectories of structural disease progression in knee osteoarthritis. Arthritis Care Res (Hoboken) 2021;73(9):1354–62.
39. Deveza LA, Downie A, Tamez-Peña JG, et al. Trajectories of femorotibial cartilage thickness among persons with or at risk of knee osteoarthritis: development of a prediction model to identify progressors. Osteoarthritis Cartilage 2019;27(2): 257–65.
40. Liukkonen MK, Mononen ME, Klets O, et al. Simulation of subject-specific progression of knee osteoarthritis and comparison to experimental follow-up data: data from the osteoarthritis initiative. Sci Rep 2017;7(1):9177.
41. LaValley MP, Lo GH, Price LL, et al. Development of a clinical prediction algorithm for knee osteoarthritis structural progression in a cohort study: value of adding measurement of subchondral bone density. Arthritis Res Ther 2017;19(1):95.
42. Zhang W, McWilliams DF, Ingham SL, et al. Nottingham knee osteoarthritis risk prediction models. Ann Rheum Dis 2011;70(9):1599–604.
43. Riddle DL, Stratford PW, Perera RA. The incident tibiofemoral osteoarthritis with rapid progression phenotype: development and validation of a prognostic prediction rule. Osteoarthritis Cartilage 2016;24(12):2100–7.
44. Roemer FW, Collins JE, Neogi T, et al. Association of knee OA structural phenotypes to risk for progression: a secondary analysis from the Foundation for National Institutes of Health Osteoarthritis Biomarkers study (FNIH). Osteoarthritis Cartilage 2020;28(9):1220–8.
45. Roemer FW, Collins J, Kwoh CK, et al. MRI-based screening for structural definition of eligibility in clinical DMOAD trials: rapid OsteoArthritis MRI Eligibility Score (ROAMES). Osteoarthritis Cartilage 2020;28(1):71–81.
46. Collins JE, Katz JN, Dervan EE, et al. Trajectories and risk profiles of pain in persons with radiographic, symptomatic knee osteoarthritis: data from the osteoarthritis initiative. Osteoarthritis Cartilage 2014;22(5):622–30.
47. Bastick AN, Wesseling J, Damen J, et al. Defining knee pain trajectories in early symptomatic knee osteoarthritis in primary care: 5-year results from a nationwide prospective cohort study (CHECK). Br J Gen Pract 2016;66(642):e32–9.
48. Holla JF, van der Leeden M, Heymans MW, et al. Three trajectories of activity limitations in early symptomatic knee osteoarthritis: a 5-year follow-up study. Ann Rheum Dis 2014;73(7):1369–75.
49. Deveza LA, Melo L, Yamato TP, et al. Knee osteoarthritis phenotypes and their relevance for outcomes: a systematic review. Osteoarthritis Cartilage 2017; 25(12):1926–41.
50. Lee AC, Harvey WF, Han X, et al. Pain and functional trajectories in symptomatic knee osteoarthritis over up to 12 weeks of exercise exposure. Osteoarthritis Cartilage 2018;26(4):501–12.
51. Allen KD, Choong PF, Davis AM, et al. Osteoarthritis: models for appropriate care across the disease continuum. Best Pract Res Clin Rheumatol 2016;30(3): 503–35.
52. Knoop J, van der Leeden M, Thorstensson CA, et al. Identification of phenotypes with different clinical outcomes in knee osteoarthritis: data from the Osteoarthritis Initiative. Arthritis Care Res (Hoboken) 2011;63(11):1535–42.
53. Knoop J, Ostelo RWJG, van der Esch M, et al. Construct validity of the OCTOPuS stratification algorithm for allocating patients with knee osteoarthritis into subgroups. BMC Musculoskelet Disord 2021;22(1):633.
54. Lentz TA, Hellkamp AS, Bhavsar NA, et al. Assessment of common comorbidity phenotypes among older adults with knee osteoarthritis to inform integrated care models. Mayo Clin Proc Innov Qual Outcomes 2021;5(2):253–64.

55. Mullaji A, Shah R, Bhoskar R, et al. Seven phenotypes of varus osteoarthritic knees can be identified in the coronal plane. Knee Surg Sports Traumatol Arthrosc 2021. [Epub ahead of print].
56. Radojčić MR, Arden NK, Yang X, et al. Pain trajectory defines knee osteoarthritis subgroups: a prospective observational study. Pain 2020;161(12):2841–51.
57. Arden NK, Cro S, Sheard S, et al. The effect of vitamin D supplementation on knee osteoarthritis, the VIDEO study: a randomised controlled trial. Osteoarthritis Cartilage 2016;24(11):1858–66.
58. Hochberg MC, Carrino JA, Schnitzer TJ, et al. Long-term safety and efficacy of subcutaneous tanezumab versus nonsteroidal Antiinflammatory drugs for hip or knee osteoarthritis: a randomized trial. Arthritis Rheumatol 2021;73(7):1167–77.
59. Rajkomar A, Dean J, Kohane I. Machine learning in medicine. N Engl J Med 2019; 380(14):1347–58.
60. Du Y, Almajalid R, Shan J, et al. A novel method to predict knee osteoarthritis progression on MRI using machine learning methods. IEEE Trans Nanobioscience 2018;17(3):228–36.
61. Huang C, Shan L, Charles HC, et al. Diseased region detection of longitudinal knee magnetic resonance imaging data. IEEE Trans Med Imaging 2015;34(9): 1914–27.
62. Lazzarini N, Runhaar J, Bay-Jensen AC, et al. A machine learning approach for the identification of new biomarkers for knee osteoarthritis development in overweight and obese women. Osteoarthritis Cartilage 2017;25(12):2014–21.
63. Nelson AE, Fang F, Arbeeva L, et al. A machine learning approach to knee osteoarthritis phenotyping: data from the FNIH biomarkers consortium. Osteoarthritis Cartilage 2019;27(7):994–1001.
64. Mobasheri A, van Spil WE, Budd E, et al. Molecular taxonomy of osteoarthritis for patient stratification, disease management and drug development: biochemical markers associated with emerging clinical phenotypes and molecular endotypes. Curr Opin Rheumatol 2019;31(1):80–9.
65. Namiri NK, Lee J, Astuto B, et al. Deep learning for large scale MRI-based morphological phenotyping of osteoarthritis. Sci Rep 2021;11(1):10915.

Best Evidence Osteoarthritis Care

What Are the Recommendations and What Is Needed to Improve Practice?

Bimbi Gray, BClinSci, BNat, MOstMed[a,b,1],
Jillian P. Eyles, BAppSc(Physiotherapy), PhD[a,b,2],
Sandra Grace, BA, MSc, PhD[c,1], David J. Hunter, MBBS, FRACP, PhD[a,b,2],
Nina Østerås, BSc Physiotherapy, MSc, PhD[d],
Jonathan Quicke, BSc(Hons) Physiotherapy, MSc, PhD[e],
Dieuwke Schiphof, BSc Physiotherapy, MSc, PhD[f],
Jocelyn L. Bowden, BLA, BHMSc, BSc(Hons), PhD[a,b,*]

KEYWORDS

- Osteoarthritis • Chronic disease • Evidence-based practice • Primary care
- Guideline-informed care • Quality indicators

KEY POINTS

- There is agreement on a core set of osteoarthritis (OA) treatment recommendations in leading clinical practice guidelines, although guidelines differ in adjunct treatment recommendations, which can cause confusion for clinicians and people with OA.
- Different Models of Care, Models of Service Delivery, and Osteoarthritis Management Programs have been used internationally as implementation strategies to increase the uptake of best evidence care for OA.
- Evaluating the quality of OA service delivery using quality indicators may improve OA management by identifying elements of care requiring improvement at the consumer, system, and organizational levels.

[a] Institute of Bone and Joint Research, Kolling Institute, University of Sydney, Sydney; [b] Department of Rheumatology, Royal North Shore Hospital, Sydney, New South Wales, Australia; [c] Faculty of Health, Southern Cross University, Lismore, New South Wales, Australia; [d] Division of Rheumatology and Research, Diakonhjemmet Hospital, PO Box 23 Vinderen, Oslo 0319, Norway; [e] School of Medicine/ Impact Accelerator Unit, Keele University, Keele, Staffordshire ST5 5BG, UK; [f] Department of General Practice, Erasmus MC University Medical Center, PO Box 2400, Rotterdam 3000 CA, the Netherlands
[1] Present address: Level 2, Z Block, Military Rd, Lismore, New South Wales 2480, Australia.
[2] Present address: Level 10, Kolling Building, Reserve Road, St Leonards, New South Wales 2065, Australia.
* Corresponding author. Level 10, Kolling Building, Reserve Road, St Leonards, New South Wales 2065, Australia.
E-mail address: jocelyn.bowden@sydney.edu.au

Clin Geriatr Med 38 (2022) 287–302
https://doi.org/10.1016/j.cger.2021.11.003
0749-0690/22/© 2021 Elsevier Inc. All rights reserved.

geriatric.theclinics.com

INTRODUCTION AND BACKGROUND

Osteoarthritis (OA) has an estimated prevalence of 20% to 30% of the population with the burden increasing, driven by factors including aging populations, and increasing incidence of obesity and joint injuries.[1] OA is the most common musculoskeletal condition in older adults worldwide, with significant and emergent societal and economic costs.[2,3] At an individual level, OA can impact well-being, quality-of-life, physical functioning, and work capacity, resulting in substantial personal economic costs.[2] People with OA often have multimorbidities that further impair health outcomes and are costly to manage.[4,5] Yet, despite the availability of OA clinical practice guidelines, the management of OA within health care services is often suboptimal[6] and discordant with recommended care.[7] Although there are many factors contributing to suboptimal OA care, variations in the recommendations between the guidelines can cause confusion among health care practitioners when implementing evidence-based care.[8]

A person with OA, also referred to as a "consumer" in some countries, typically presents to primary care providers for advice on pain, stiffness, or functional impairments. In many countries, general practitioners (GPs), physiotherapists,[9] and other health care professionals (eg, osteopaths and chiropractors) are the first points of contact. Optimally, primary care should focus on delivering the recommended "core" interventions to everyone with OA.[10] These interventions are consistently recommended in OA practice guidelines because of their effectiveness and safety, low-cost and high accessibility,[11] and include education for self-management, physical activity, therapeutic exercise (eg, strengthening, aerobic exercise), and weight-loss when indicated.[12–17]

Adjunctive treatments can be provided in addition to core treatments, if needed.[17] However, their evidence base is often less clear than for core treatments. Adjunctive treatments may incorporate a combination of modalities such as local assistive devices (eg, braces and splints) or psychological support, tailored to meet individual needs and circumstances. They may also be recommended for a person with more severe or complex OA, for example, for those presenting with very high pain, depression, or sleep impairment.[18] Appropriate evidence-based pharmacologic interventions can also be used alongside core interventions, although, this is an area where guideline advice also differs.[10,12,14] Surgical interventions are also an option but should only be considered for people with end-stage OA, with symptoms that have a substantial impact on quality of life, and who have not responded to core treatments.[18]

Reasons for suboptimal care are multifaceted,[7,19,20] with barriers to uptake occurring at the consumer, practitioner, and system levels.[8] For people with OA, barriers include a lack of understanding of the role of lifestyle treatments, consequently resulting in poor adherence to those treatments.[21] Another major barrier is limited access to allied health services, because of both geographic location and poor referral to those services from general practice.[22] For health care practitioners, reported barriers include: (i) gaps in the knowledge, confidence, and attitudes of health care practitioners to deliver core interventions; (ii) insufficient time and low prioritization of holistic assessments, diagnosis, and treatment planning; and (iii) confusion about the recommended adjunctive therapies resulting from guideline discrepancies.[6,8]

It has been shown that improved uptake of OA guidelines in clinical care can be supported by different strategies at distinct levels of the care pathway.[23] From a clinical and service delivery perspective, strategies such as Osteoarthritis Management Programs (OAMPs) and coordinated interdisciplinary Models of Care (MOC) can facilitate translation of knowledge and improve uptake of best-evidence care.[21,24]

In this narrative review, we synthesize the treatment recommendations from 7 current international OA clinical guidelines, and briefly discuss the underpinning evidence. We will also discuss strategies to improve uptake and implementation of the guidelines in primary care, including considerations for health care practitioners and in reference to consumer needs.

SUMMARY OF KEY OSTEOARTHRITIS CLINICAL PRACTICE GUIDELINES AND RECOMMENDATIONS
What are the Core Interventions?

There is an international consensus on a recommended core set of OA interventions. The American College of Rheumatology (ACR),[12] European Society for Clinical and Economic Aspects of Osteoporosis, Osteoarthritis and Musculoskeletal Diseases (ESCEO),[16] European League Against Rheumatism (EULAR),[13] EULAR recommendations for the management of hand osteoarthritis,[17] National Institute for Health and Clinical Excellence (NICE),[15] OA Research Society International (OARSI),[14] and the Royal Australian College of General Practitioners (RACGP)[10] strongly recommend a core set of interventions, including self-management education, physical activity, therapeutic exercise, and weight management with weight loss when indicated.

Self-management education: OA education should be the first step in any OA treatment, and include information on the nature and course of the condition, with explanation of benefits, likely outcomes, and potential risks of all treatment options.[10,12–16,25] OA education alone has little effect on OA pain and function, but has been shown to influence self-efficacy for OA self-management, especially when paired with other treatments.[26] OA self-management education is also suggested to increase treatment adherence.[12,13] Examples of available resources for patient self-education, which meet current guideline recommendations, include the online self-paced modules from *MyJointPain* (Australia),[27] *Versus Arthritis* (UK),[28] and the *OA Action Alliance* (USA).[29]

Physical activity: Maintaining recommended levels of physical activity is essential for anyone with OA. It typically refers to activities of daily living and other exercises undertaken in daily life (eg, walking or cycling to the shops or work).[10,12–16] Maintaining physical activity levels has shown to be important for managing OA clinical outcomes (eg, reducing pain) and is essential for overall well-being and general health.[10,12–16] EULAR recommends people with OA undertake physical activity for a minimum of 30 minutes, 5 days per week or vigorous-intensity aerobic activity for a minimum of 20 minutes, 3 days per week.[30] However, there is no "one size fits all" physical activity prescription, and practitioners are encouraged to adapt the recommendations to suit the individual circumstances of the person with OA.[31]

Therapeutic exercise: Therapeutic exercise is any type of prescribed exercise that targets OA symptoms. It is often prescribed by a health care professional (eg, physiotherapist, osteopath) and typically includes functional and/or neuromuscular goals.[32] Prescribed therapeutic exercises, particularly land-based exercises, feature strongly in the clinical practice guidelines,[10,12–17] with a broad range of exercise types, frequencies, and intensities shown to be clinically effective. For example, the NICE guidelines endorse therapeutic exercise comprising local muscle strengthening and general aerobic exercise,[15] whereas structured land-based exercise is recommended by OARSI as a core treatment for polyarticular and knee OA.[14] Water-based exercise programs are also specifically recommended in the OARSI and RACGP guidelines as low impact options.[10,14] Aerobic, strength-based and specific neuromuscular/balance exercises are also of benefit.[10,12] Regardless, prescription of therapeutic exercise should account for personal preferences, ability and accessibility for the person with OA to promote greater adherence.[12]

Weight management and weight loss

Exercise and weight loss show the greatest clinical effect for improving pain and functional outcomes, particularly for knee OA.[33] Consequently, weight loss is recommended in all clinical guidelines for anyone above a healthy weight (body mass index [BMI] $\geq$25 kg/m^2).[10,12–16] As a starting point, the OARSI guidelines[14] recommend a minimum weight loss of 5%, whereas the RACGP guidelines[10] recommend between 5% and 7.5%. However, greater weight loss that brings the person closer to a healthy weight range is optimal (BMI 18.5–24.9 kg/m^2). The mechanism by which weight loss improves OA symptoms is poorly understood; however, it is thought to act through reducing both the biomechanical load and the inflammatory stressors that contribute to the OA process.[34] In hand OA, weight loss is not a specific recommendation.[17]

Adjunctive treatments

Adjunctive treatments are second-level therapies that can be added to individual OA management plans, in response to clinical needs. These treatments should ideally be tailored to individual circumstances and delivered supplementary to, and pending response from, the core interventions. Adjunctive therapy recommendations show greater variability than core interventions. The evidence is often conflicting between guidelines for the same therapy, with recommendations often ranging from strong support though to recommendations against (**Table 1**). Adjunctive treatments may include assistive devices, footwear, mind/body therapies, psychological support, and other therapies as indicated (**Box 1**). Similarly, pain-relieving pharmacologic treatments should be used judiciously, in combination with core interventions, and with full consideration of the benefits and harms before prescription. **Box 1** summarizes the current recommendations for lifestyle, psychosocial, mind-body, and pharmacologic treatments and highlights current variations between guidelines.

Recommendations differ between guidelines, both in the adjunctive therapies included and the strength of the recommendations. The lack of stakeholder engagement, potential lack of editorial independence, and potentially biased representation of committee members in the development of some leading practice guidelines have received criticism.[37,38] This lack of consensus potentially influences the interpretation and application of guidelines at the practitioner and consumer levels. Interpretation of evidence is particularly controversial for manual therapy, acupuncture, intra-articular hyaluronic acid injections, and many pharmacologic treatments[39] (see **Box 1**).

STRATEGIES TO SUPPORT MOVING FROM CLINICAL GUIDELINES TO CLINICAL CARE

Strategies to mobilize best evidence into clinical care for OA require a pragmatic approach at all levels of care delivery. In Australia, the "Living Well with OA" component of the National Osteoarthritis Strategy[21] provides an organizational framework to support the uptake of evidence-informed approaches by health care practitioners for the management of OA. Implementation of guidelines through applicable MOC frameworks can facilitate practitioner and consumer access to training, resources, support networks, and platforms to facilitate remote access to Web-based tools and clinical guidelines.[40] For example, Web-based systems can support clinician decision-making by providing easy access to evidence-based clinical algorithms and decision aids that present treatment options in real-time based on patients' individual presentations.[41] Ensuring guidelines are presented in a stepwise, logical, and visible format using algorithms may be one way to address the evidence-to-practice gap and help clinicians to contextualize best care pathways.[42]

Table 1
Summary of key osteoarthritis clinical practice guidelines and recommendations

Core interventions

	ACR 2020[12]			ESCEO 2019[16]	OARSI 2019[14]		EULAR-Hand 2019[17]	EULAR 2018[13]			RACGP 2018[10]		NICE[a] 2014[15]		
	Knee	Hip	Hand	Knee	Knee	Hip	Hand	Knee	Hip	Hand	Knee	Hip	Knee	Hip	Hand
Education and self-management strategies	✓	✓	✓	✓	✓	✓	✓	✓	✓	✓	✓	✓	✓	✓	✓
Physical Activity	✓	✓		✓	✓	✓		✓	✓		✓	✓	✓	✓	✓
Therapeutic Exercise	✓	✓	✓	✓	✓	✓	✓	✓	✓	✓	✓	✓	✓	✓	✓
Weight-loss	✓	✓		✓	✓	□		✓	✓		✓	✓	✓	✓	✓

Adjunctive treatments

	ACR 2020[12]			ESCEO 2019[16]	OARSI 2019[14]		EULAR-Hand 2019[17]	EULAR 2018[13]			RACGP 2018[10]		NICE[a] 2014[15]		
	Knee	Hip	Hand	Knee	Knee	Hip	Hand	Knee	Hip	Hand	Knee	Hip	Knee	Hip	Hand
Assistive devices	✓	✓		X			✓			✓			□		□
Bracing			✓		X	X	✓	□	□	✓	X		□	□	
Orthotic Footwear/insoles	X	X						✓	□		X		✓	✓	
Mind Body (Tai Chi/yoga)	✓	✓			□	□		□		□					
Psychological therapies	□	□					X	□	□	□					
Manual therapies	X	X								□	□	□	□		
TENS	X	X								□	□	□	□		
Acupuncture	□	□			X	X					□	□	X	X	X

Pharmacologic treatments

	ACR 2020[12]			ESCEO 2019[16]	OARSI 2019[14]		EULAR-Hand 2019[17]	EULAR 2018[13]			RACGP 2018[10]		NICE[a] 2014[15]		
	Knee	Hip	Hand	Knee	Knee	Hip	Hand	Knee	Hip	Hand	Knee	Hip	Knee	Hip	Hand
Topical NSAIDs	✓		✓	✓	✓		✓				□	□	✓	✓	✓
Oral NSAIDs	✓	✓		✓	□	✓	□		✓		□	□	✓	✓	✓
Paracetamol / acetaminophen	□	□		✓	X	X	□	✓	✓	✓			✓	✓	✓
Tramadol	□	□													
Opioids	X	X	X	□	X	X					X	X	□	□	
Duloxetine	□	□		□							□	□			
Glucosamine	X	X	X	X	X	X					X	X	X	X	X
Chondroitin	X	X	X	✓	X	X	✓			✓	X	X	X	X	X
Glucocorticoid injection	✓	✓		□	□	□	□	✓	✓		□	□	✓	✓	
Hyaluronic acid injection	X	X			□	X					X	X	X	X	X
Topical capsaicin	□				X	X	□	✓		✓	□	□	✓		✓
Fish oil	X	X	X								X	X			
Vitamin D	X	X	X				X				X	X			

✓ recommended, □ conditionally recommended, X recommended <u>against.</u>
Abbreviations: ACR, American College of Rheumatology; ESCEO, European Society for Clinical and Economic Aspects of Osteoporosis, Osteoarthritis and Musculoskeletal Diseases; EULAR Hand, EULAR recommendations for the management of hand osteoarthritis; EULAR, European League Against Rheumatism; NICE, National Institute for Health and Clinical Excellence. NSAIDs = Non-steroidal anti-inflammatory drugs; RACGP, Royal Australian College of General Practitioners; TENS, transcutaenous electrical nerve stimulation.
Blank cells = not included in clinical practice guideline
[a] 2014 NICE guidelines were not stratified by joint.

Data from Refs.[10,12–17]

Box 1
Summary of adjunctive treatment variations

Lifestyle, Psychosocial and Mind-Body Treatments

Assistive devices, joint braces, and joint taping	*Hand OA:* ACR and EULAR guidelines provide a strong recommendation for the use of hand orthoses in carpometacarpal joint OA.[12,17] The use of assistive devices for hand OA (eg, jar-openers, ergonomic grip utensils) is also recommended by EULAR.[17] *Lower Limb OA:* The ACR provides a strong recommendation for tibiofemoral bracing for knee OA.[12] Similarly, NICE and EULAR conditionally recommend bracing and strapping in knee and hand OA where required.[13,15] Where knee and hip OA significantly affects ambulation, including balance, cane use is also strongly recommended.[12] However, OARSI recommends against patella taping, patellofemoral braces, soft knee braces, or varus/valgus braces as there is insufficient evidence to support efficacy.[14]
Footwear	*Lower Limb OA:* Orthotic footwear and shock-absorbing insoles are recommended by NICE and EULAR.[13,15] Conversely, the RACGP and ACR recommend against the use of footwear marketed for OA because of the lack of high-quality evidence.[12,14]
Mind/body therapies (eg, Tai Chi, Yoga)	*Lower Limb OA:* Although not unanimously recommended across all clinical practice guidelines, Tai Chi and other mind/body exercises are gaining popularity. ACR strongly recommends Tai Chi for people with hip and knee OA for the positive mind-body impacts on balance, strength, and emotional well-being.[12] Likewise, although conditionally, the ACR recommends yoga for knee OA.[12] OARSI guidelines conditionally recommend mind-body interventions such as Tai Chi and yoga as part of structured self-management programs because of the favorable efficacy and good safety profile for this intervention.[14]
Psychological therapies	Conditional recommendations are made by ACR, EULAR, and NICE for psychological therapies for persons with knee, hip, and/ or hand OA. Cognitive behavioral therapies in particular are recommended as strategies to improve emotional well-being, encourage appropriate positive behavioral change, and learn pain coping skills.[12,13,15] Psychological therapies that target mood, sleep, stress, and anxiety are also recommended.[10,12]
Other	Other adjunctive therapies are more cautiously recommended in different clinical guidelines, primarily due to the relatively low level of evidence or quality of evidence available. NICE recommends the consideration of adjunctive therapies such as thermal interventions (heat/cold

	application), manipulation and stretching (particularly for hip OA), and transcutaneous electrical stimulation (TENS).[15] ACR also provides a conditional recommendation for thermal interventions (heat/cold application) and acupuncture.[12] TENS has a conditional recommendation for use in the RACGP guideline.[10]
	However, ACR conditionally recommends against massage and manual therapy in people with hip and knee OA and TENS is strongly recommended against hip and knee OA.[12]
Pharmacologic treatments	
Nonsteroidal anti-inflammatory drugs (NSAIDs)	Topical NSAIDs feature strongly as preferred treatments in all clinical practice guidelines and are especially appropriate for people with underlying gastrointestinal or cardiovascular conditions.[12–17]
	Oral NSAIDs are recommended for persons with knee, hip, and/or hand OA, although they should only be used for a short period and in conjunction with gastric protection from a proton pump inhibitor.[10,12–16] Topical NSAIDs are recommended before oral NSAIDs because of their superior safety profile.[14,15]
Paracetamol/acetaminophen	The efficacy and safety of paracetamol for OA pain relief is not clearly defined in the guidelines and remains a controversial issue.[35] The ACR gives a conditional recommendation for the use of acetaminophen (paracetamol). Likewise, low-dose, short-term acetaminophen use is a recommended first-line treatment in the ESCEO, EULAR, and NICE guidelines.[13,15,16] However, paracetamol is no longer recommended by the OARSI guideline as first-line therapy due to greater risk of adverse effects (gastrointestinal adverse effects and multiorgan failure) compared with analgesic benefit.[14] Any use of paracetamol requires careful consultation with the patient.
Opioids	The use of tramadol (and other opioids) is highly controversial and while the ACR guidelines recommend it (when NSAIDs are contraindicated and other therapies are ineffective),[12] and most other guidelines recommend against their use.
Duloxetine	The ACR guidelines recommend duloxetine, commonly used to treat major depressive disorders, as appropriate for people with knee, hip, and/or hand OA.[12] OARSI provides recommendations for the prescription of duloxetine for the management of OA if associated with widespread pain and/or depression.[14]

Injectable therapies	Viscosupplements (eg, hyaluronic acid injections) and other injectable therapies are other areas of debate. For viscosupplements, meta-analyses have found little additional benefit over saline injections.[36] Conversely, the ACR, EULAR, NICE, and OARSI guidelines recommend intra-articular glucocorticoid injection for relief of moderate-to-severe knee and hip OA pain,[12–15] although the RACGP guidelines caution against repeated use because of the associated risk of harm and decreasing effectiveness.[10]
Other	The use of topical capsaicin for knee and hand OA is endorsed in the RACGP, NICE, and EULAR guidelines,[12,13,15] whereas the ACR is conditionally recommended for knee OA only.[12] For other supplements, the ACR and RACGP recommend against fish oil, vitamin D, glucosamine, and chondroitin for people with knee, hip, and/or hand OA,[10,12] whereas chondroitin is recommended for use in hand OA by EULAR.[17]

MODELS AND PROGRAMS TO IMPROVE THE DELIVERY OF OA CARE

Internationally, several MOC and OAMPs are used to facilitate the translation of evidence into practice across primary, secondary, and tertiary settings.[40] These models and programs, although similar in the key aspects of OA care (the "what"), vary in how the care is delivered (the "how"), and ideally reflect the different health care systems in which they operate.[43] A strength of these models is the ability to deliver the tailored, multidisciplinary care needed for OA, while adapting to different patient volumes. However, although there is evidence to support the effectiveness of different models and programs to improve the health outcomes of people with OA (**Box 2**), this is still an emerging area. More research is needed to determine the best models to use, how

---

Box 2
Clinical trial evidence for OA care pathways

Examples of recent large-scale clinical trials that have tested new models to improve uptake of evidence-based OA care include the *"Primary care management on knee pain and function in patients with osteoarthritis"* (PARTNER, Australia),[44] the *"Structured model for osteoarthritis care in primary healthcare"* (SAMBA, Norway),[45] and the *"Management of osteoarthritis in consultations"* (MOSAICS, UK).[46] These clinical trials were underpinned by frameworks for encouraging behavioral change and promotion of OA self-management that could be delivered in primary care and community-based settings. Key findings from the MOSAICS trial evaluation highlighted the important role that multidisciplinary primary care practitioners play in the implementation of OA guidelines. The MOSAICS trial was described as a knowledge brokering service for people with OA, that facilitates adherence to core and adjunctive guideline-endorsed treatments.[47] The authors suggested successful implementation of the MOSAICS MOC in a real-world setting requires adequate resources, and appropriate infrastructure and institutional support.[47] Encouragingly, the results from the SAMBA trial showed that the MOC led to OA care that was more in line with current care recommendations, with better patient-reported quality of care and greater satisfaction compared with usual care.[48]

Table 2
Models of care

	OACCP[45]	JIGSAW-E[43]	GLA:D[27]	BOA/ Joint Academy[46]	AktivA[47]
			OA Programs Implemented Internationally		
Population/problem	OA of hip and knee	OA of hip, knee, hand, and/or foot	OA of hip and knee	OA of hip, knee, hand, and shoulder	OA of hip and knee
Intervention	Patient education, physical activity, therapeutic exercise, dietary advice/weight management (if needed), adjunctive therapies via multidisciplinary team as needed, eg, review of medications by medical practitioner, assistive devices and sleep with occupational therapist, psychosocial support with social worker, bracing with orthotist. Physiotherapist led	Patient education, physical activity, therapeutic exercise, weight management, pharmaceutical analgesia. Different models including: GP & nurse; GP & physiotherapist; Community pharmacy.	Patient education, therapeutic exercise program Physiotherapist & "expert patient" led	Patient education, physical activity, (optional) therapeutic exercise program Physiotherapist or occupational therapist & "expert patient" led	Patient education, therapeutic exercise program Physiotherapist led with "peer support"
Setting	Outpatient in public hospital	Outpatient, primary care	Private practice	Outpatient, primary care Online (Joint Academy)	Private practice
Duration of program for participants	12 mo with personalized plan adjusted every 3/12	Up to 3 mo	3 mo with follow-up at 12 mo	3 mo with follow-up at 12 mo	3 mo with follow-up at 12 and 24 mo

(continued on next page)

Table 2
(continued)

	OA Programs Implemented Internationally				
	OACCP[45]	**JIGSAW-E[43]**	**GLA:D[27]**	**BOA/ Joint Academy[46]**	**AktivA[47]**
Outcome measures	Among others: Pain VAS, HOOS/KOOS, DASS, TUG, 40MWT, AQoL, BMI & hip/ waist ratio, willingness for surgery, surgical waitlist removal/ acceleration	OA-QI Electronic medical record template capturing pain, BMI, and QIs	Among others: Pain VAS, KOOS/HOOS, QOL UCLA Activity Score EQ-5D, SF-12, ASES, BMI, & hip/waist ratio	Among others: EQ-5D, pain rating (numeric rating scale, pain frequency), ASES, Charnley comorbidity index	Among others: OA-QI, HOOS/KOOS sports/recreational activities disease-specific quality of life AQoL, ASES, PSFS, fear of physical activity questionnaire.
Practitioner training	OACCP site manual	Four practitioner training sessions (2 h × 3 h; 1 h) Four-day practice nurse training Online module physiotherapy and pharmacy training	Two-day course on the diagnosis and management of OA in accordance with guidelines.	One- or 2-day training course with access to digital resources	One-day certification course for physiotherapists
Web site	https://aci.health.nsw. gov.au/resources/ musculoskeletal/ osteoarthritis_ chronic_care_ program/ osteoarthritis-chronic-care-program	https://jigsaw-e.com/	https://www.glaid.dk/ https:// gladinternational. org/	https://boa. registercentrum.se/	www.aktivmedartrose. no

Comparative summary of 5 international Models of Care (MOC), Web site links are provided for further detail.
MOC—AktivA, Active with Osteoarthritis; BOA, Better Management of Patients with Osteoarthritis and its online counterpart Joint Academy; GLA:D, Good Life with Osteoarthritis: Denmark; JIGSAW-E, Joint Implementation for Guidelines for Osteoarthritis in Western Europe; OACCP, Osteoarthritis Chronic Care Program.
Outcome measures—40MWT, 40-m walk test; AQoL, Assessment of Quality of life questionnaire; ASES, Arthritis Self-Efficacy Scale; BMI, body mass index; DASS, Depression Anxiety Stress Scale; EQ-5D, European Quality of Life Five Dimension questionnaire; HOOS, Hip Disability and Osteoarthritis Outcome Score; KOOS, Knee Injury and Osteoarthritis Outcome Score; OA-QI, OsteoArthritis Quality Indicator questionnaire; Pain VAS, visual analog scale/ pain intensity; PSFS, patient-specific functional scale; SF-12, 12-item short form survey; TUG, Timed Up and Go Test; UCLA Activity Score, University of California at Los Angeles Activity Score.

they perform in real-world settings, and the benefits of remotely delivered versus traditional face-to-face care. Furthermore, longitudinal evaluations of long-term patient health outcomes and the economic impact of different MOCs are warranted.

OA PROGRAMS IMPLEMENTED IN THE REAL WORLD

Examples of programs developed and successfully implemented in real-world settings (ie, not via a clinical trial) are summarized in **Table 2**. These programs include the *Osteoarthritis Chronic Care Program* (OACCP, Australia),[49] the *Joint Implementation for Guidelines for Osteoarthritis in Western Europe* (JIGSAW-E),[46] *Good Life with Osteoarthritis: Denmark* (GLA:D, international),[32] *Better Management of Patients with Osteoarthritis* (BOA) and its online counterpart *Joint Academy* (Sweden),[50] and *Active with Osteoarthritis* (AktivA, Norway).[51]

All these programs deliver person-centered education, promote self-management strategies, and provide exercise therapy; however, the mode, delivery, and intensity of interventions vary. Of note, only the OACCP and JIGSAW-E include weight management, dietary, or psychological support.[46,49] In addition, GLA:D, BOA, and AktivA are mainly physiotherapy-led programs and do not routinely refer for pharmacologic treatment, orthoses, or joint replacement surgery.[32,50,51] The BOA also has an associated eHealth delivery option, *Joint Academy*.[50] There are other stand-alone eHealth models and support programs for OA. The *MyJointPain*[27] in Australia and the *Join2-move*[41] in the Netherlands are 2 examples that provide remote access to resources and interventions in a self-help format for people with OA. *Join2move*[41] provides education to improve physical activity and decrease pain with structured goal setting over 8 modules. *MyJointPain*[27] incorporates a series of video resources and fact sheets to provide education on OA prognosis, treatment options, and long-term management. It is designed to promote greater understanding and awareness of the condition for both practitioners and people with OA.[27]

There are no studies comparing patient or economic outcomes across the various OA models or care pathways, primarily due to the expense and difficulty of doing so. However, there are some parallels in studies looking at the barriers and enablers for these individual programs. Eyles and colleagues investigated perceived barriers and enablers to implementing the OACCP in public hospitals, from the perspective of the clinicians delivering the program.[51] The OACCP was found to empower consumers through the provision of self-supported management strategies and resources, whereas staff were supported to establish strong therapeutic alliances and shared case-loads with a focus on discrete multidisciplinary skills.

Implementation and evaluation of OAMPs and MOCs across international and multisector health care systems are required if the full potential of OAMPs is to be realized.[52] However, the optimal methods for achieving widespread implementation in a format compatible with complex health care systems has not yet been determined. Effective implementation of OAMPs and MOCs may need to incorporate recommendations for the setting-based redesign of service delivery, including changes to clinical information systems (eg, electronic medical records) and development of more consumer or community-led initiatives. Ongoing education and training for health care providers delivering OA care has also been identified as a priority for optimizing implementation to ensure that reform and sustainability of OAMPs and MOC continue to keep pace with clinical guidelines.[52–54]

EVALUATING THE QUALITY OF OA CARE

Evaluation of the effectiveness of any program is essential to determine if guideline-informed care has been delivered by health care practitioners or health care services.[55] One method is routine monitoring of care using OA quality indicators (QIs) that target clinician-delivered care. Alternatively, process and structural indicators, which refer to where and how OA care is delivered in the broader context, can also be used to measure if guideline translation into the operational and service delivery mechanisms has been successful.

Determining the most appropriate QIs, however, is reliant on the setting and context of care delivery. Earlier research has indicated that QIs developed in one country are not always comparable for use across borders because of cultural and structural differences within the health care systems.[56] Furthermore, measuring care is complex as assessing individual impact needs to be carefully considered to ensure the correct outcome is measured. For example, QIs target different joints (eg, hip vs knee OA), whereas others target the type or frequency of treatment,[57] or are for use by different health professions (eg, GP or physiotherapist[58]).

QI assessments can be undertaken through an audit of medical records, although QI results based on medical records should be treated with caution as consumer perceptions of their treatment outcome may be different from that of their health care practitioner.[59] Therefore, consumer-reported QI sets developed from OA clinical practice guidelines are considered a better option to effectively monitor and evaluate care than medical records.[60] One example is the OsteoArthritis Quality Indicator (OA-QI) questionnaire.[60] This tool is based on international clinical practice guidelines and has been validated to assess the patient-reported quality of OA care within OAMPs.[60] Another example is the Quality Indicators for Physiotherapy Management of Hip and Knee Osteoarthritis (QUIPA) tool, developed for use in physiotherapy.[61] Both tools are used to assess and determine service delivery and outcomes of OA care.[60,61]

Standardization across QI sets and therefore better direction for their usage is needed. No clear synthesis or guidelines for the use of QIs currently exist, although QIs have been used effectively to evaluate care concordance in OAMPs and other service delivery models.[57] Qualitative investigations into reasons underlying practice concordance with clinical guidelines are warranted to provide this direction.[6]

SUMMARY

Translation of clinical guidelines into practice is essential to ensure care is delivered in concordance with current best-practice evidence.[34] Although strategies to mobilize best evidence into OA clinical care have been identified, an evidence-to-practice gap still exists with many people not receiving recommended care.[62] The implementation of clinical practice guidelines for OA is a challenging task with many barriers at the practitioner and clinical management level still to be addressed.[47] Development of guidelines that accurately represent the best available evidence, are free from industry bias, and cognizant of consumer needs, are needed to ensure clinicians can be confident in the care they recommend. There are leading international examples of MOCs and OAMPs that can be used as the basis to implement evidence-based care for people with OA[32,46,49-51] and QIs can be used in practice settings to evaluate the quality of care delivered.[56,57]

CLINICS CARE POINTS

- Core interventions should be offered to everyone with OA, with adjunctive therapies used as needed.
- When prescribing adjunctive therapies, individual circumstances of the person with OA should be taken into consideration to weigh up the cost and benefit of treatment.

- Implementation of clinical practice guidelines using different validated service delivery models can facilitate evidence-based treatments in all OA care pathways.
- Quality indicators are useful to evaluate evidence-based service delivery and quality of care.
- Models of care incorporating remote access, web-based delivery of OA care is a feasible and effective strategy to facilitate best outcomes for people with OA and provide support for health care practitioners.

DISCLOSURE

D.J. Hunter provides consulting advice for Pfizer, Lilly, Biobone, Novartis, Tissuegene. JGQ was partly funded by an NIHR Clinical Research Network West Midlands, Research Scholar Fellowship. The views expressed in this publication are those of the author and not necessarily those of the NHS, NICE, NIHR, or the Department of Health and Social Care. The other authors declare no conflicts of interest.

REFERENCES

1. Vina ER, Kwoh CK. Epidemiology of osteoarthritis: literature update. Curr Opin Rheumatol 2018;30(2):160–7.
2. Plotnikoff R, Karunamuni N, Lytvyak E, et al. Osteoarthritis prevalence and modifiable factors: a population study. BMC Public Health 2015;15:1195.
3. Safiri S, Kolahi AA, Smith E, et al. Global, regional and national burden of osteoarthritis 1990-2017: a systematic analysis of the Global Burden of Disease Study 2017. Ann Rheum Dis 2020;79(6):819–28.
4. Briggs AM, Shiffman J, Shawar YR, et al. Global health policy in the 21st century: challenges and opportunities to arrest the global disability burden from musculoskeletal health conditions. Best Pract Res Clin Rheumatol 2020;34(5):101549.
5. Zambon S, Siviero P, Denkinger M, et al. Role of osteoarthritis, comorbidity, and pain in determining functional limitations in older populations: european project on osteoarthritis. Arthritis Care Res (Hoboken) 2016;68(6):801–10.
6. Egerton T, Diamond LE, Buchbinder R, et al. A systematic review and evidence synthesis of qualitative studies to identify primary care clinicians' barriers and enablers to the management of osteoarthritis. Osteoarthr Cartil 2017;25(5):625–38.
7. Basedow M, Esterman A. Assessing appropriateness of osteoarthritis care using quality indicators: a systematic review. J Eval Clin Pract 2015;21(5):782–9.
8. Egerton T, Nelligan RK, Setchell J, et al. General practitioners' views on managing knee osteoarthritis: a thematic analysis of factors influencing clinical practice guideline implementation in primary care. BMC Rheumatol 2018;2(1):30.
9. Allen KD, Choong PF, Davis AM, et al. Osteoarthritis: models for appropriate care across the disease continuum. Best Pract Res Clin Rheumatol 2016;30(3):503–35.
10. Royal Australian College of General Practitioners. Guideline for the management of knee and hip osteoartthritis. South Melbourne, Victoria, Australia: RACGP; 2018. Available at: https://www.racgp.org.au/download/Documents/Guidelines/Musculoskeletal/guideline-for-the-management-of-knee-and-hip-oa-2nd-edition.pdf. Accessed 2021.
11. Bierma-Zeinstra S, van Middelkoop M, Runhaar J, et al. Nonpharmacological and nonsurgical approaches in OA. Best Pract Res Clin Rheumatol 2020;34(2):101564.
12. Kolasinski SL, Neogi T, Hochberg MC, et al. 2019 American College of Rheumatology/arthritis Foundation guideline for the management of osteoarthritis of the hand, hip, and knee. Arthritis Care Res (Hoboken) 2020;72(2):149–62.

13. Geenen R, Overman CL, Christensen R, et al. EULAR recommendations for the health professional's approach to pain management in inflammatory arthritis and osteoarthritis. Ann Rheum Dis 2018;77(6):797–807.
14. Bannuru RR, Osani MC, Vaysbrot EE, et al. OARSI guidelines for the non-surgical management of knee, hip, and polyarticular osteoarthritis. Osteoarthr Cartil 2019; 27(11):1578–89.
15. National Institute for Health and Clinical Excellence. Osteoarthritis: the care and management of osteoarthritis in adults. London: Royal College of Physicians (UK): National Collaborating Centre for Chronic Conditions; 2014.
16. Bruyere O, Honvo G, Veronese N, et al. An updated algorithm recommendation for the management of knee osteoarthritis from the European society for clinical and economic aspects of Osteoporosis, osteoarthritis and musculoskeletal Diseases (ESCEO). Semin Arthritis Rheum 2019;49(3):337–50.
17. Kloppenburg M, Kroon FP, Blanco FJ, et al. 2018 update of the EULAR recommendations for the management of hand osteoarthritis. Ann Rheum Dis 2019; 78(1):16–24.
18. Kongsted A, Kent P, Quicke JG, et al. Risk-stratified and stepped models of care for back pain and osteoarthritis: are we heading towards a common model? Pain Rep 2020;5(5):e843.
19. Bennell KL, Bayram C, Harrison C, et al. Trends in management of hip and knee osteoarthritis in general practice in Australia over an 11-year window: a nationwide cross-sectional survey. Lancet Reg Health West Pac 2021;12:100187.
20. Hagen KB, Smedslund G, Osteras N, et al. Quality of community-based osteoarthritis care: a systematic review and meta-analysis. Arthritis Care Res (Hoboken) 2016;68(10):1443–52.
21. Eyles JP, Hunter DJ, Briggs AM, et al. National Osteoarthritis Strategy brief report: living well with osteoarthritis. Aust J Gen Pract 2020;49(7):438–42.
22. Briggs AM, Houlding E, Hinman RS, et al. Health professionals and students encounter multi-level barriers to implementing high-value osteoarthritis care: a multi-national study. Osteoarthr Cartil 2019;27(5):788–804.
23. Briggs AM, Page CJ, Shaw BR, et al. A model of care for osteoarthritis of the hip and knee: development of a system-wide plan for the health sector in Victoria, Australia. Healthc Policy 2018;14(2):47–58.
24. Bowden JL, Hunter DJ, Deveza LA, et al. Core and adjunctive interventions for osteoarthritis: efficacy and models for implementation. Nat Rev Rheumatol 2020;16(8):434–47.
25. Bichsel D, Liechti FD, Schlapbach JM, et al. Cross-sectional analysis of recommendations for the treatment of hip and knee osteoarthritis in clinical guidelines. Arch Phys Med Rehabil 2021. https://doi.org/10.1016/j.apmr.2021.07.801.
26. Kroon FP, van der Burg LR, Buchbinder R, et al. Self-management education programmes for osteoarthritis. Cochrane Database Syst Rev 2014;(1):CD008963.
27. Arthritis Australia. MyJointPain. 2021. Available at: https://www.myjointpain.org.au/. Accessed October 1, 2021.
28. Versus arthritis. Versus arthritis. 2018. Available at: https://www.versusarthr-itis.org/. Accessed October 6, 2021.
29. Osteoarthritis action alliance. Osteoarthritis (OA) action alliance resource library. OAAA. 2019. Available at: https://oaaction.unc.edu/resource-library/. Accessed October 6, 2021.
30. Rausch Osthoff A-K, Niedermann K, Braun J, et al. 2018 EULAR recommendations for physical activity in people with inflammatory arthritis and osteoarthritis. Ann Rheum Dis 2018;77(9):1251–60.

31. Daste C, Kirren Q, Akoum J, et al. Physical activity for osteoarthritis: Efficiency and review of recommandations. Joint Bone Spine 2021;88(6):105207.
32. Skou ST, Roos EM. Good Life with osteoArthritis in Denmark (GLA:D): evidence-based education and supervised neuromuscular exercise delivered by certified physiotherapists nationwide. BMC Musculoskelet Disord 2017;18(1):72.
33. McAlindon TE, Bannuru RR, Sullivan MC, et al. OARSI guidelines for the non-surgical management of knee osteoarthritis. Osteoarthr Cartil 2014;22(3):363–88.
34. Nelson AE, Allen KD, Golightly YM, et al. A systematic review of recommendations and guidelines for the management of osteoarthritis: the chronic osteoarthritis management initiative of the U.S. bone and joint initiative. Semin Arthritis Rheum 2014;43(6):701–12.
35. Leopoldino AO, Machado GC, Ferreira PH, et al. Paracetamol versus placebo for knee and hip osteoarthritis. Cochrane Database Syst Rev 2019;2(2):CD013273.
36. Phillips M, Bhandari M, Grant J, et al. A systematic review of current clinical practice guidelines on intra-articular hyaluronic acid, corticosteroid, and platelet-rich plasma injection for knee osteoarthritis: an international perspective. Orthop J Sports Med 2021;9(8). 23259671211030272.
37. Zhang W, Moskowitz RW, Nuki G, et al. OARSI recommendations for the management of hip and knee osteoarthritis, Part II: OARSI evidence-based, expert consensus guidelines. Osteoarthr Cartil 2008;16(2):137–62.
38. Dieppe P, Doherty M. Contextualizing osteoarthritis care and the reasons for the gap between evidence and practice. Clin Geriatr Med 2010;26(3):419–31.
39. Dziedzic KS, Allen KD. Challenges and controversies of complex interventions in osteoarthritis management: recognizing inappropriate and discordant care. Rheumatology (Oxford) 2018;57(suppl_4):iv88–98.
40. Costa D, Cruz EB, Rodrigues AM, et al. Models of care for patients with knee osteoarthritis in primary healthcare: a scoping review protocol. BMJ Open 2021;11(6):e045358.
41. Bossen D, Veenhof C, Dekker J, et al. The usability and preliminary effectiveness of a web-based physical activity intervention in patients with knee and/or hip osteoarthritis. BMC Med Inform Decis Mak 2013;13(1):61.
42. Meneses SR, Goode AP, Nelson AE, et al. Clinical algorithms to aid osteoarthritis guideline dissemination. Osteoarthr Cartil 2016;24(9):1487–99.
43. Briggs AM, Chan M, Slater H. Extending evidence to practice: implementation of Models of Care for musculoskeletal health conditions across settings. Best Pract Res Clin Rheumatol 2016;30(3):357–8.
44. Hunter DJ, Hinman RS, Bowden JL, et al. Effectiveness of a new model of primary care management on knee pain and function in patients with knee osteoarthritis: protocol for THE PARTNER STUDY. BMC Musculoskelet Disord 2018;19(1):132.
45. Osteras N, van Bodegom-Vos L, Dziedzic K, et al. Implementing international osteoarthritis treatment guidelines in primary health care: study protocol for the SAMBA stepped wedge cluster randomized controlled trial. Implement Sci 2015;10:165.
46. Dziedzic KS, Healey EL, Porcheret M, et al. Implementing the NICE osteoarthritis guidelines: a mixed methods study and cluster randomised trial of a model osteoarthritis consultation in primary care–the Management of OsteoArthritis in Consultations (MOSAICS) study protocol. Implement Sci 2014;9(1):95.
47. Swaithes L, Paskins Z, Dziedzic K, et al. Factors influencing the implementation of evidence-based guidelines for osteoarthritis in primary care: a systematic review and thematic synthesis. Musculoskeletal Care 2020;18(2):101–10.

48. Osteras N, Moseng T, van Bodegom-Vos L, et al. Implementing a structured model for osteoarthritis care in primary healthcare: a stepped-wedge cluster-randomised trial. PLoS Med 2019;16(10):e1002949.
49. Agency for Clinical Innovation. Osteoarthritis chronic care program model of care ACI. 2020. Available at: https://aci.health.nsw.gov.au/networks/musculoskeletal. Accessed 2021.
50. Better management of patients with Osteoarthritis (BOA). Better Care of Patients with Osteoarthritis; 2019. Available at: https://boa.registercentrum.se/boa-in-english/better-management-of-patients-with-osteoarthritis-boa/p/By_o8GxVg. [Accessed 6 October 2021].
51. Holm I, Pripp AH, Risberg MA. The Active with OsteoArthritis (AktivA) physio-therapy implementation model: a patient education, supervised exercise and self-management program for patients with mild to moderate osteoarthritis of the knee or hip joint. a national register study with a two-year follow-up. J Clin Med 2020;9(10):3112.
52. Briggs AM, Chan M, Slater H. Models of Care for musculoskeletal health: moving towards meaningful implementation and evaluation across conditions and care settings. Best Pract Res Clin Rheumatol 2016;30(3):359–74.
53. Wallis JA, Ackerman IN, Brusco NK, et al. Barriers and enablers to uptake of a contemporary guideline-based management program for hip and knee osteoar-thritis: a qualitative study. Osteoarthr Cartil Open 2020;2(4):100095.
54. Eyles JP, Bowden JL, Redman S, et al. Barriers and enablers to the implementa-tion of the Australian osteoarthritis chronic care program (OACCP). Osteoarthr Cartil 2020;28:S446.
55. Petrosyan Y, Sahakyan Y, Barnsley JM, et al. Quality indicators for care of osteo-arthritis in primary care settings: a systematic literature review. Fam Pract 2018; 35(2):151–9.
56. Arslan IG, Rozendaal RM, van Middelkoop M, et al. Quality indicators for knee and hip osteoarthritis care: a systematic review. RMD Open 2021;7(2):e001590.
57. Edwards JJ, Khanna M, Jordan KP, et al. Quality indicators for the primary care of osteoarthritis: a systematic review. Ann Rheum Dis 2015;74(3):490–8.
58. Teo PL, Hinman RS, Egerton T, et al. Patient-reported quality indicators to eval-uate physiotherapy care for hip and/or knee osteoarthritis- development and evaluation of the QUIPA tool. BMC Musculoskelet Disord 2020;21(1):202.
59. Jordan K, Jinks C, Croft P. Health care utilization: measurement using primary care records and patient recall both showed bias. J Clin Epidemiol 2006;59(8): 791–7.
60. Osteras N, Tveter AT, Garratt AM, et al. Measurement properties for the revised patient-reported OsteoArthritis Quality Indicator questionnaire. Osteoarthr Cartil 2018;26(10):1300–10.
61. Teo PL, Hinman RS, Egerton T, et al. Identifying and prioritizing clinical guideline recommendations most relevant to physical therapy practice for hip and/or knee osteoarthritis. J Orthop Sports Phys Ther 2019;49(7):501–12.
62. Rice D, McNair P, Huysmans E, et al. Best evidence rehabilitation for chronic pain part 5: osteoarthritis. J Clin Med 2019;8(11):1769.

The Role of Nutrition in Osteoarthritis
A Literature Review

Ni Wei, PhD, MS[a],*, Zhaoli Dai, PhD, MS, MA[b,c]

KEYWORDS

- Osteoarthritis • Obesity • Nutrition • Fatty acids • Vitamin D • Vitamin K
- Antioxidant • Fiber • Supplements

KEY POINTS

- Evidence on polyunsaturated fatty acids, vitamin D, vitamin K, and antioxidants (vitamin C, E, selenium) has suggested some health benefits on cartilage, pain symptoms, and structural parameters related to osteoarthritis (OA), whereas high levels of iron and copper may be harmful to synovial membrane and cartilage, as suggested in animal studies.
- Given that the body of evidence on the role of nutrients in OA is generally low in quality, and the long-term effects of supplementation remain to be determined, clinicians should be cautious when recommending these supplements to manage OA.
- The significant causal relationship between weight loss and OA suggests that a well-balanced diet focusing on foods that are high in dietary fiber or the Mediterranean diet rich in polyunsaturated fats, fruits, and vegetables may provide benefits to prevent and manage OA in addition to metabolic health.

INTRODUCTION
Epidemiology of Osteoarthritis

Osteoarthritis (OA) is a common joint disorder that affects the knees, hips, hands, spine, and feet,[1] resulting in pain, stiffness, and function loss. Contributing to the global disease burdens,[2,3] OA has a significant impact on mental health, quality of life, and occupational activities.[4] Currently, more than 250 million people worldwide live with hip OA and/or knee OA,[5] with an increasing prevalence of OA largely caused by the growth of global aging populations and the high prevalence of obesity.[6] In

[a] Department of Rheumatology, Dongfang Hospital, Beijing University of Chinese Medicine, No. 6 Fangxingyuan 1st Block, Fengtai District, Beijing 100078, China; [b] Sydney Pharmacy School and the Charles Perkins Centre, Faculty of Medicine and Health, The University of Sydney, Sydney, Australia; [c] Centre for Health Systems and Safety Research, Australian Institute of Health Innovation, Macquarie University, Level 6 |75 Talavera Road, Sydney, NSW 2109, Australia
* Corresponding author.
E-mail address: whinny_pooh@yeah.net

Clin Geriatr Med 38 (2022) 303–322
https://doi.org/10.1016/j.cger.2021.11.006
0749-0690/22/© 2021 Elsevier Inc. All rights reserved.

addition, individuals with OA are at greater risk of all-cause mortality than the general population.[7]

There is a substantial economic burden of OA to both patients and society.[8] In high-income countries, the medical cost related to OA is estimated to be between 1% and 2.5% of the gross domestic product.[9] Among treatment options, total knee replacement (TKR) and total hip replacement (THR) represent the most direct medical expenses.[6] Furthermore, the indirect costs caused by low productivity, absence at work, and early retirement are also high.[10] Other invisible costs include diminished quality of life and potential comorbidities with depression and anxiety.[11]

The Importance of Nutrition in Osteoarthritis

Although OA was previously considered a passive degenerative (or so-called wear-and-tear) disease,[12] an increasing number of studies have shown that OA is a whole-joint disease, involving structural alterations in articular cartilage, subchondral bone, ligaments, capsule, synovium, and muscles.[13] Mechanical, inflammatory, and metabolic factors play a vital role in the pathogenesis of OA, which can ultimately lead to structural destruction and failure of the synovial joint.[6] At present, a growing body of evidence indicates that obesity and several nutritional factors are involved in the development or progression of OA.[14]

The objective of this review was to summarize the evidence on how nutrition affects knee OA, including animal studies to illustrate the potential mechanisms and human studies that imply the role of nutrition. This literature review was based on the current evidence, using keyword search on OA, obesity, fatty acids, vitamins, antioxidants, and minerals in the PubMed database from inception until March 2020. The review included randomized controlled trials (RCTs) and observational studies (cohort, case-control, and cross-sectional studies). Because nutrition plays a direct role in obesity, we first reviewed obesity and OA.

Obesity and Osteoarthritis

Obesity is closely related to the imbalance between physical activity and caloric intake. Obesity is widely acknowledged as the most significant risk factor for the incidence and progression of OA.[15] It is estimated that every 5 kg of weight gain increases the risk of knee OA by 36%, whereas weight loss of at least 10% can significantly relieve pain, enhance physical function, and improve health-related quality of life.[16] Obesity accelerates the progression of OA by increasing the load on weight-bearing joints.[17] For example, every 1 kg of body weight is equivalent to adding 4 kg of load to the knee joint,[18] but the association between obesity and OA in non–weight-bearing joints is unclear.[19]

Globally, it is estimated that there will be nearly 1.3 billion overweight and 573 million obese adults by 2030.[20] Obesity increases the burden on weight-bearing joints, which, in turn, increases the risk of arthroplasty among overweight or obese adults.[21] Several large cohort studies have consistently shown a strong association between body mass index (BMI) and the prevalence and incidence of OA. A recent meta-analysis showed that for every 5-unit increase in BMI, there was a 35% increase in the risk of knee OA (relative risk [RR], 1.35; 95% confidence interval [CI], 1.21 to 1.51).[22] After 10-year follow-up, a higher BMI (>30) was significantly associated with knee OA (odds ratio [OR], 2.81; 95% CI, 1.32–5.96) and hand OA (OR, 2.59; 95% CI, 1.08–6.19).[19] Cooper and colleagues[23] found that patients aged 55 years and older with higher BMI at baseline had a significantly increased risk for developing radiographic knee OA (OR, 18.3; 95% CI, 5.1–65.1), comparing the highest versus the lowest tertile of

BMI.[24] Consistent with this, Raud and colleagues[25] found a significant dose-response relationship between BMI and clinical and functional consequences of knee OA, including pain, physical disability, level of physical activity, fears, and beliefs concerning knee OA.

Furthermore, current research strongly suggests a higher likelihood of TKR or THR procedures as a treatment option in individuals who are obese with OA.[26] A literature review from the workgroup of the American Association of Hip and Knee Surgeons Evidence-Based Committee reported that more than 90% of patients with OA undergoing TKR and THR were overweight or obese.[27] A case-control study found higher odds of having TKR in overweight men (OR, 1.7; 95% CI, 1.1–2.6), obese men (5.3; 95% CI, 2.8–10.1), overweight women (1.6; 95% CI, 1.1–2.2), and obese women (4.0; 95% CI, 2.6–6.1) after adjusting for age and occupation, although there was no association with THR.[28] However, another study showed that patients with OA with higher BMI are 8.5 times more likely to undergo THR than normal-weight patients.[29] Owing to the need for longer operative time and the complexity of surgical access, arthroplasty may be technically more challenging in obese patients with OA, and the risk of perioperative complications is high.[30] A prospective cohort study following 105,189 participants for 2.5 years has suggested that those overweight or obese compared with those with normal weight were at greater risk of having TKR by 40% or 2-fold, respectively.[21]

Additionally, venous thromboembolism and deep infection are the most common surgical complications for obese patients with OA in arthroplasty. Previous studies found that the risk of venous thromboembolism in TKR or THR increased by 50% ($P = .031$; OR, 1.5) for every 5 kg/m^2 increase in BMI.[31] Another meta-analysis has also shown that infection occurred more frequently in obese patients with OA who underwent TKR (OR, 2.38; 95% CI, 1.28–4.55).[32]

Besides mechanical loading, other mechanisms, such as dyslipidemia, inflammation, and adipokines,[33] have also been suggested to link with obesity-induced OA.[34,35] For instance, obesity may enhance adipokine production from the adipose tissue,[36] which further induces a state of low-grade systemic inflammation to promote the progression of OA. In previous evidence, leptin, one of the main adipokines, has showed proinflammatory and procatabolic actions on the cartilage[37] and decreased the expression of primary fibroblast growth factor and proteoglycan depletion in animal models.[38] Furthermore, leptin has been shown to mediate the association between adiposity and OA partially.[39] Furthermore, those with OA and metabolic syndrome had higher levels of synovial leptin.[40] Because of the potential catabolic effect of leptin on synovial fibroblasts, leptin has the potential to damage joints by inducing synovial inflammation.[33]

Clinical effects of weight loss on osteoarthritis

Weight loss through lifestyle modifications is a safe and effective way for patients with OA to reduce pain, restore joint function, and delay articular cartilage degradation without serious adverse effects,[41] for which multiple studies can provide supportive evidence. For example, data from the Osteoarthritis Initiative and the Multicenter Osteoarthritis Study have suggested a significant dose-response relationship between weight loss and improvement in the Western Ontario and McMaster University Osteoarthritis Index (WOMAC) pain and function.[42] Foy and colleagues[43] reported similar results among 2203 obese diabetic patients with coexisting symptomatic knee OA with a mean BMI of 37 kg/m^2 for 1 year. The participants in the weight-loss group had lower WOMAC pain, function, and stiffness scores than those in the stable-weight group.[43] Messier and colleagues[44] also found that, in persons with knee OA, weight loss of at least 20% of the baseline weight was associated with 25% lower pain and 20% improvement in function than weight loss of 10% to 20%. A similar effect of pain and function improvement was observed in those who had at least 10% weight loss than in those who had less than 10% weight loss.

Effective weight-management program in osteoarthritis

Weight loss is recognized as a promising therapeutic intervention in OA, and dietetic advice and physical activity have suggested effective and sustainable interventions.[45] Low-energy diet is an effective treatment of weight loss and symptomatic improvements in patients with knee OA. However, its short-term results are not inferior to arthroplasty.[46] A 16-week pragmatic RCT showed that low-energy diets resulted in rapid and effective weight loss without adverse events and significantly improved the symptoms of overweight or obese patients with knee OA. There were no clinically significant differences between these 2 types of low-energy diets (415 kcal/d and 810 kcal/d).[47] However, the long-term effect, ranging from 1 to 5 years, of a low-energy diet on weight loss remains to be determined.[48]

As another weight-loss strategy, physical activity offers successful interventions for the management of OA, especially for patients who are overweight or obese. Earlier studies suggest that physical activity has a series of short-term and long-term benefits, including weight control, maintaining muscle mass, and improving bone and functional health. A meta-analysis also shows that interventions that combine reinforcement, flexibility, and aerobic exercise are likely to more effective in losing weight and improvement of pain and function for persons with OA.[49] Barrow and colleagues[50] proposed an evidence-based exercise prescription for weight management in obese adults at risk of OA. The regimens include (1) exercise safely until reaching a vigorous intensity of approximately 70% to 80% of maximal heart rate to optimize weight management and improve physical function; (2) exercise 2 to 3 times a week for 30 to 60 minutes each time and gradually increasing the frequency to maintain weight loss; (3) maintain weight loss through multiple exercise modes. Because of the limited mobility and a lack of adherence, weight-management programs can be challenging for overweight or obese patients with OA in general. The Intensive Diet and Exercise for Arthritis (IDEA) trial has shown that a combined intervention of intensive diet plus exercise had the most significant benefit on improving joint function, relieving pain, reducing knee compressive forces, and alleviating inflammation compared with either diet or exercise alone.[51] In clinical practice, successful weight loss and maintenance programs also depend on a series of factors, including behavior change strategies, extended treatment, and increased intervention exposure time, which will enhance long-term adherence to the programs.[52]

Weight management is one of the key nonpharmacological recommendations in preventing and managing knee or hip OA in several clinical guidelines.[53,54] However, weight loss remains a challenge to many individuals as well as clinicians. Understanding the barriers will aid a better outcome on initiating and sustaining weight loss to benefit persons with OA. Earlier research has suggested some of the barriers to weight loss at the patient and clinician levels.

At the patient level, persons with OA may lack the motivation to exercise or modify their diets; furthermore, they also mentioned that joint pain was a primary barrier to weight loss.[55,56] For clinicians, some have expressed a lack of time, capacity, or skills to address effective strategies, such as exercise, nutrition, or other clinical procedures on weight loss, to their patients.[57,58]

Nutritional Influences in Osteoarthritis

Polyunsaturated fatty acids

Most studies have focused on adipokines as a systemic mediator of obesity-related OA,[59] but the role of lipids as inflammatory regulators in the pathogenesis of OA should not be ignored. Some findings indicate that articular cartilage and chondrocytes can interact with lipids, leading to inflammation and degradation of cartilage.[60] Data from the Osteoarthritis Initiative have reported an association between higher intakes of total and saturated fat and increased structural knee OA progression, whereas higher intakes of monounsaturated fatty acids (MUFAs) and polyunsaturated fatty acids (PUFAs) may reduce radiographic progression.[61] Eicosanoids, as mediators and regulators of inflammation, are the critical link between PUFAs and inflammation. This may be because eicosanoids are generated from 20-carbon PUFAs, whose precursors are n-6 PUFAs and n-3 PUFAs.[62] For example, arachidonic acid (ARA), a major n-6 PUFA, promotes inflammation after conversion to proinflammatory eicosanoids.[63] Conversely, eicosapentaenoic acid (EPA) and docosahexaenoic acid (DHA), the major n-3 PUFAs, suppress inflammation and accelerate the subsidence of inflammation. In vitro studies have shown that a higher ARA intake increased the content of ARA in inflammatory cells, leading to a higher production of inflammatory eicosanoids.[64]

Furthermore, research has found slight differences in mechanisms underlying the antiinflammatory actions of EPA and DHA. The upregulation of eicosanoid synthesis depends on enzyme activation and increased expression of genes encoding enzymes.[65] EPA has been shown to inhibit ARA metabolism,[66] whereas DHA plays a primary role in decreasing the expression of adhesion molecules on macrophages and lymphocytes.[67]

Eicosapentaenoic acid/docosahexaenoic acid supplementation

Dietary sources of EPA and DHA primarily include flaxseed oil, walnuts, Chia seeds, and oily fish such as salmon, tuna, anchovies, sardines, and shellfish. Western diets, characterized by high-fat dairy products, refined grains, and high consumption of red meat, contain higher levels of n-6 PUFAs than n-3 PUFAs. The ratio of n-6 to n-3 PUFAs could reach 20:1 to 30:1, which predisposes to inflammation.[68] In fact, the use of n-3 PUFAs as dietary supplements has increased significantly in the past few decades. In Australia, 80.3% of general practitioners and 90.2% of community pharmacists recommend n-3 PUFAs supplements to their patients.[69] Another cross-sectional study of 260,000 Australians also suggested that 32.6% of the participants used n-3 PUFA supplements, among whom those with OA used them more frequently.[70] Although there is evidence linking dietary supplementation of EPA/DHA to the improvement in arthritis in dogs with OA,[71] EPA/DHA supplementation has limited clinical efficacy in patients with OA.[72]

Clinical studies have indicated that daily doses of EPA plus DHA greater than 2.7 g may exert antiinflammatory effects.[73] However, most people who self-medicate with EPA/DHA generally take a much lower dose than this amount. In a double-blind RCT involving 202 patients with symptomatic knee OA for 2 years, there was no additional benefit of a high, antiinflammatory dose of fish oil (4.5 g of n-3 PUFAs) compared with low-dose fish oil (0.45 g of n-3 PUFAs) in WOMAC pain and function scores.[74] In a systematic review of studies testing the effects of EPA/DHA supplementation on OA, the overall effect was not satisfactory because of the insufficient number of conducted trials and high heterogeneity in study design and implementation protocols.[75] Another systematic review of marine oil supplements for arthritis pain in human patients also reports that the quality of evidence was low for OA and moderate for rheumatoid arthritis.[76] More well-designed trials are needed to fully evaluate the potential benefits of EPA/DHA supplements for OA.

Vitamin D and osteoarthritis

The primary functions of vitamin D are regulations of bone metabolism and maintenance of calcium and phosphate homeostasis.[77] The vitamin D receptors (VDRs), the active form of vitamin D, are responsible for most of the biological activity of vitamin D.[78] VDRs have been demonstrated in human chondrocytes and osteoblasts. Through these receptors, vitamin D regulates chondrocyte hypertrophy, osteoblastic bone proliferation, and mineralization.[79] Because of the overexpression of VDRs in hypertrophic and proliferating chondrocytes, inadequate vitamin D status has been speculated to influence the development and progression of OA via its direct impact on the cartilage. Upregulated expression of VDRs is also associated with matrix metalloproteinase (MMP) expression, specifically MMP-1, MMP-3, and MMP-9, which leads to cartilage degradation at increased rates.[80] Furthermore, vitamin D could help to prevent the progression of OA by enhancing bone remodeling and muscle strength.[81]

In addition to a possible contributory role in the etiopathogenesis of OA, vitamin D deficiency is also thought to be associated with pain, diminished joint function, impaired quality of life, cartilage loss, and high risk of radiological progression in patients with OA.[82] These can be explained by the direct effects of vitamin D on chondrocytes in OA cartilage and the indirect effects on subchondral bone, synovium, and periarticular muscles.[83] Pain is a common symptom of OA. A large population-based cohort study containing 877 participants in the United Kingdom showed a significant association between the lower serum vitamin D concentration and knee pain.[84] Another population-based cohort study in older patients with OA with a mean age of 74.2 ± 7.1 years indicated low 25-hydroxyvitamin D levels are associated with OA-related pain, particularly in female patients with OA.[85] Laslett and colleagues[86] found an association between moderate vitamin D deficiency [serum $25(OH)D_3$ range 12.5–25 nmol/L] and the occurrence and exacerbation of knee pain within 5 years. However, the result did not reach statistical significance. A similar situation has been found in the study on the correlation between vitamin D and cartilage thickness. Malas and colleagues[87] reported that distal femoral cartilage was thinner in patients with OA with low vitamin D levels (<10 ng/mL) compared with patients with OA with higher vitamin D levels (>10 ng/mL). In one longitudinal study with more than 2.9 years of follow-up, serum levels of vitamin D positively predicted changes in both medial and lateral tibial cartilage volume assessed by MRI.[88] By contrast, the study conducted by Felson and colleagues[89] indicated that vitamin D status was unrelated to cartilage loss assessed by MRI. Additionally, several studies showed inconsistent results regarding the association between vitamin D deficiency and the increased risk of OA progression.[90–92]

Vitamin D supplementation

Epidemiologic evidence suggests inconsistent results on vitamin D deficiency in association with the predisposition to OA. Furthermore, the efficacy of vitamin D supplementation as a treatment for OA also remains uncertain, with conflicting results. An RCT of 107 persons with knee OA and deficient in vitamin D ($25(OH)D \leq 50$ nmol/L) has shown visual analog scale pain and WOMAC pain decreased significantly after the intervention of vitamin D in the treatment group.[93] The authors indicate that vitamin D supplementation at a dose of 60,000 IU of vitamin D_3 monthly for 1 year may alleviate knee pain. Another RCT also found short-term vitamin D supplementation

(50,000 IU of cholecalciferol weekly for 2 months) had a beneficial effect on knee pain and quadriceps muscle strength in patients with knee OA who were deficient in vitamin D.[94] However, based on several reviews on the effect of vitamin D supplementation on the OA, evidence is lacking to support the beneficial effect of vitamin D supplementation on knee pain, radiographic OA, or cartilage volume in longitudinal studies or clinical trials.[95,96]

Vitamin K and osteoarthritis

Vitamin K is a fat-soluble vitamin, consisting of 3 different forms, namely vitamin K_1 (phylloquinone), K_2 (menaquinone), and K_3 (menadione). Vitamin K_1 is abundant in leafy green vegetables, and vitamin K_2, predominantly produced by gut bacteria, is contained in fermented foods.[97] Vitamin K is an essential cofactor of γ-glutamyl carboxylase, which is responsible for the activation of γ-carboxyglutamate(Gla)–containing proteins that negatively regulate calcification.[98] Because vitamin K–dependent Gla proteins have a high affinity for calcium, phosphate, and hydroxyapatite crystals, vitamin K, as a regulator, plays a vital role in bone and cartilage mineralization.[99] Aside from the biological roles discussed earlier, vitamin K is also involved in the process of converting inactive uncarboxylated matrix Gla protein (MGP) to active carboxylated MGP.[100] Inadequate vitamin K intake leading to undercarboxylation of MGP and other Gla proteins may decrease the functioning of these proteins, and ultimately influence chondrocyte differentiation and endochondral bone formation.[101] Thus, vitamin K deficiency is thought to play a potential role in the pathophysiology of OA.

The evidence on the relationship between vitamin K status and OA in human observational studies and clinical trials is limited. In a case-controlled study, patients with knee OA deficient in vitamin K were reported to have a higher WOMAC total score, suggesting that vitamin K may be an indicator for OA severity.[102] A longitudinal study involving 1180 subjects from the Multicenter Osteoarthritis Study showed subclinical vitamin K deficiency (plasma phylloquinone <0.5 nmol/L) was associated with an increased risk of developing radiographic knee OA and cartilage lesions assessed by MRI rather than osteophytes.[103] Neogi and colleagues[104] also found an association between low plasma levels of vitamin K and increased incidence of osteophytes and joint space narrowing in patients with hand and knee OA. Oka and colleagues[105] reported similar results in a cross-sectional study, suggesting that vitamin K supplementation may be a disease-modifying therapy in knee OA. Boer and colleagues[106] found an increased overall OA incidence and risk of progression in users of the vitamin K antagonist anticoagulants; this risk was higher in carriers of VKORC1 BB - haplotype and MGP risk alleles. Their findings suggest the importance of vitamin K and vitamin K-dependent Gla proteins in the pathogenesis of OA.

Vitamin K supplementation

Despite the likelihood of vitamin K deficiency as a potential risk factor for the development of OA, the only study in hand OA suggests no overall effect of vitamin K supplementation on radiographic OA.[107] Because vitamin K level decreases with age, elderly patients with OA are more susceptible to vitamin K deficiency. Therefore, vitamin K supplementation could be another alternative to alleviate OA progression for elderly patients, like vitamin D supplementation. However, further research is needed to understand the efficacy, doses, and form of vitamin K.

Antioxidants and osteoarthritis

In the biological system, free radicals involving oxygen are called reactive oxygen species (ROS). Normal physiologic processes leading to ROS production at a deficient concentration are beneficial to the human body.[108] At high concentrations, ROS can cause damage to various molecules in the system. This is possible because high levels of oxidative stress may destroy osteoblasts and chondrocytes by oxidizing lipids and changing the DNA and protein structures.[109] Therefore, ROS may participate in the pathophysiology of OA, whereas antioxidants could delay this process. The currently available evidence focuses on antioxidants, such as vitamins C and E. In animal models, vitamin C not only has a chondroprotective effect on articular cartilage but also stimulates chondrocyte metabolism, collagen, and proteoglycan synthesis.[110] Similar metabolic effects have been reported for vitamin E. Vitamin E may reduce oxidative stress in the cartilage explants or chondrocyte cultures caused by mechanical stress or free radicals.[111] Angthong and colleagues[112] also found that the concentration of vitamin E in synovial fluid was inversely related to the severity of knee OA.

Antioxidant supplementation

Although existing studies support the potential protective effect of antioxidants in the pathophysiology of OA, there is no consensus on whether antioxidant supplements can delay the disease process. In the Framingham Osteoarthritis Cohort Study, McAlindon and colleagues[113] reported a lower risk of cartilage loss, joint pain, and disease progression in patients with OA who had a higher intake of vitamin C equivalent to more than 75 mg per day. Another RCT also found that vitamin C supplementation in patients with hip or knee OA resulted in pain reduction compared with placebo.[114] Vitamin E supplementation may also relieve clinical symptoms and improve joint function in patients with OA. In an RCT by Tantavisut and colleagues,[115] oral vitamin E of 400 IU daily or placebo was given to patients with knee OA scheduled for TKR. Two months later, those on the vitamin E supplements had improved WOMAC scores in different domains and reduced oxidative stress.[115]

Selenium

Selenium is one of the essential trace elements. In the form of selenoproteins, selenium plays a crucial role in tissue development and homeostasis of articular cartilage.[116] Selenium may play a role in the occurrence and progression of Kachin-Beck disease (KBD).[117] In one study, although the plasma concentration of selenium was lower in patients with OA than in their healthy counterparts, this difference was not statistically significant.[118] Moreover, accumulated evidence has supported that selenium supplementation is beneficial for preventing and treating KBD,[119] but no clinical trial has shown the effect in treating OA.

Micronutrients and osteoarthritis

Magnesium. Magnesium is a cofactor of hundreds of enzymes in the human body. It is predominantly found within cartilage and bone. Notably, magnesium shows a chondroprotective action on OA by increasing cell proliferation, protein expression, and growth factor efficacy.[120] Therefore, the depletion of magnesium during cartilage development has been speculated to result in cartilage lesions. Additionally, it shows that magnesium deficiency induces an inflammatory response that leads to the release of inflammatory cytokines and excessive production of free radicals.[121] Therefore, magnesium deficiency may be involved in OA development through inflammation and/or alterations of chondrocyte metabolism.[122] Furthermore, a study by Musik and colleagues[123] has suggested an association between a lower level of magnesium and a higher incidence of OA in women. Similarly, Hunter and colleagues[124] observed a significant reduction in serum magnesium of female twins with OA. In a cross-sectional study, serum magnesium concentration was inversely associated with radiographic knee OA.[125] Another cross-sectional study also suggests that a higher magnesium intake was associated with a lower risk to develop radiographic knee OA.[126] Despite the results reported on a protective association between magnesium and knee OA in observational studies, no clinical trials have investigated this aspect.

Iron. The relationship between iron and OA development has not been fully understood, and current evidence mainly comes from studies on hereditary hemochromatosis (HH). HH is a disease characterized by a systemic iron overload phenotype related primarily to mutations in the human hemochromatosis protein (high-Fe [HFe]) gene. Arthropathy in OA is the most prevalent and often the earliest clinical manifestation of HH.[127] HH-related arthropathy is considered a progression of OA, with an onset at younger age and involvement of typical and atypical joints, huge osteophytes, and rapid progression of cartilage loss.[128] Simão and colleagues[129] found that after exposure to 50 M iron, chondrocytes isolated from the Hfe-KO mice joint tissue developed an OA-related phenotype, suggesting higher iron levels may be detrimental to the cartilage. Another study by Camacho and colleagues[130] found similar results and suggested that high iron exposure may compromise chondrocyte metabolism, suggesting a synovial iron overload may affect the progression of HH-related OA. Treatments for HH include phlebotomy and oral deferiprone or deferasirox to remove excess iron from the body.[131] In terms of diet, patients with HH are advised to maintain a diet low in iron and reduce red meat and alcohol intake.[131]

Copper. In healthy tissues, especially cartilage, copper is an essential component of cellular enzyme synthesis. Lysyl oxidase, a copper-dependent amine oxidase, is a crucial enzyme for collagen crosslinking, which plays a vital role in cartilage formation.[132] Therefore, copper deficiency may result in cartilage lesions and increase the incidence of OA.[133] However, an excessive copper accumulation can impair the joints, such as in Wilson disease. In patients with this disease, copper accumulation in the synovial membrane and cartilage has been suggested as the primary cause of OA and accelerated degenerative changes with deformities affecting the larger joints.[133] Also, in patients with Wilson disease, large amounts of copper accumulate in the synovium and cartilage and may accelerate the process of cartilage and joint degeneration leading to joint deformity.[134] A dietary copper restriction may improve joint symptoms in patients with Wilson disease. Foods that contain high copper contents, such as shellfish, nuts, chocolate, and mushrooms, should be limited in these patients.[135]

Dietary fiber. As the commonly shared and beneficial nondigestible carbohydrate, earlier studies using data from 2 population-based longitudinal cohorts have shown the health benefits of fiber-rich foods in reducing the risk of symptomatic knee OA and knee pain severity but not with radiographic knee OA.[136,137] Both cohorts, the Osteoarthritis Initiative (OAI) and the Framingham Offspring Study, show consistent results of a statistically significant lower risk to develop knee OA in those who consumed the highest quartile of total fiber compared with the lowest quartile. Furthermore, a 5-g daily increment of dietary fiber was also associated with a lower risk of incident symptomatic OA (OR, 0.85 per 5-g increment; 95% CI, 0.76, 0.94; $P<.002$ for total fiber) and the results of cereal fiber suggest a protective association against the risk of symptomatic knee OA. Similarly, in the Framingham Offspring Study, even after adjustment for other dietary factors and diet quality, dietary fiber intake was suggested to have a strong protective association against the development of incident symptomatic OA. However, statistically significant results were found in this cohort for total fiber intake and fiber from nuts and legumes.[136]

Table 1
Summary of potential benefits and mechanisms of obesity and nutrients in the prevention and management of osteoarthritis

Intervention/ Exposures	Observed Benefits in OA		Potential Mechanisms
	Observational Studies	Clinical Trials	
Weight loss	Reduced pain and improved joint function[17,18,42]	Reduced pain and improved joint function[43,44]	Reduce mechanical loadings; inflammation
Polyunsaturated fatty acids	Likely reduced pain[61,72]	Reduced pain[74]	Possibly caused by its antiinflammatory property
Vitamin C	Likely reduced the risk of cartilage loss and disease progression[108]	Reduced pain[113]	Possibly caused by its function in stimulating chondrocyte metabolism; reducing oxidative stress
Vitamin D	It likely reduced pain and improved joint function. However, Systematic reviews did not suggest this[84–86,94]	Reduced pain[93]	Possibly caused by its enhancement of bone remodeling and muscle strength
Vitamin E	Likely delayed the disease progression[112]	Relieved clinical symptoms and improved joint function[115]	Likely caused by reduced oxidative stress
Vitamin K	Likely reduced cartilage loss[103–105]	No overall effect[107]	Vitamin K may likely regulate bone and cartilage mineralization
Selenium	Possible protective role in chondrocytes[117–119]	NA	Likely caused by maintaining tissue development and homeostasis of articular cartilage
Magnesium	Possible protective role in chondrocytes[122–125]	NA	Magnesium might regulate the metabolism of chondrocytes and reduce inflammation to affect OA
Iron	High iron exposure may compromise chondrocyte metabolism.[129,130]	NA	Uncertain
Copper	Copper deficiency or accumulation impairs cartilage or synovial membrane[133,134]	NA	Copper might promote articular cartilage formation

(continued on next page)

Table 1 *(continued)*			
Intervention/ Exposures	**Observed Benefits in OA**		**Potential Mechanisms**
	Observational Studies	**Clinical Trials**	
Dietary fiber	Higher intake of dietary fiber or 5 g/ d increments reduced the risk of symptomatic knee OA or knee pain[136,137]	NA	Dietary fiber reduces body weight and inflammation and promotes a healthy microbiome to reduce pain and symptoms

Abbreviation: NA, not available.

This protective association was partly explained by the mechanism where fiber reduced body weight preceding the effect on symptomatic knee OA and potentially by reducing inflammation, such as C-reactive protein (although the mediation analysis did not reach statistical significance).[138] Because many plant-based foods are generally high in dietary fiber, adopting healthy dietary patterns such as the Mediterranean diet or a plant-based vegetarian diet pattern can be feasible to increase fiber intake in general. In line with this, a systematic review on the Mediterranean diet[139] has suggested a beneficial association with knee OA in observational studies and clinical trials. However, meta-analysis was not conducted in this review because the heterogeneity of the included studies was high. Therefore, to determine whether dietary fiber has a causal effect on knee OA and related OA pain, well-designed clinical trials are needed to confirm the beneficial associations found in observational studies.

The evidence mentioned earlier is summarized in **Table 1** to outline the beneficial effects or associations and their potential mechanisms. The table also provides the evidence rating by strength based on the reported statistically significant results in the hierarchy of evidence in **Fig. 1**.

Intervention/exposure tested	Knee OA	Hip OA	Hand OA
Weight loss	5	5	2
Polyunsaturated fatty acids	2.5	N/A	N/A
Vitamin C	2	N/A	N/A
Vitamin D	2.5	2.5	2.5
Vitamin E	3	N/A	N/A
Vitamin K	3	N/A	2
Selenium	1	N/A	N/A
Magnesium	2	N/A	N/A
Iron	N/A	N/A	N/A
Copper	N/A	N/A	N/A
Dietary fiber	3	N/A	N/A

Fig. 1. Nutritional components/interventions and their potential effects on OA. A Likert scale ranging from 1 to 5 was used to rate the strength of the evidence for each intervention/exposure on knee, hip, or hand OA by 2 reviewers. If there is a statistically significant effect estimate reported in the hierarchy of evidence: 5 represents significant results in a systematic review; 4 represents significant results in RCTs; 3 represents significant results in a longitudinal cohort; 2 represents significant results in a cross-sectional or case-control study; 1 represents no significant results in any of the preceding. NA represents no studies available in the included studies in the review.

DISCUSSION

OA is the most common form of arthritis in older adults, affecting individuals' ability to work and independent living.[140] Because of the lack of an effective treatment to relieve pain and other symptoms related to OA, safe and effective alternative options are sought by many with OA. Weight loss is considered one of the core nonpharmacological interventions. Besides physical activity, diet and nutrition also provide long-term health benefits to prevent and manage chronic diseases, including OA.[141]

As a well-established risk factor for OA,[142] body-weight loss reduces joint loads and reduces the levels of inflammatory adipokines. Although dietary modification can offer a safe and effective strategy to manage weight, long-term weight-loss maintenance can be challenging. Hence, a weight-management program should be person-centered and consider personal mobility, comorbidities, and preferences. If possible, referral to a registered dietitian can be helpful to overcome these barriers.[16] An ideal goal of weight loss is recommended at 10% loss of the baseline body weight.[42]

The health benefits of nutrients in the management of OA also include their antiinflammatory properties and antioxidant capacities. However, there is limited evidence supporting the use of EPA/DHA in managing OA.[143] Although some studies suggest that vitamin or micronutrient supplementation may have some benefits, the most widely used supplements, such as glucosamine, chondroitin, vitamin D, and vitamin E, have not been shown to provide clinically meaningful long-term effects to improve pain symptoms in a systematic review.[144] With the health benefits in weight control, reduced inflammation, and reducing the risk of symptomatic knee OA, dietary fiber or a fiber-rich diet has the potential to be a dietary regimen to prevent and manage OA, which will require confirmation in clinical trials.

In summary, this review on different nutritional components concerning the prevention and management of OA indicates that consuming a balanced diet may benefit individuals with OA, particularly through interventions on weight control and reduced systemic inflammation, to improve quality of life in people living with OA.[145]

CLINICS CARE POINTS

- Weight loss
  Numerous studies have suggested a strong association between obesity and OA, in which obesity increases the risk of OA and total joint replacement.
  Weight control is vital to reduce the risk of developing and progression of OA for people who are overweight or obese.

- Nutrition
  Accumulating evidence has shown that several nutritional factors may be involved in the development or progression of OA. Therefore, consuming a healthy diet high in dietary fiber or the Mediterranean diet should be considered for OA prevention and pain management.

- Nutritional supplements
  There is no consensus about using nutritional supplements to prevent or manage OA. As a result, clinicians need to be cautious when recommending supplements to individuals with OA because of the uncertainty of their clinically meaningful effects to improve pain long-term.

ACKNOWLEDGMENT

We thank Rosie Venman for her help with the literature search.

DISCLOSURE

N. Wei is supported by a scholarship from the China Scholarship Council. Z. Dai has nothing to disclose.

REFERENCES

1. Global Burden of Disease Study 2013 Collaborators. Global, regional, and national incidence, prevalence, and years lived with disability for 301 acute and chronic diseases and injuries in 188 countries, 1990-2013: a systematic analysis for the Global Burden of Disease Study 2013. Lancet 2015;386:743–800.
2. Vos T, Flaxman AD, Naghavi M, et al. Years lived with disability (YLDs) for 1160 sequelae of 289 diseases and injuries 1990-2010: a systematic analysis for the Global Burden of Disease Study 2010. Lancet 2012;380:2163–96.
3. Woolf AD, Pfleger B. Burden of major musculoskeletal conditions. Bull World Health Organ 2003;81:646–56.
4. Cross M, Smith E, Hoy D, et al. The global burden of hip and knee osteoarthritis: estimates from the Global Burden of Disease 2010 Study. Ann Rheum Dis 2014; 73:1323–30.
5. Hawker GA. Osteoarthritis is a serious disease. Clin Exp Rheumatol 2019; 37(Suppl 120):3–6.
6. Hunter DJ, Bierma-Zeinstra S. Osteoarthritis. Lancet 2019;393:1745–59.
7. Palazzo C, Nguyen C, Lefevre-Colau MM, Rannou F, Poiraudeau S. Risk factors and burden of osteoarthritis. Ann Phys Rehabil Med 2016;59:134–8.
8. Berenbaum F, Walker C. Osteoarthritis and inflammation: a serious disease with overlapping phenotypic patterns. Postgrad Med 2020;132:377–84.
9. Hunter DJ, Schofield D, Callander E. The individual and socioeconomic impact of osteoarthritis. Nat Rev Rheumatol 2014;10:437–41.
10. Loza E, Lopez-Gomez JM, Abasolo L, et al. Economic burden of knee and hip osteoarthritis in Spain. Arthritis Rheum 2009;61:158–65.
11. Chen A, Gupte C, Akhtar K, et al. The global economic cost of osteoarthritis: how the UK Compares. Arthritis 2012;2012:698709.
12. Fu K, Robbins SR, McDougall JJ. Osteoarthritis: the genesis of pain. Rheumatology (Oxford) 2018;57:iv43–50.
13. Lambova SN, Müller-Ladner U. Osteoarthritis-current insights in pathogenesis, diagnosis and treatment. Curr Rheumatol Rev 2018;14:91–7.
14. Li Y, Luo W, Deng Z, et al. Diet-intestinal microbiota axis in osteoarthritis: a possible role. Mediators Inflamm 2016;2016:3495173.
15. Sun AR, Udduttula A, Li J, et al. Cartilage tissue engineering for obesity-induced osteoarthritis: physiology, challenges, and future prospects. J Orthop Translat 2020;26:3–15.
16. Bliddal H, Leeds AR, Christensen R. Osteoarthritis, obesity and weight loss: evidence, hypotheses and horizons-a scoping review. Obes Rev 2014;15:578–86.
17. Teichtahl AJ, Wluka AE, Tanamas SK, et al. Weight change and change in tibial cartilage volume and symptoms in obese adults. Ann Rheum Dis 2015;74: 1024–9.

18. Messier SP, Gutekunst DJ, Davis C, et al. Weight loss reduces knee-joint loads in overweight and obese older adults with knee osteoarthritis. Arthritis Rheum 2005;52:2026–32.

19. Grotle M, Hagen KB, Natvig B, et al. Obesity and osteoarthritis in knee, hip and/or hand: an epidemiological study in the general population with 10 years follow-up. BMC Musculoskelet Disord 2008;9:132.

20. Kelly T, Yang W, Chen CS, et al. Global burden of obesity in 2005 and projections to 2030. Int J Obes (Lond) 2008;32:1431–7.

21. Leyland KM, Judge A, Javaid MK, et al. Obesity and the relative risk of knee replacement surgery in patients with knee osteoarthritis: a prospective cohort study. Arthritis Rheumatol 2016;68:817–25.

22. Reyes C, Leyland KM, Peat G, et al. Association between overweight and obesity and risk of clinically diagnosed knee, hip, and hand osteoarthritis: a population-based cohort study. Arthritis Rheumatol 2016;68:1869–75.

23. Cooper C, Snow S, McAlindon TE, et al. Risk factors for the incidence and progression of radiographic knee osteoarthritis. Arthritis Rheum 2000;43:995–1000.

24. Niu J, Zhang YQ, Torner J, et al. Is obesity a risk factor for progressive radiographic knee osteoarthritis? Arthritis Rheum 2009;61:329–35.

25. Raud B, Gay C, Guiguet-Auclair C, et al. Level of obesity is directly associated with the clinical and functional consequences of knee osteoarthritis. Sci Rep 2020;10:3601.

26. Jackson MP, Sexton SA, Yeung E, et al. The effect of obesity on the mid-term survival and clinical outcome of cementless total hip replacement. J Bone Joint Surg Br 2009;91:1296–300.

27. Workgroup of the American Association of Hip and Knee Surgeons Evidence Based Committee. Obesity and total joint arthroplasty: a literature based review. J Arthroplasty 2013;28:714–21.

28. Franklin J, Ingvarsson T, Englund M, et al. Sex differences in the association between body mass index and total hip or knee joint replacement resulting from osteoarthritis. Ann Rheum Dis 2009;68:536–40.

29. Singh JA, Lewallen DG. Increasing obesity and comorbidity in patients undergoing primary total hip arthroplasty in the US: a 13-year study of time trends. BMC Musculoskelet Disord 2014;15:441.

30. Salih S, Sutton P. Obesity, knee osteoarthritis and knee arthroplasty: a review. BMC Sports Sci Med Rehabil 2013;5:25.

31. Mantilla CB, Horlocker TT, Schroeder DR, et al. Risk factors for clinically relevant pulmonary embolism and deep venous thrombosis in patients undergoing primary hip or knee arthroplasty. Anesthesiology 2003;99:552–60.

32. Kerkhoffs GM, Servien E, Dunn W, et al. The influence of obesity on the complication rate and outcome of total knee arthroplasty: a meta-analysis and systematic literature review. J Bone Joint Surg Am 2012;94:1839–44.

33. Thijssen E, van Caam A, van der Kraan PM. Obesity and osteoarthritis, more than just wear and tear: pivotal roles for inflamed adipose tissue and dyslipidaemia in obesity-induced osteoarthritis. Rheumatology (Oxford) 2015;54:588–600.

34. Rosa Cde O, Dos Santos CA, Leite JI, et al. Impact of nutrients and food components on dyslipidemias: what is the evidence? Adv Nutr 2015;6:703–11.

35. Minihane AM, Vinoy S, Russell WR, et al. Low-grade inflammation, diet composition and health: current research evidence and its translation. Br J Nutr 2015; 114:999–1012.

36. Kershaw EE, Flier JS. Adipose tissue as an endocrine organ. J Clin Endocrinol Metab 2004;89:2548–56.

37. Abella V, Scotece M, Conde J, et al. Leptin in the interplay of inflammation, metabolism and immune system disorders. Nat Rev Rheumatol 2017;13:100–9.

38. Bao JP, Chen WP, Feng J, et al. Leptin plays a catabolic role on articular cartilage. Mol Biol Rep 2010;37:3265–72.

39. Kroon FPB, Veenbrink AI, de Mutsert R, et al. The role of leptin and adiponectin as mediators in the relationship between adiposity and hand and knee osteoarthritis. Osteoarthritis Cartilage 2019;27:1761–7.

40. Liu B, Gao YH, Dong N, et al. Differential expression of adipokines in the synovium and infrapatellar fat pad of osteoarthritis patients with and without metabolic syndrome. Connect Tissue Res 2019;60:611–8.

41. DeRogatis M, Anis HK, Sodhi N, et al. Non-operative treatment options for knee osteoarthritis. Ann Transl Med 2019;7:S245.

42. Riddle DL, Stratford PW. Body weight changes and corresponding changes in pain and function in persons with symptomatic knee osteoarthritis: a cohort study. Arthritis Care Res (Hoboken) 2013;65:15–22.

43. Foy CG, Lewis CE, Hairston KG, et al. Intensive lifestyle intervention improves physical function among obese adults with knee pain: findings from the look AHEAD trial. Obesity (Silver Spring) 2011;19:83–93.

44. Messier SP, Resnik AE, Beavers DP, et al. Intentional weight loss for overweight and obese knee osteoarthritis patients: is more better? Arthritis Care Res (Hoboken) 2018;70:1569–75.

45. Kushner RF, Ryan DH. Assessment and lifestyle management of patients with obesity. JAMA 2014;312:943–52.

46. Christensen P, Bliddal H, Riecke BF, et al. Comparison of a low-energy diet and a very low-energy diet in sedentary obese individuals: a pragmatic randomised controlled trial. Clin Obes 2011;1:31–40.

47. Riecke BF, Christensen R, Christensen P, et al. Comparing two low-energy diets for the treatment of knee osteoarthritis symptoms in obese patients: a pragmatic randomised clinical trial. Osteoarthritis Cartilage 2010;18:746–54.

48. Saris WH. Very-low-calorie diets and sustained weight loss. Obes Res 2001;9: 295S–301S.

49. Uthman OA, van der Windt DA, Jordan JL, et al. Exercise for lower limb osteoarthritis: systematic review incorporating trial sequential analysis and network meta-analysis. BMJ 2013;347:f5555.

50. Barrow DR, Abbate LM, Paquette MR, et al. Exercise prescription for weight management in obese adults at risk for osteoarthritis: synthesis from a systematic review. BMC Musculoskelet Disord 2019;20:610.

51. Messier SP, Mihalko SL, Legault C, et al. Effects of intensive diet and exercise on knee joint loads, inflammation, and clinical outcomes among overweight and obese adults with knee osteoarthritis: the IDEA randomised clinical trial. JAMA 2013;310:1263–73.

52. Messier SP. Obesity and osteoarthritis: disease genesis and nonpharmacologic weight management. Rheum Dis Clin North Am 2008;34:713–29.

53. Kolasinski SL, Neogi T, Hochberg MC, et al. 2019 American College of Rheumatology/Arthritis Foundation Guideline for the Management of Osteoarthritis of the Hand, Hip, and Knee. Arthritis Rheumatol 2020;72:220–33.

54. McAlindon TE, Bannuru RR, Sullivan MC, et al. OARSI guidelines for the nonsurgical management of knee osteoarthritis. Osteoarthritis Cartilage 2014;22: 363–88.

55. Bunzli S, O'Brien P, Ayton D, et al. Misconceptions and the acceptance of evidence-based nonsurgical interventions for knee osteoarthritis. a qualitative study. Clin Orthop Relat Res 2019;477:1975–83.

56. Howarth D, Inman D, Lingard E, et al. Barriers to weight loss in obese patients with knee osteoarthritis. Ann R Coll Surg Engl 2010;92:338–40.

57. Briggs AM, Houlding E, Hinman RS, et al. Health professionals and students encounter multi-level barriers to implementing high-value osteoarthritis care: a multi-national study. Osteoarthritis Cartilage 2019;27:788–804.

58. Selten EMH, Vriezekolk JE, Nijhof MW, et al. Barriers impeding the use of non-pharmacological, non-surgical care in hip and knee osteoarthritis: the views of general practitioners, physical therapists, and medical specialists. J Clin Rheumatol 2017;23:405–10.

59. Sellam J, Berenbaum F. Is osteoarthritis a metabolic disease? Joint Bone Spine 2013;80:568–73.

60. Masuko K, Murata M, Suematsu N, et al. A metabolic aspect of osteoarthritis: lipid as a possible contributor to the pathogenesis of cartilage degradation. Clin Exp Rheumatol 2009;27:347–53.

61. Lu B, Driban J, Xu C, et al. Dietary fat and progression of knee osteoarthritis dietary fat intake and radiographic progression of knee osteoarthritis: data from the Osteoarthritis Initiative. Arthritis Care Res (Hoboken) 2017;69:368–75.

62. Baker KR, Matthan NR, Lichtenstein AH, et al. Association of plasma n-6 and n-3 polyunsaturated fatty acids with synovitis in the knee: the MOST Study. Osteoarthritis Cartilage 2012;20:382–7.

63. Cai A, Hutchison E, Hudson J, et al. Metabolic enrichment of omega-3 polyunsaturated fatty acids does not reduce the onset of idiopathic knee osteoarthritis in mice. Osteoarthritis Cartilage 2014;22:1301–9.

64. Calder PC. n-3 polyunsaturated fatty acids, inflammation, and inflammatory diseases. Am J Clin Nutr 2006;83:1505S–19S.

65. Calder PC. Omega-3 fatty acids and inflammatory processes: from molecules to man. Biochem Soc Trans 2017;45:1105–15.

66. Calder PC. Marine ω-3 fatty acids and inflammatory processes: effects, mechanisms and clinical relevance. Biochim Biophys Acta 2015;1851:469–84.

67. Miles EA, Wallace FA, Calder PC. Dietary fish oil reduces intercellular adhesion molecule 1 and scavenger receptor expression on murine macrophages. Atherosclerosis 2000;152:43–50.

68. Simopoulos AP. The importance of the omega-6/omega-3 fatty acid ratio in cardiovascular disease and other chronic diseases. Exp Biol Med (Maywood) 2008;233:674–88.

69. Brown J, Morgan T, Adams J, et al. Complementary medicines information use and needs of health professionals: general practitioners and pharmacists. Sydney (Australia): National Prescribing Service; 2008.

70. Adams J, Sibbritt D, Lui CW, et al. Ω-3 fatty acid supplement use in the 45 and up Study Cohort. BMJ Open 2013;3:e002292.

71. Mehlera SJ, Maya LR, King C, et al. A prospective, randomised, double blind, placebo-controlled evaluation of the effects of eicosapentaenoic acid and docosahexaenoic acid on the clinical signs and erythrocyte membrane polyunsaturated fatty acid concentrations in dogs with osteoarthritis. Prostaglandins Leukot Essent Fatty Acids 2016;109:1–7.

72. Loef M, Schoones JW, Kloppenburg M, et al. Fatty acids and osteoarthritis: different types, different effects. Joint Bone Spine 2019;86:451–8.

73. Cleland LG, James MJ, Proudman SM. Fish oil: what the prescriber needs to know. Arthritis Res Ther 2006;8:202.
74. Hill CL, March LM, Aitken D, et al. Fish oil in knee osteoarthritis: a randomised clinical trial of low dose versus high dose. Ann Rheum Dis 2016;75:23–9.
75. Akbar U, Yang M, Kurian D, et al. Omega-3 fatty acids in rheumatic diseases: a critical review. J Clin Rheumatol 2017;23:330–9.
76. Senftleber NK, Nielsen SM, Andersen JR, et al. Marine oil supplements for arthritis pain: a systematic review and meta-analysis of randomised trials. Nutrients 2017;9:42.
77. Mabey T, Honsawek S. Role of vitamin D in osteoarthritis: molecular, cellular, and clinical perspectives. Int J Endocrinol 2015;2015:383918.
78. Anderson PH, Turner AG, Morris HA. Vitamin D actions to regulate calcium and skeletal homeostasis. Clin Biochem 2012;45:880–6.
79. Wang Y, Zhu J, Deluca HF. Identification of the vitamin D receptor in osteoblasts and chondrocytes but not osteoclasts in mouse bone. J Bone Miner Res 2014;29:685–92.
80. Tetlow LC, Woolley DE. Expression of vitamin D receptors and matrix metalloproteinase in osteoarthritic cartilage and human articular chondrocytes in vitro. Osteoarthritis Cartilage 2001;9:423–31.
81. Holick MF. High prevalence of vitamin D inadequacy and implications for health. Mayo Clin Proc 2006;81:353–73.
82. Heidari B, Babaei M. Therapeutic and preventive potential of vitamin D supplementation in knee osteoarthritis. ACR Open Rheumatol 2019;1:318–26.
83. Jin X, Antony B, Wang X, et al. Effect of vitamin D supplementation on pain and physical function in patients with knee osteoarthritis (OA): an OA Trial Bank protocol for a systematic review and individual patient data (IPD) meta-analysis. BMJ Open 2020;10:e035302.
84. Muraki S, Dennison E, Jameson K, et al. Association of vitamin D status with knee pain and radiographic knee osteoarthritis. Osteoarthritis Cartilage 2011;19:1301–6.
85. Veronese N, Maggi S, Noale M, et al. Serum 25-hydroxyvitamin D and osteoarthritis in older people: the progetto veneto anziani study. Rejuvenation Res 2015;18:543–53.
86. Laslett LL, Quinn S, Burgess JR, et al. Moderate vitamin deficiency is associated with changes in knee and hip pain in older adults: a 5-year longitudinal study. Ann Rheum Dis 2014;73:697–703.
87. Malas FU, Kara M, Aktekin L, et al. Does vitamin D affect femoral cartilage thickness? An ultrasonographic study. Clin Rheumatol 2014;33:1331–4.
88. Ding C, Cicuttini F, Parameswaran V, et al. Serum levels of vitamin D, sunlight exposure, and knee cartilage loss in older adults: the Tasmanian older adult cohort study. Arthritis Rheum 2009;60:1381–9.
89. Felson DT, Niu J, Clancy M, et al. Low levels of vitamin D and worsening of knee osteoarthritis: results of two longitudinal studies. Arthritis Rheum 2007;56:129–36.
90. Zhang FF, Driban JB, Lo GH, et al. Vitamin D deficiency is associated with progression of knee osteoarthritis. J Nutr 2014;144:2002–8.
91. Heidari B, Heidari P, Hajian-Tilaki K. Association between serum vitamin D deficiency and knee osteoarthritis. Int Orthop 2011;35:1627–31.
92. Konstari S, Kaila-Kangas L, Jääskeläinen T, et al. Serum 25-hydroxyvitamin D and the risk of knee and hip osteoarthritis leading to hospitalisation: a cohort study of 5274 Finns. Rheumatology(Oxford) 2014;53:1778–82.

93. Sanghi D, Mishra A, Sharma AC, et al. Does vitamin D improve osteoarthritis of the knee: a randomised controlled pilot trial. Clin Orthop Relat Res 2013;471: 3556–62.

94. Heidari B, Javadian Y, Babaei M, et al. Restorative effect of vitamin D deficiency on knee pain and quadriceps in knee osteoarthritis. Acta Med Iran 2015;53: 466–70.

95. BerGink AP, Trajanoska K, Uitterlinden AG, et al. Mendelian randomisation study on vitamin D levels and osteoarthritis risk: a concise report. Rheumatology (Oxford) 2021;60:3409–12.

96. Yu Y, Liu D, Feng D, et al. Association between vitamin D and knee osteoarthritis: a PRISMA-compliant meta-analysis. Z Orthop Unfall 2021;159:281–7.

97. Tarvainen M, Fabritius M, Yang B. Determination of vitamin K composition of fermented food. Food Chem 2019;275:515–22.

98. Chin KY. The Relationship between vitamin K and osteoarthritis: a review of current evidence. Nutrients 2020;12:1208.

99. Fusaro M, Mereu MC, Aghi A, et al. Vitamin K and bone. Clin Cases Miner Bone Metab 2017;14:200–6.

100. Theuwissen E, Smit E, Vermeer C. The role of vitamin K in soft-tissue calcification. Adv Nutr 2012;3:166–73.

101. Azuma K, Inoue S. Multiple modes of vitamin K actions in aging-related musculoskeletal disorders. Int J Mol Sci 2019;20:2844.

102. El-Brashy AEWS, El-Tanawy RM, Hassan WA, et al. Potential role of vitamin K in radiological progression of early knee osteoarthritis patients. Egypt Rheumatol 2016;38:217–23.

103. Misra D, Booth SL, Tolstykh I, et al. Vitamin K deficiency is associated with incident knee osteoarthritis. Am J Med 2013;126:243–8.

104. Neogi T, Booth SL, Zhang YQ, et al. Low vitamin K status is associated with osteoarthritis in the hand and knee. Arthritis Rheum 2006;54:1255–61.

105. Oka H, Akune T, Muraki S, et al. Association of low dietary vitamin K intake with radiographic knee osteoarthritis in the Japanese elderly population: dietary survey in a population-based cohort of the ROAD study. J Orthop Sci 2009;14: 687–92.

106. Boer CG, Szilagyi I, Nguyen NL, et al. Vitamin K antagonist anticoagulant usage is associated with increased incidence and progression of osteoarthritis. Ann Rheum Dis 2021;80:589–604.

107. Neogi T, Felson DT, Sarno R, et al. Vitamin K in hand osteoarthritis: results from a randomised clinical trial. Ann Rheum Dis 2008;67:1570–3.

108. Fridovich I. Oxygen: how do we stand it? Med Princ Pract 2013;22:131–7.

109. Grover AK, Samson SE. Benefits of antioxidant supplements for knee osteoarthritis: rationale and reality. Nutr J 2016;15:1.

110. Clark AG, Rohrbaugh AL, Otterness I, et al. The effects of ascorbic acid on cartilage metabolism in Guinea pig articular cartilage explants. Matrix Biol 2002;21: 175–84.

111. Tiku ML, Shah R, Allison GT. Evidence linking chondrocyte lipid peroxidation to cartilage matrix protein degradation: possible role in cartilage aging and the pathogenesis of osteoarthritis. J Biol Chem 2000;275:20069–76.

112. Angthong C, Morales NP, Sutipornpalangkul W, et al. Can levels of antioxidants in synovial fluid predict the severity of primary knee osteoarthritis: a preliminary study. Springerplus 2013;2:652.

113. McAlindon TE, Jacques P, Zhang Y, et al. Do antioxidant micronutrients protect against the development and progression of knee osteoarthritis? Arthritis Rheum 1996;39:648–56.

114. Jensen NH. Reduced pain from osteoarthritis in hip joint or knee joint during treatment with calcium ascorbate. a randomised, placebo-controlled crossover trial in general practice. Ugeskr Laeger 2003;165:2563–6.

115. Tantavisut S, Tanavalee A, Honsawek S, et al. Effect of vitamin E on oxidative stress level in blood, synovial fluid, and synovial tissue in severe knee osteoarthritis: a randomised controlled study. BMC Musculoskelet Disord 2017;18:281.

116. Avery JC, Hoffmann PR. Selenium, selenoproteins, and immunity. Nutrients 2018;10:1203.

117. Zhao ZJ, Li Q, Yang PZ, et al. Selenium: a protective factor for Kaschin-beck disease in qing-tibet plateau. Biol Trace Elem Res 2013;153:1–4.

118. Yazar M, Sarban S, Kocyigit A, et al. Synovial fluid and plasma selenium, copper, zinc, and iron concentrations in patients with rheumatoid arthritis and osteoarthritis. Biol Trace Elem Res 2005;106:123–32.

119. Shi CH, Tian HL, Tian JH, et al. A Systematic review regarding the effects of different kinds of selenium supplementations on Kaschin-Beck Disease. Zhong hua Liu Xing Bing Xue Za Zhi 2013;34:507–14.

120. Baker JF, Byrne DP, Walsh PM, et al. Human chondrocyte viability after treatment with local anesthetic and/or magnesium: results from an in vitro study. Arthroscopy 2011;27:213–7.

121. Nielsen FH. Magnesium deficiency and increased inflammation: current perspectives. J Inflamm Res 2018;11:25–34.

122. Coşkun Benlidayı İ, Gökçen N, Sarpel T. Serum magnesium level is not associated with inflammation in patients with knee osteoarthritis. Turk J Phys Med Rehabil 2017;63:249–52.

123. Musik I, Kurzepa J, Luchowska-Kocot D, et al. Correlations among plasma silicon, magnesium and calcium in patients with knee osteoarthritis-analysis in consideration of gender. Ann Agric Environ Med 2019;26:97–102.

124. Hunter DJ, Hart D, Snieder H, et al. Evidence of altered bone turnover, vitamin D and calcium regulation with knee osteoarthritis in female twins. Rheumatology (Oxford) 2003;42:1311–6.

125. Zeng C, Wei J, Li H, et al. Relationship between serum magnesium concentration and radiographic knee osteoarthritis. J Rheumatol 2015;42:1231–6.

126. Qin B, Shi X, Samai PS, et al. Association of dietary magnesium intake with radiographic knee osteoarthritis: results from a population-based study. Arthritis Care Res (Hoboken) 2012;64:1306–11.

127. Braner A. Haemochromatosis and arthropathies. Dtsch Med Wochenschr 2018; 143:1167–73.

128. Kiely PD. Haemochromatosis arthropathy - a conundrum of the celtic curse. J R Coll Physicians Edinb 2018;48:233–8.

129. Simão M, Gavaia PJ, Camacho A, et al. Intracellular iron uptake is favored in Hfe-KO mouse primary chondrocytes mimicking an osteoarthritis-related phenotype. Biofactors 2019;45:583–97.

130. Camacho A, Simão M, Ea HK, et al. Iron overload in a murine model of hereditary hemochromatosis is associated with accelerated progression of osteoarthritis under mechanical stress. Osteoarthritis Cartilage 2016;24:494–502.

131. Milman NT, Schioedt FV, Junker AE, et al. Diagnosis and treatment of genetic HFE-Hemochromatosis: the Danish Aspect. Gastroenterol Res 2019;12:221–32.

132. Alshenibr W, Tashkandi MM, Alsaqer SF, et al. Anabolic role of lysyl oxidase like-2 in cartilage of knee and temporomandibular joints with osteoarthritis. Arthritis Res Ther 2017;19:179.
133. Medeiros DM. Copper, iron, and selenium dietary deficiencies negatively impact skeletal integrity: a review. Exp Biol Med (Maywood) 2016;241:1316–22.
134. Czlonkowska A, Litwin T, Dusek P, et al. Wilson disease. Nat Rev Dis Primers 2018;4:21.
135. Russell K, Gillanders LK, Orr DW, et al. Dietary copper restriction in Wilson's disease. Eur J Clin Nutr 2018;72:326–31.
136. Dai Z, Niu J, Zhang Y, et al. Dietary intake of fibre and risk of knee osteoarthritis in two US prospective cohorts. Ann Rheum Dis 2017;76:1411–9.
137. Dai Z, Lu N, Niu J, et al. Dietary fiber intake in relation to knee pain trajectory. Arthritis Care Res (Hoboken) 2017;69:1331–9.
138. Dai Z, Jafarzadeh SR, Niu J, et al. Body mass index mediates the association between dietary fiber and symptomatic knee osteoarthritis in the osteoarthritis initiative and the framingham osteoarthritis study. J Nutr 2018;148:1961–7.
139. Morales-Ivorra I, Romera-Baures M, Roman-Viñas B, et al. Osteoarthritis and the mediterranean diet: a systematic review. Nutrients 2018;10:1030.
140. Nüesch E, Dieppe P, Reichenbach S, et al. All cause and disease specific mortality in patients with knee or hip osteoarthritis: population based cohort study. BMJ 2011;342:d1165.
141. World Health Organization. Diet, nutrition, and the prevention of chronic diseases. World Health Organ Tech Rep Ser 2003;916(i-viii):1–149.
142. Funck-Brentano T, Nethander M, Movérare-Skrtic S, et al. Causal factors for knee, hip, and hand osteoarthritis: a mendelian randomization study in the UK Biobank. Arthritis Rheumatol 2019;71:1634–41.
143. Kuszewski JC, Wong RHX, Howe PRC. Fish oil supplementation reduces osteoarthritis-specific pain in older adults with overweight/obesity. Rheumatol Adv Pract 2020;4:rkaa036.
144. Liu X, Machado GC, Eyles JP, et al. Dietary supplements for treating osteoarthritis: a systematic review and meta-analysis. Br J Sports Med 2018;52:167–75.
145. Castrogiovanni P, Trovato FM, Loreto C, et al. Nutraceutical supplements in the management and prevention of osteoarthritis. Int J Mol Sci 2016;17:2042.

Towards a Communication Framework for Empowerment in Osteoarthritis Care

Naomi Simick Behera, MPhys[a],*, Samantha Bunzli, PhD[b]

KEYWORDS

- Osteoarthritis • Education • Communication • Empowerment

KEY POINTS

- Misconceptions and prominent discourses around osteoarthritis perpetuate beliefs that individuals have little control over their symptoms and depend on experts to fix their worn-out joints.
- Best practice guidelines recommend education as a first-line treatment for osteoarthritis and identify communication skills as a core clinical capability for health professionals involved in osteoarthritis care.
- Empowerment models in health communication and chronic disease are based on a clinician–patient partnership involving mutual behavior change and on prioritizing patient needs and preferences in an on-going cyclical pattern of education and action.
- There are no existing empowerment models or frameworks for osteoarthritis education or communication documented in literature.
- This narrative review identifies essential characteristics of an empowerment model in health, and proposes a framework for empowerment-based communication in osteoarthritis.

BACKGROUND

Osteoarthritis (OA) is one of the most prevalent chronic conditions and the leading cause of disability in older adults.[1] Affecting approximately 343 million people worldwide,[2] OA is a growing physical, psychological, and economic burden on individuals and health care systems worldwide.[1,3,4] The prevalence of OA continues to increase owing to the combined effects of an aging population, increasing obesity, a higher incidence of joint injuries, physical inactivity, and chronic stress.[1,4]

[a] University of Sydney, New South Wales, Australia; [b] Department of Surgery, The University of Melbourne, St Vincent's Hospital, Level 2, Clinical Sciences Building, 29 Regent St, Fitzroy, Victoria 3065, Australia
* Corresponding author. Kolling Institute, Level 10, Royal North Shore Hospital, Reserve Road, St Leonards, New South Wales 2065, Australia.
E-mail address: nsim2829@uni.sydney.edu.au

Clin Geriatr Med 38 (2022) 323–343
https://doi.org/10.1016/j.cger.2021.11.004
0749-0690/22/© 2021 Elsevier Inc. All rights reserved.
geriatric.theclinics.com

OA directly impedes healthy aging, which is a global priority.[5] The main symptom of OA is joint pain, which can lead to mobility restrictions with profound impacts on physical and psychosocial well-being.[6] People with OA often present with comorbidities like diabetes, heart disease, stroke, and depression[7] and have a shorter life expectancy (by 10 years) than those without OA.[8] Physical limitations also put people with OA at an increased risk of social isolation[6] and poorer mental health, with anxiety, depression, and psychological distress seen 1.3 times more commonly in people with OA than those without.[3,9] The burden of OA seems to disproportionately affect communities that are often already disempowered by other factors. Women are twice as likely to be affected by OA than men.[10] The prevalence of OA is greater and outcomes are poorer among those already disadvantaged by geography, socioeconomic status, and low health literacy levels, specifically those living in rural and remote areas.[10,11] People living in these disadvantaged communities often have less access to health care, a higher burden of comorbidities and greater risk factors for OA (eg, obesity, sedentary lifestyles, and older populations in rural areas).[10,11]

OA has historically been conceptualized as a degenerative joint disease associated with cartilage loss owing to mechanical wear and tear.[12] The history of OA is checkered with confusion with other forms of arthritis, and its very name is a misnomer because it implies an inflammatory process.[13] Although often described as wear and tear on the joint,[14–17] this description of OA as a passive erosion of the joint is inaccurate. Instead, evidence suggests that OA is an active, dynamic alteration of joint tissue caused by an imbalance between injury and repair.[12,18] The observation that pain severity is poorly associated with structural changes seen on imaging[18] has shifted the focus away from the articular cartilage alone; OA is now considered a complex whole person condition associated with comorbidities[7] and influenced by epigenetic factors,[19] psychosocial factors,[20] and the central nervous system.[21]

There is strong evidence that OA symptoms and disease risk are affected by modifiable biopsychosocial factors that can be within an individual's control.[20,22] Through weight management, maintaining a healthy diet, managing comorbidities (eg, diabetes, cardiovascular disease, and depression), modifying occupational stressors, and improving physical activity, strength, and fitness levels, people can gain control over their symptoms and live active, healthy lives with OA.[22] As such, contemporary best practice guidelines endorse a personalized holistic approach to OA management with education and self-management as the first lines of treatment, along with exercise and weight management where indicated.[23–25] Education in this context is defined as the provision of information or advice that is aimed at influencing the health-related knowledge, beliefs, perceptions, and self-management skills or behaviors of individuals.[26] The strategies used to connect to other people and provide information or advice are referred to as health communication.[27]

Evidence from western countries, including Australia, the UK, and the United States points to the underuse of recommended self-management and lifestyle modifications[28] with clinical decisions often favoring analgesia and surgery.[29] Widespread misconceptions about OA seem to play a role in treatment decision-making.[14] People commonly perceive a linear pathway from diagnosis to treatment to cure, and believe imaging is a prerequisite to enter this pathway.[30,31] However, imaging findings are poorly associated with pain severity and unnecessary joint imaging can lead to dependence on passive analgesic treatments and interventions purporting to reverse cartilage loss or damage, which have been shown to have no clinically meaningful benefits over placebo (eg, glucosamine, opioids, viscosupplements, electrotherapy, massage, and arthroscopy).[32,33] People commonly believe that exercise and activity will harm a joint that shows evidence of cartilage loss resulting in bone-on-bone changes, and the experience of joint pain during movement can lead to feelings of frustration (**Fig. 1**).[14,15] However, exercise has been found to be safe for people with OA[34] and is associated with a lower occurrence of OA.[35] Appropriately dosed exercise provides the mechanical loading required by the joint to prevent cartilage atrophy and can lead to improvements in pain, function, quality of life, depression, and self-efficacy.[34–37] The common belief that OA always follows a fixed downward trajectory leads to the assumption that the surgical replacement of worn-out joint is inevitable.[14] The dependence on passive interventions can leave people with OA feeling helpless and disempowered to control their symptoms.[15,16]

These misconceptions are perpetuated in part by the dominant narrative of OA. Discourse analyses exploring ways of talking about OA have exposed a strong impairment discourse.[17,38] According to this discourse, the body is viewed as an inert machine that wears out over time. The inevitable decline of the body is a normal process that one does not have the power to stop. By focusing on irreversible structural changes, the impairment discourse implies that the individuals cannot fix the diseased joint by themselves and that the only solution is to seek out an expert to repair or replace worn out joints (**Fig. 2**).[17] The impairment discourse characterizes clinicians as experts who know best and patients as passive recipients of prescribed health advice.[38] However, health information framed this way can lead to feelings of guilt among people are unable to, or choose not to, follow the advice.[39]

The dominant OA discourse contrasts with the shift in health communication away from impairment toward participation, as advocated by The International

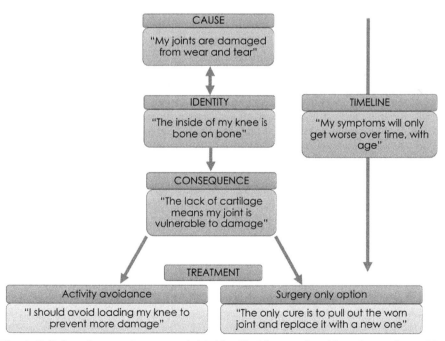

Fig. 1. Beliefs and perceptions around OA identified by people with end-stage knee OA. (*Adapted from* Bunzli S, O'Brien P, Ayton D, et al. Misconceptions and the Acceptance of Evidence-based Nonsurgical Interventions for Knee Osteoarthritis. A Qualitative Study. Clin Orthop Relat Res. 2019;477(9):1975-1983. https://doi.org/10.1097/CORR.0000000000000784; with permission)

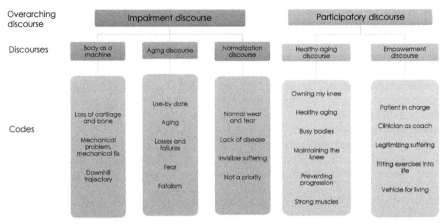

Fig. 2. Details of a discourse analysis in OA. (*Adapted from* Bunzli S, Taylor N, O'Brien P, et al. How Do People Communicate About Knee Osteoarthritis? A Discourse Analysis. Pain Med. 2021;22(5):1127-1148. https://doi.org/10.1093/pm/pnab012; with permission)

Classification of Functioning, Disability and Health (ICF). The ICF is a biopsychosocial framework for measuring health and disability that integrates medical and social models of health and disability.[40] According to the ICF, even in severe health conditions where there is a focus on curing disease, psychosocial and environmental factors remain important considerations. Participation (which is defined as "involvement in a life situation"), is the ultimate health outcome.[41] In the context of OA management, this focus on participation turns attention to what individuals can do despite OA, rather than what they are unable to do. According to the ICF, the role of the clinician is to empower individuals with strategies that support them to live active, engaged lives where possible, rather than only focusing on fixing the joint.

The paternalistic model of clinician knows best also contrasts with shifts toward an empowerment model of health education in the wider health communication literature. Empowering patients with the knowledge, skills, resources, and authority they require to make evidence-based decisions and get control over their symptoms is considered to be a fundamental component of chronic disease management.[42–45] The shift away from a paternalistic, didactic model of health education toward an empowerment model has been associated with improved health outcomes, including a decrease in the inappropriate use of medication, surgery, and diagnostics by 25% to 40%[46] and improved compliance with best practice by 33% to 60%.[47]

AIMS AND METHODS

A key objective of the clinical encounter for OA is to address misconceptions, promote healthy behaviors, and equip people with self-management strategies so they can get control over the symptoms and live active, healthy lives with OA. The core capability framework for health professionals involved in the clinical care of people with OA identifies communication as a key competency, but does not provide detail on how to convey information in a way that avoids jargon that perpetuates misconceptions, optimizes understanding and adapts communication styles to meet individual needs.[48] Indeed, many clinicians feel that they lack the skills to effectively communicate with people seeking care.[49,50] To build capabilities among clinicians, there is a need for a clinically useful OA communication framework.

To inform an empowerment-based communication framework for OA, the aim of this narrative review was to review empowerment models of health education. A literature search of electronic databases (MEDLINE, Scopus, CINAHL) was conducted to gain an overview of empowerment models of education in the wider health communication, aging, and chronic disease literature. Reference lists of seminal articles were also reviewed. From the retrieved models, essential characteristics were identified and potential application of these characteristics in the context of OA education were considered to inform a preliminary empowerment-based communication framework for OA.

WHAT IS EMPOWERMENT?

Empowerment is a complex construct and its meaning can vary from individual to individual and from one situation to another. It can be defined as a dynamic 2-way process that is an outcome of a partnership where individuals are enabled to change a situation through the sharing of knowledge, skills, resources and the authority to do so.

The individual seeking care has the power and freedom to make informed choices about their health and to accept responsibility for their actions.[42,43,51,52] Empowerment can be considered both a process as well as an outcome.[53] The process or outcome can be analyzed at 3 levels: individual, organizational, and community (**Fig. 3**).[54]

Although empowerment has its roots at the individual level, it is a mutual process and requires the active participation of all parties that can hinder or facilitate the process. In health, the 2 main requirements for the empowerment process to be set into motion are a clinician with a raised consciousness about the need to empower their patient and a patient who seeks to be empowered.[55]

Empowerment theory[54] suggests that people need opportunities to become active in shared decision-making to improve their lives, organizations, and communities. Even when wrong decisions are made, individuals can develop a sense of

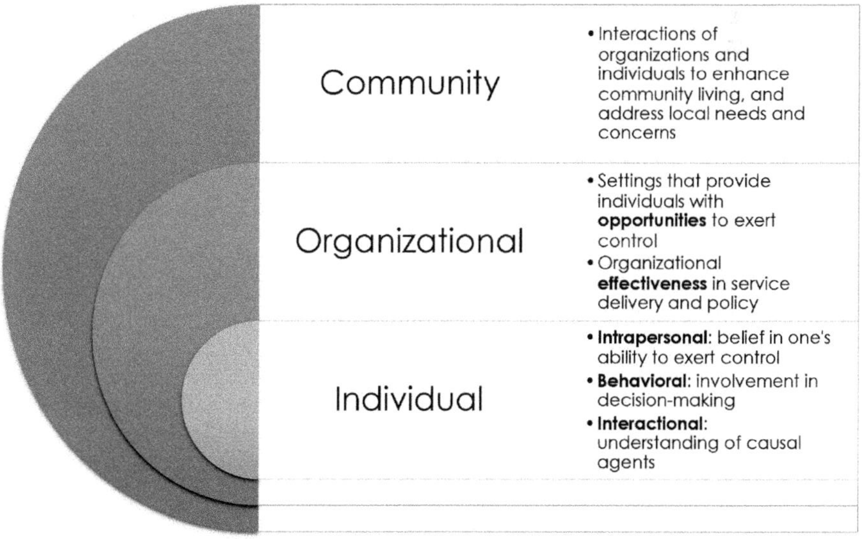

Fig. 3. Levels of empowerment according to Zimmerman's empowerment theory. (*Adapted from* Zimmerman M.A. (2000) Empowerment Theory. In: Rappaport J., Seidman E. (eds) Handbook of Community Psychology. Springer, Boston, MA. https://doi.org/10.1007/978-1-4615-4193-6_2; with permission)

empowerment by developing a greater understanding of the decision-making process, developing the confidence to make decisions that affect their lives, and communicating their concerns. Similarly, even in the absence of policy change, organizations and communities can be empowered by providing settings in which individuals can attempt to take control of their own lives. Individuals can empower communities by engaging in activities that maintain or improve their collective quality of life. Research that delves deeper into the contexts and processes in which empowerment takes place can assist in developing greater opportunities to help empowered and empowering systems flourish and grow.[53,54]

MODELS OF EMPOWERMENT IN HEALTH

Several models of empowerment can be identified in the health communication, aging, and chronic disease literature. **Table 1** presents an overview of these models and notes how they differ from the dominant traditional biomedical model that views disease from a medical or mechanistic angle focused on physical impairment.

Although empowerment research is nascent in the field of OA and empowerment models specific to the context of OA education are currently lacking, 2 recent studies have especially targeted empowerment in OA populations. Using a making, telling, and enacting framework of participatory action research to empower women with hand OA, Flinn and colleagues[56] conceived an innovative adaptive equipment design and generated new ideas to overcome functional challenge. More recently, Egerton and colleagues[57] developed a brief video of empowering education that enabled people with knee OA to construct their own understanding of health and disease as active participants in communication with choice and individual perspectives. The researchers found that the video could provide positive messaging, improve knowledge and lead to the adoption of intentions to self-manage knee OA.[57]

PRINCIPLES OF EMPOWERMENT

Based on the theories, frameworks and models presented in this article, key characteristics of empowerment approaches that set them apart from the traditional models of health communication and care can be identified. Each of these characteristics is explained in this section.

Empowerment Is Active and Intentional

Empowerment is a process that is initiated and sustained by individuals who seek power or self-determination—others, such as clinicians, can only aid in this process.[55] Patients themselves can shift the balance of power from being passive receivers of help (the clinician knows best) to active agents in the management of their own care.[55] This process also involves the active participation of informed, motivated clinicians and health settings that make a deliberate decision to put patient needs front and center.[58] In OA, the prevalent impairment discourse and misconceptions surrounding OA such as, "I need an expert to fix my worn out joint,"[14–16] can make it hard for people to realize that they can seek and attain power in this situation. Clinicians, therefore, play a crucial role in creating awareness among people with OA that they can be empowered in the management of their own care.

Empowerment Is Individual

An empowerment approach pivots around the individual's goals and issues of concern. These issues can vary from one individual to the next and, therefore, requires a sensitivity to each situation and the resources to customize education delivery for

Table 1			
An overview of empowerment models in chronic disease and health communication			
Empowerment Model	**Model Focus/Target Group**	**Key Concepts**	**Differences From Traditional Biomedical Model**
EMPATHiE model[60]	Older people with chronic conditions	Considers empowerment at 3 levels—micro (individual, center), meso (local, regional, national), and macro (high-level policy at national or international level)	Requires behavior shift in both patients and health professionals
Kayser etal. (2014, 2019) Country: Denmark		Identifies 3 main dimensions of patient empowerment strategies: Education, information provision and health literacy interventions— self-management Joint decision-making	Prioritizes well-being over traditional clinical outcomes
Chronic care model[74,75] Funnel and Anderson (1991, 2004) Country: United States of America	Diabetes education and self-management	Involves a 5-step protocol for behavior change toward empowerment in diabetes Step I: Explore the Problem or Issue (Past) Step II: Clarify Feelings and Meaning (Present) Step III: Develop a Plan (Future) —Long and short term Step IV: Commit to Action (Future) Step V: Experience and Evaluate the Plan (Future)	Listening is as important as offering advice in health education Clinician as coach or partner in the care process Patient as primary decision-maker

(continued on next page)

			Differences From
Empowerment Model	**Model Focus/Target Group**	**Key Concepts**	**Traditional Biomedical Model**
Ongoing diabetes self-management support interventions Tang et al,[70] 2005 Country: United States	Diabetes education and self-management	Presents a framework for clinicians to empower patients composed of 5 components: 1. Reflecting on relevant experiences 2. Discussing the emotional impacts of living with the condition 3. Engaging in systematic problem solving of issues that are relevant and meaningful to the individual 4. Answering questions about the condition and its management 5. Choosing a self-management experiment or strategy to achieve one of their short-term goals	Patient centered rather than content based Community rather than clinic based On-going process of education that re-evaluates outcomes and modifies the next cycle according to patient needs
Languages of empowerment and strengths Greene et al,[64] 2005 Country: United States	Clinical social work	An empowerment framework of clinical language to identify and amplify existing patient strengths, competencies, assets, resources and personal agency comprising: Language of collaboration in place of the language of help Language of ownership that allows the possibility for the client to be the source for change	Goes beyond patient deficiencies, inadequacies and pathology to accessing, the creative, resourceful parts of themselves

Table 1 (continued)

(continued on next page)

Empowerment Model	Model Focus/Target Group	Key Concepts	Differences From Traditional Biomedical Model
Table 1 *(continued)*			
		Language of possibilities that positively reframes reality to include more alternatives and perceive challenges as being resources rather than deficits	
		Language of solutions, shifting from problem-talk to solution-talk	
		Language of elaboration and clarification to encourage the speaker to consider if their language is limiting them from discovering resources and options and work toward effective interventions	
Chronic care model McCorkle et al,[45] 2011 Country: USA	Self-management in people with cancer and their families	A cyclic empowerment model for the cancer care continuum from treatment to end of life that includes: Patient–provider partnerships Productive interactions Mutually determined care plan, including self-management Goal setting Self-management interventions Goal attainment	Patient–provider relationships fostered through partnerships Individual's management preferences are prioritized— changes in priorities are respected

each person.[59] This practice is particularly important to ensure that people with different health literacy levels or those from diverse linguistic backgrounds are not left behind. It also fits with best practice guidelines in OA that recommend individualized, patient-centered care.[25] Modifiable biopsychosocial factors implicated in the pain experience are unique to each individual and warrant the use of management strategies that are in accordance with individual preferences, habits, environment, history, and overall health condition.[22]

Empowerment Is Mutual

Empowerment-based education involves a process of teaching and learning and involves an interdependent relationship between clinician and client. It fosters the development of health literacy, both among clinicians as well as the people that they serve.[60] People seeking care are empowered with evidence-based knowledge to meet their health needs and clinicians are empowered with accurate knowledge about the individual, their story, and their circumstances, which then offers a framework to interpret clinical findings and find the right course of management for that individual.[61] This finding highlights the need to shift from paternalistic communication methods and a didactic, 1-way education delivery in OA, for the empowerment of both the clinician and the patient.

Empowerment Is about Choice and Responsibility

Although freedom of choice seems to indicate power and opportunity for the patient in their own health care, when patients are insufficiently informed or supported about the actual benefits, limitations, possibilities, and consequences, the ability to make a choice loses its significance. Freedom without knowledge disempowers patients, rather than empowering them to make evidence-based decisions about their health.[62] In the context of OA, the overuse of low-value care (including passive treatments like analgesia and surgery for inappropriate candidates) by both patients and clinicians has been well-documented.[29,63] Education that empowers, produces informed, self-aware individuals who are able and motivated to take action in daily life to the extent that they wish to do so.[64] With the power to choose comes responsibility. The empowerment approach recognizes the rights of the individual to be involved in their health decisions, but also realizes that they must accept responsibility for their health choices and behaviors.[65] Empowerment results in a sense of personal agency that replaces learned helplessness.[64] This new sense of ownership is demonstrated in the individual, organization, or community's ability to accept responsibility for the actions they take.

Empowerment Requires Critical Thinking

Critical consciousness is a basic outcome of empowerment. It is the process by which people acquire a greater understanding of themselves and the organizational, cultural, and social conditions that shape their lives and affect their ability to create change.[66] Successful empowerment interventions enable people to improve their knowledge, change their outlook on themselves and their world, and feel confident to question the status quo.[66] This process often begins by building self-efficacy for the individual, and ultimately progresses to taking community action, for example, working together to share accurate information and build support systems.[67] For coconstructive change to occur in patients and clinicians, new ideas and information need to be presented as food for thought to be discussed and considered in dialogue with each other.[68] In the context of OA, misconceptions are widespread and have been reinforced by clinicians, family, friends, and the media.[15,65] Questioning these beliefs, which are often deeply engrained, is challenging, but essential for empowerment to be achieved.

Empowerment Is Multidimensional

Empowerment is a multidimensional construct that needs to occur at the individual, organizational, and community levels to be truly successful.[67] Although empowerment stimulates a sense of personal control, it also creates a sense of power at the communal or collective levels.[53] Activated and empowered community members not only participate more, but feel confident to take on leadership roles to drive positive change in their own lives and in the community.[67] Likewise, empowerment at the individual level would not be sustainable without resource mobilization and participatory opportunities at the organizational level, or without a sociopolitical structure and social culture that did not support empowerment.[54] For example, community-based management strategies like education in a community setting and social support have been seen to reinforce positive health behaviors and improve compliance in OA management,[69] thereby enabling individuals to be more in control of their disease.

Empowerment Is Constant and On-going

The process of empowerment does not follow a linear path, but is organic and cyclical,[70,71] reflecting the changing needs and challenges faced by the individual. Clinical discourses and therapeutic conversations need to be modified to continue this adapting, coconstructing process of empowerment.[64] OA is a chronic condition that is experienced over a long period of time in the changing contexts of an individual's life.[18,20] Beliefs about OA (of patients and clinicians) are constantly updated and may vary at different time points, resulting in different behavioral responses and management choices.[72,73] The empowerment process, therefore, goes beyond the successful delivery of knowledge and information and needs to keep up with these changing conditions.

PROPOSED FRAMEWORK FOR EMPOWERMENT IN OSTEOARTHRITIS PRACTICE

Models of empowerment have been proposed and used in various fields of health and chronic disease to guide empowerment-based communication, education and interventions, however such models are lacking in the field of OA. Drawing on the key principles of empowerment identified elsewhere in this article, in this section, we propose a preliminary empowerment framework on which communication in OA may be structured to enable to shift from a traditional, didactic format to one that empowers individuals and communities with OA. This proposed framework comprises of 3 main domains that each have a strong participatory theme (**Fig. 4**). These domains are described, supported by a clinical application guide containing discussion prompts (**Table 2**).

Past: "What Is This Person's Story?"

This domain involves the patient and the clinician working together to identify the problem from the patient's perspective and gain an understanding of it. It involves looking at the issue at hand through a historical lens, discovering the origin story of the problem, the ways it has impacted life, and the levels of disempowerment that have been faced by the individual. Looking at the past should also aim to investigate how the individual has adapted and coped with the stresses of OA in the past and what has made them resilient, as this is the foundation for building empowerment and self-efficacy. Furthermore, it is important to understand what beliefs are harbored by patients and clinicians that could facilitate or hinder the process of empowerment.

Present: "How Does This Person Make Sense of Their Osteoarthritis?"

Reflecting on the present involves asking, answering, and discussing questions that are relevant to the current issues faced by the patient. It is important to understand how the patient's present health status, socioeconomic background, ethnicity, culture, competence, environment, and motivations affect their experience of OA. Identifying and

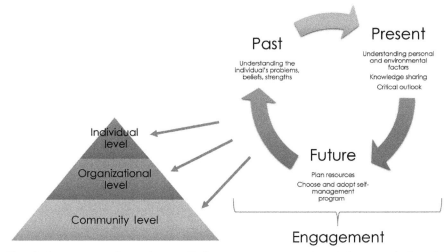

Fig. 4. A representation of a preliminary empowerment-based framework for OA communication.

coming to terms with the factors that promote disempowerment, without being judgmental of them, can be confronting, but is critical to moving ahead. Instead of using a didactic approach, individuals should be invited to ask questions to clarify knowledge about OA and share what that knowledge means to them. It is critical to understand what empowerment means to the patient and what level of empowerment they are ready and willing to work toward. Clinicians need to ensure that they are armed with evidence-based information and be able to present facts and explanations that are relevant to the immediate needs of the patient (**Box 1**). The present needs to be viewed through a critical lens, taking into account the facts as they stand, but ready to question the status quo. This process can be challenging for both the patient and the clinician, and so needs to be approached with patience and an open mind.

Future: "How Can This Person Be Empowered to Live Well with Osteoarthritis?"

The next phase comprises collaboratively devising a plan, tools, and strategies to tackle the challenges and reach the goals identified. The construction of resources should draw and build on the resources, both internal and external, that already exist in the patient's life and environment. This process of dialogue and collaborative planning culminates in the adoption of a self-management experiment that is most relevant to the patient and their personal goals. A culture of questioning and reflection is maintained throughout, to ensure knowledge has the opportunity to expand at all points and the that plan is able to be modified to suit the best interests of the patient and the clinical relationship. Moving into the future also involves going beyond the individual level of empowerment to the organizational and community levels.

This process does not end here, but circles back to reflection on the past (evaluating the strategies and self-management experiment undertaken), the present (the results of the changes on the individual's current condition and what that means to them), and further planning for the future.[70,74]

CHALLENGES TO EMPOWERMENT EDUCATION AND DIRECTIONS FOR FUTURE RESEARCH

Sometimes patients may choose to decline power and transfer it back to the clinician for a more directive or prescriptive approach.[75] Empowerment education respects

Table 2
Clinical application of the OA communication framework

Framework Domain	Overarching Question	Discussion Prompts	Application
Past	What is this person's story?	What has it been like living with OA? What has it been like to live with the physical impact of OA? What has it been like to live with the emotional impact of OA? How have you coped with the impacts of OA? Why? What has worked well? Why do you think this? What treatments have you taken part in? How did it go? What did you learn?	This information is gathered overtime, with more meaningful knowledge surfacing as the therapeutic alliance develops and health/life conditions evolve. This information changes with changing beliefs, life and health situations. Clinician empowerment affects how this knowledge is interpreted and used to aid clinical decisions
Present	How does this person make sense of their OA?	What does having OA mean to you? Can you explain to me what OA is? Why do you think this? What do you think causes your symptoms? Why do you think this? What do you think the future looks like for you? Why do you think this?	The clinician listens for gaps in understanding that need to be filled or misconceptions that need to be addressed. The person's understanding of any jargon they use, for example, "degeneration" or "bone on bone" should be explored. Filling gaps in understanding/ addressing misconceptions can be done through various modes of education delivery (verbal/pictorial/ written material/ multimedia/behavioral experimentation) are trialed and evaluated for greatest impact on the individual. Discussions and feedback are the mainstay of delivering new information and advice.

(continued on next page)

Table 2
(continued)

Framework Domain	Overarching Question	Discussion Prompts	Application
Future	How can this person be empowered to live well with OA?	What are the things you love doing in life? What will it take to get you doing the things you love? What are some steps you could take? What support do you need to take these steps? How will you know if you have succeeded? When are you going to take these steps? What will you do when you leave here today?	Management strategies are decided on collaboratively after all options have been discussed. A plan is developed and resources are cultivated in partnership with the individual seeking care. The aim of adopting management strategies is to enable the person with OA to reach their goals and participate in meaningful activities through self-efficacy and the ability to self-manage.

that the choice to decline or delay power is also a choice that the patient has the right to exercise. Responsibility for choices made and their consequences ultimately lie with the individual.[75] Although the individual's values and beliefs need to be taken into consideration, clinicians need to be aware that patients can sometimes make injudicious choices that may result in overuse of health care or declining a beneficial intervention.[76] In most cases, it is appropriate for clinicians to attempt to persuade competent individuals and give them opportunities to reconsider their choices. The meaning of these decisions should be explored with the individual, keeping their beliefs and value system in clear sight, so as not to confuse their philosophy with irrationality.[75]

The presence of illness, impairments, socioeconomic, language, and cultural barriers can often make it hard for the patient to participate in the decision-making process.[77] For example, someone with distressing levels of pain may simply want to be told what to do to find some relief instead of sitting down with a clinician to reflect on and discuss their condition. Where barriers cannot be addressed by the clinician (eg, by decreasing pain levels, arranging for language or culturally appropriate support), it is important to respect the individual's position and continue to look for ways to support them.

Box 1
Example explanation of OA

OA is a condition that makes your joints hurt, but it actually affects, and is affected by, your general health and lifestyle factors, such as physical activity, diet, stress, and sleep. The good news is that we can support you to get control over these. By making some changes, you may find your symptoms improve over time. In particular, through exercising and maintaining a healthy weight, you can improve your general health as well as the health of your joints. You can become stronger and cope better with your symptoms so you can do more of the activities that you love. How do you feel about this?

Health professionals themselves may not attempt to engage patients in the self-management process owing to barriers like time and knowledge. The empowerment process may be perceived by clinicians to be time consuming and, therefore, impractical. Many clinicians may worry that an empowerment approach can disengage patients by challenging their expectations about the care they will receive.[77] This point calls into question the structuring of clinical training and care provision. The transition from an outdated biomedical model to empowerment-based communication needs to be introduced at the rudimentary training levels for all clinicians involved in OA care (**Table 3**). Future research is needed to inform how clinicians deliver adaptable, individualized empowerment-based approaches and communication strategies in the context of OA care. However, upskilling clinicians in patient empowerment is not enough. Clinicians need to be able to reflect on their own biases and clinical culture that could be hindering the sharing of power and authority. Importantly, making resources available to clinicians to undertake this process is key to success, for example, by putting funding models in place to support empowerment and disincentivize low-value care and compliance-oriented models. It is important to note that, even among people with advanced OA who require surgical intervention, these principles of empowerment still apply. Surgical candidates can be empowered during

Table 3
A shift toward empowerment-based communication in OA care

Traditional Education Model	Empowerment-Based Communication Model
1. OA is a physical illness.	1. OA is a complex biopsychosocial condition.
2. The clinician is viewed as the teacher and problem solver, and responsible for outcomes.	2. The person with OA is viewed as problem solver and self- manager. The clinician acts as a resource and shares responsibility for outcomes.
3. The relationship between clinician and patient is authoritarian and based on clinician expertise.	3. The relationship between clinician and patient is an equal partnership based on shared expertise.
4. Learning needs are usually identified by the professional.	4. Problems and learning needs are identified by participants.
5. Education is primarily didactic.	5. Patient experiences and emotional impacts of the disease are used as learning opportunities for problem. Patients are encouraged to think critically about information.
6. Goals and action plans are used to help patients reach recommended targets.	6. Goals and action plans are codesigned to help individuals reach self-selected goals.
7. Behavioral strategies are externally motivated and are used to increase compliance with recommended treatments.	7. Individuals are coached to adopt behavioral strategies to enable them to change behaviors that are meaningful to them.
8. The goal of education is compliance and adherence with recommendations.	8. The goal is to enable patients to make informed choices.
9. Not achieving goals is viewed as a failure on the part of patient and clinician.	9. Not achieving goals is viewed as feedback and informs the modification of future goals and action plans.

Adapted from Funnell M, Anderson R. Patient Co-operation and Empowerment. *Treatment Strategies - Diabetes 2011*, 98-103.

the decision-making process, in preparation for surgery, and postoperatively to promote participation in valued life activities.[78]

Finally, empowerment is hard to quantify, making it difficult to evaluate the effectiveness of empowerment-based approaches. As this review has highlighted, empowerment is a multidimensional construct and it can be problematic to adequately capture multiple domains in a single snapshot.[79] Arvidsson and colleagues[80] modified a diabetes empowerment scale to be relevant for rheumatic disease covering factors like goal achievement, self-knowledge, stress management, readiness to change, and support. A recent Empowerment Score attempted to quantify the empowerment an individual feels by asking them questions around choice, values, and social norms on a topic.[81] To date, no measure of empowerment has been validated in the context of OA. To determine how to assess empowerment as an outcome, future research is needed to define what empowerment in OA means to patients, clinicians, and other key stakeholders. The effect of empowerment on specific outcomes needs to be clearly articulated for it to be acceptable and meaningful to patients and clinicians to adopt.

For empowerment approaches to be sustainable in the clinical environment, clinicians need to be supported to be empowered in their own personal and professional roles to set it in motion and keep it going. What changes are required in clinical culture, health policy, and community mindsets needs to be investigated. Patients, too, need to be supported to become active participants and informed consumers, and further research is required to understand how this can be done most efficiently. The ultimate outcome of empowerment is to create agents of change within health systems and communities. Further research is required to determine what changes are needed at individual, organizational and community levels to aid individuals and collectives to be empowered to engage in transformative action and drive change.[82]

SUMMARY

Empowerment is a complex multidimensional concept that is essential for long-term self-management in OA. Although future research is needed to better understand empowerment and the implementation of empowerment-based communication in the context of OA care, the proposed empowerment framework may function as a preliminary guide for clinicians to shift away from the traditional passive approach focused on fixing OA toward an approach that empowers people to live active, healthy lives with OA.

CLINICS CARE POINTS

- Clinicians play a crucial role in communicating to people with OA about their ability to be empowered to take control of their symptoms and live healthy lives with OA

- A communication framework is needed to assist clinicians empower people with OA.

- Based on existing empowerment models in the wider health communication and chronic disease literature, empowerment can be characterized as intentional, individualized, mutual, multidimensional, on-going, and involving critical thinking, choice, and responsibility.

- A preliminary empowerment-based framework for communication in OA is proposed consisting of 3 main domains (past, present and future) that span across 3 levels (individual, organizational, community).

- Future research is needed to define what empowerment in OA means to individuals and communities, to clearly articulate the effect of empowerment on meaningful outcomes and specify what changes are required in community mindsets, clinical culture and health policy to achieve empowerment in OA.

DISCLOSURE

The authors declare no conflicts of interest and no funding source.

REFERENCES

1. Hunter DJ, Bierma-Zeinstra S. Osteoarthritis. Lancet 2019;393(10182):1745–59.
2. Chronic Diseases and Health Promotion. World Health Organisation. 2020. Available at: http://www.who.int/chp/topics/rheumatic/en/. Accessed September 24, 2021.
3. Sharma A, Kudesia P, Shi Q, et al. Anxiety and depression in patients with osteoarthritis: impact and management challenges. Open Access Rheumatol 2016;8: 103–13.
4. Osteoarthritis. Australian Institute of Health and Welfare. Cat. no. PHE 232 Web site.. 2020. Available at: https://www.aihw.gov.au/reports/chronic-musculoskeletal-conditions/osteoarthritis. Accessed September 24, 2021.
5. World Health Organization. (2015). World report on ageing and health. World Health Organization. Available at: https://apps.who.int/iris/handle/10665/186463.
6. Hunter DJ, Schofield D, Callander E. The individual and socioeconomic impact of osteoarthritis. Nat Rev Rheumatol 2014;10(7):437–41.
7. Swain S, Sarmanova A, Coupland C, et al. Comorbidities in osteoarthritis: a systematic review and meta-analysis of observational studies. Arthritis Care Res (Hoboken) 2020;72(7):991–1000.
8. Nüesch E, Dieppe P, Reichenbach S, et al. All cause and disease specific mortality in patients with knee or hip osteoarthritis: population based cohort study. BMJ 2011;342:d1165.
9. Stubbs B, Aluko Y, Myint PK, et al. Prevalence of depressive symptoms and anxiety in osteoarthritis: a systematic review and meta-analysis. Age Ageing 2016; 45(2):228–35.
10. Australian Institute of Health and Welfare 2021. Australian Burden of Disease Study: impact and causes of illness and death in Australia 2018. Australian Burden of Disease Study series no. 23. Cat. no. BOD 29. Canberra: AIHW.
11. Callahan LF, Cleveland RJ, Allen KD, et al. Racial/ethnic, socioeconomic, and geographic disparities in the epidemiology of knee and hip osteoarthritis. Rheum Dis Clin North Am 2021;47(1):1–20.
12. Dobson GP, Letson HL, Grant A, et al. Defining the osteoarthritis patient: back to the future. Osteoarthritis Cartilage 2018;26(8):1003–7.
13. Dequeker J, Luyten FP. The history of osteoarthritis-osteoarthrosis. Ann Rheum Dis 2008;67(1):5–10.
14. Bunzli S, O'Brien P, Ayton D, et al. Misconceptions and the acceptance of evidence-based nonsurgical interventions for knee osteoarthritis. A qualitative study. Clin Orthop Relat Res 2019;477(9):1975–83.
15. Darlow B, Brown M, Thompson B, et al. Living with osteoarthritis is a balancing act: an exploration of patients' beliefs about knee pain. BMC Rheumatol 2018; 2(1):15.
16. Wallis J, Taylor N, Bunzli S, et al. Experience of living with knee osteoarthritis: a systematic review of qualitative studies. BMJ Open 2019;9:e030060.
17. Bunzli S, Taylor N, O'Brien P, et al. How do people communicate about knee osteoarthritis? A discourse analysis. Pain Med 2021;22(5):1127–48.
18.. Hunter DJ, Pietro-Alhambra D, Arden N. Osteoarthritis: the facts. 2nd edition. Oxford: Oxford University Press; 2014.

19. Fathollahi A, Aslani S, Jamshidi A, et al. Epigenetics in osteoarthritis: novel spotlight. J Cell Physiol 2019;234(8):12309–24.
20. Hunt MA, Birmingham TB, Skarakis-Doyle E, et al. Towards a biopsychosocial framework of osteoarthritis of the knee. Disabil Rehabil 2008;30(1):54–61.
21. Murphy S, Phillips K, Williams D, et al. The role of the central nervous system in osteoarthritis pain and implications for rehabilitation. Curr Rheumatol Rep 2012;14:576–82.
22. Georgiev T, Angelov AK. Modifiable risk factors in knee osteoarthritis: treatment implications. Rheumatol Int 2019;39(7):1145–57.
23. Guideline for the management of knee and hip osteoarthritis. 2018. Published 2nd edition.
24. 45 Clinical Guideline C. National Institute for Health and Clinical Excellence: Guidance. In: Osteoarthritis: care and management in adults. London: National Institute for Health and Care Excellence
25. Bannuru RR, Osani MC, Vaysbrot EE, et al. OARSI guidelines for the non-surgical management of knee, hip, and polyarticular osteoarthritis. Osteoarthritis Cartilage 2019;27(11):1578–89.
26. Catford J, Nutbeam D. Towards a definition of health education and health promotion. Health Educ J 1984;43(2–3):38.
27. Ishikawa H, Kiuchi T. Health literacy and health communication. Biopsychosoc Med 2010;4(1):18.
28. Paskins Z, Sanders T, Hassell AB. Comparison of patient experiences of the osteoarthritis consultation with GP attitudes and beliefs to OA: a narrative review. BMC Fam Pract 2014;15(1):46.
29. Healey EL, Afolabi EK, Lewis M, et al. Uptake of the NICE osteoarthritis guidelines in primary care: a survey of older adults with joint pain. BMC Musculoskelet Disord 2018;19(1):295.
30. Hunter DJ, Neogi T, Hochberg MC. Quality of osteoarthritis management and the need for reform in the US. Arthritis Care Res (Hoboken) 2011;63(1):31–8.
31. Sherman SL, Gulbrandsen TR, Lewis HA, et al. Overuse of magnetic resonance imaging in the diagnosis and treatment of moderate to severe osteoarthritis. Iowa Orthop J 2018;38:33–7.
32. Hunter DJ. Osteoarthritis: time for us all to shift the needle. Rheumatology (Oxford) 2018;57(suppl_4):iv1–2.
33. Caneiro JP, O'Sullivan PB, Roos EM, et al. Three steps to changing the narrative about knee osteoarthritis care: a call to action. Br J Sports Med 2020;54(5):256–8.
34. Raposo F, Ramos M, Lúcia Cruz A. Effects of exercise on knee osteoarthritis: A systematic review [published online ahead of print, 2021 Mar 5]. Musculoskeletal Care; 2021. https://doi.org/10.1002/msc.1538.
35. Alentorn-Geli E, Samuelsson K, Musahl V, et al. The association of recreational and competitive running with hip and knee osteoarthritis: a systematic review and meta-analysis. J Orthop Sports Phys Ther 2017;47(6):373–90.
36. Hurley M, Dickson K, Hallett R, et al. Exercise interventions and patient beliefs for people with hip, knee or hip and knee osteoarthritis: a mixed methods review. Cochrane Database Syst Rev 2018;4(4):Cd010842.
37. Hunter DJ, Eckstein F. Exercise and osteoarthritis. J Anat 2009;214(2):197–207.
38. Dixon-Woods M. Writing wrongs? An analysis of published discourses about the use of patient information leaflets. Soc Sci Med 2001;52(9):1417–32.
39. Mackintosh N. Self-empowerment in health promotion: a realistic target? Br J Nurs 1995;4(21):1273–8.

40. The ICF: an overview. Available at: https://www.wcpt.org/sites/wcpt.org/files/files/GHICF_overview_FINAL_for_WHO.pdf. Accessed September 24, 2021.

41. Whiteneck G, Dijkers MP. Difficult to measure constructs: conceptual and methodological issues concerning participation and environmental factors. Arch Phys Med Rehabil 2009;90(11 Suppl):S22–35.

42. Rodwell CM. An analysis of the concept of empowerment. J Adv Nurs 1996;23(2):305–13.

43. Pigg K. Three faces of empowerment: expanding the theory of empowerment in community development. Community Development 2002;33:107–23.

44. Ancheta MC, Basatan TN, Maskay GP. Theory of Mutual Empowerment. TIJ's Research Journal of Social Science & Management - RJSSM 2014;4(3):105–8.

45. McCorkle R, Ercolano E, Lazenby M, et al. Self-management: enabling and empowering patients living with cancer as a chronic illness. CA Cancer J Clin 2011;61(1):50–62.

46. Sypes EE, de Grood C, Whalen-Browne L, et al. Engaging patients in de-implementation interventions to reduce low-value clinical care: a systematic review and meta-analysis. BMC Med 2020;18(1):116.

47. Couët N, Desroches S, Robitaille H, et al. Assessments of the extent to which health-care providers involve patients in decision making: a systematic review of studies using the OPTION instrument. Health Expect 2015;18(4):542–61.

48. Hinman RS, Allen KD, Bennell KL, et al. Development of a core capability framework for qualified health professionals to optimise care for people with osteoarthritis: an OARSI initiative. Osteoarthritis Cartilage 2020;28(2):154–66.

49. Egerton T, Nelligan RK, Setchell J, et al. General practitioners' views on managing knee osteoarthritis: a thematic analysis of factors influencing clinical practice guideline implementation in primary care. BMC Rheumatol 2018;2(1):30.

50. Briggs AM, Houlding E, Hinman RS, et al. Health professionals and students encounter multi-level barriers to implementing high-value osteoarthritis care: a multi-national study. Osteoarthritis Cartilage 2019;27(5):788–804.

51. Feste C, Anderson RM. Empowerment: from philosophy to practice. Patient Educ Couns 1995;26(1–3):139–44.

52. Virtanen H, Leino-Kilpi H, Salanterä S. Empowering discourse in patient education. Patient Educ Couns 2007;66(2):140–6.

53. Perkins DD, Zimmerman MA. Empowerment theory, research, and application. Am J Community Psychol 1995;23(5):569–79.

54. Zimmerman M. Empowerment theory. In: Rappaport J, ES, editors. Handbook of community psychology. Boston (MA): Springer; 2000.

55. Lee JA. The Empowerment Approach to Social Work Practice. 6th edition ed. New York: Columbia University Press; 1994.

56. Flinn SR, Sanders EB, Yen WT, et al. Empowering elderly women with osteoarthritis through hands-on exploration of adaptive equipment concepts. Occup Ther Int 2013;20(4):163–72.

57. Egerton T, McLachlan L, Graham B, et al. How do people with knee pain from osteoarthritis respond to a brief video delivering empowering education about the condition and its management? Patient Educ Couns 2021;104(8):2018–27.

58. Lord J, Hutchison P. The process of empowerment: implications for theory and practice. 2006.

59. Marcus C. Strategies for improving the quality of verbal patient and family education: a review of the literature and creation of the EDUCATE model. Health Psychol Behav Med 2014;2(1):482–95.
60. Kayser L, Karnoe A, Duminski E, et al. A new understanding of health related empowerment in the context of an active and healthy ageing. BMC Health Serv Res 2019;19(1):242.
61. Goodyear-Smith F, Buetow S. Power issues in the doctor-patient relationship. Health Care Anal 2001;9(4):449–62.
62. Nordgren L. Mostly empty words – what the discourse of 'choice' in health care does. J Health Organ Manag 2010;24:109–26.
63. Dhawan A, Mather RC 3rd, Karas V, et al. An epidemiologic analysis of clinical practice guidelines for non-arthroplasty treatment of osteoarthritis of the knee. Arthroscopy 2014;30(1):65–71.
64. Greene GJ, Lee MY, Hoffpauir S. The languages of empowerment and strengths in clinical social work: a constructivist perspective. Families Soc 2005;86(2):267–77.
65. Swire-Thompson B, Lazer D. Public health and online misinformation: challenges and recommendations. Annu Rev Public Health 2020;41:433–51.
66. Freire PRMB. Pedagogy of the oppressed. 1970.
67. Wiggins N. Popular education for health promotion and community empowerment: a review of the literature. Health Promot Int 2012;27(3):356–71.
68. Lax W. Postmodern thinking in a clinical practice. In: McNamee S, Gergen KJ, editors. Therapy as social construction. Newbury Park (CA): Sage; 1993. p. 69–85.
69. Ali S, Kokorelias K, Macdermid J, et al. Education and social support as key factors in osteoarthritis management programs: a scoping review. Arthritis 2018;2018:1–8.
70. Tang T, Gillard M, Funnell M, et al. Developing a new generation of ongoing diabetes self-management support interventions: a preliminary report. Diabetes Educ 2005;31:91–7.
71. Chen J, Mullins CD, Novak P, et al. Personalized strategies to activate and empower patients in health care and reduce health disparities. Health Educ Behav 2016;43(1):25–34.
72. Caneiro JP, Bunzli S, O'Sullivan P. Beliefs about the body and pain: the critical role in musculoskeletal pain management. Braz J Phys Ther 2021;25(1):17–29.
73. Bunzli S, Smith A, Schütze R, et al. Making sense of low back pain and pain-related fear. J Orthop Sports Phys Ther 2017;47(9):628–36.
74. Funnell MM, Anderson RM. Empowerment and self-management of diabetes. Clin Diabetes 2004;22(3):123.
75. Funnell MM, Anderson RM, Arnold MS, et al. Empowerment: an idea whose time has come in diabetes education. Diabetes Educ 1991;17(1):37–41.
76. Brock DW, Wartman SA. When competent patients make irrational choices. N Engl J Med 1990;322(22):1595–9.
77. Scott IA, Elshaug AG, Fox M. Low value care is a health hazard that calls for patient empowerment. Med J Aust 2021;215(3):101–3.e1.
78. Klem NR, Smith A, O'Sullivan P, et al. What influences patient satisfaction after TKA? A qualitative investigation. Clin Orthop Relat Res 2020;478(8):1850–66.
79. Cyril S, Smith BJ, Renzaho AM. Systematic review of empowerment measures in health promotion. Health Promot Int 2016;31(4):809–26.

80. Arvidsson S, Bergman S, Arvidsson B, et al. Psychometric properties of the Swedish rheumatic disease empowerment scale, SWE-RES-23. Musculoskeletal Care 2012;10(2):101–9.
81. Maiorano D, Shrimankar D, Thapar-Björkert S, et al. Measuring empowerment: choices, values and norms. World Development 2021;138(C). S0305750X20303478.
82. Funnell MM, Anderson RM. Patient empowerment: a look back, a look ahead. Diabetes Educ 2003;29(3):454–8, 460, 462 passim.

Predictors and Measures of Adherence to Core Treatments for Osteoarthritis

Vicky Duong, DPT[a], David J. Hunter, PhD[a],
Philippa J.A. Nicolson, PhD[a,b,*]

KEYWORDS

- Osteoarthritis • Adherence • Physical activity • Exercise

KEY POINTS

- Adherence to core treatments for OA remains a challenge and is influenced by many intrinsic and extrinsic factors.
- Measurement of adherence to core treatments for OA needs to be standardized in trials, and developing a tool to measure adherence is a priority.
- Strategies to improve and maintain long-term adherence should be implemented in the research and clinical settings.
- A patient-centered approach considering patients' goals, abilities, and barriers with long-term monitoring should be adopted to maximize adherence in OA populations.

INTRODUCTION

Adherence, or the extent to which treatments are completed as prescribed, is a worldwide issue compromising healthcare outcomes.[1] The World Health Organization (WHO) stated in 2003 that "across diseases, adherence is the single most important modifiable factor that compromises treatment outcomes."[2] In the context of core osteoarthritis (OA) management, poor adherence has been proposed as one of the main barriers to achieving and maintaining the benefits of treatments.[3] Core OA management refers to the subset of treatments that form the basis of OA management plans and are recommended for OA, prior to pharmacologic or surgical interventions. These treatments are deemed high-value treatments, which are cost-effective and the benefits or probable benefits outweigh the harms of the treatment.[4] Core OA treatments comprise education, exercise, physical activity, and weight management/

[a] Department of Rheumatology, Institute of Bone and Joint Research, Kolling Institute, Royal North Shore Hospital and Northern Clinical School, University of Sydney, NSW 2065, Australia;
[b] Nuffield Department of Orthopaedics, Rheumatology and Musculoskeletal Sciences, University of Oxford, UK
* Corresponding author. Botnar Research Centre, Windmill Road, Headington, Oxford OX37LD.
E-mail address: philippa.nicolson@ndorms.ox.ac.uk

Clin Geriatr Med 38 (2022) 345–360
https://doi.org/10.1016/j.cger.2021.11.007
0749-0690/22/© 2021 Elsevier Inc. All rights reserved.

loss, and are supported by all clinical guidelines.[5–7] These treatments require significant and sustained behavior modifications, as opposed to passive treatments such as a one-off injection, making them particularly challenging for clinicians to implement and for patients to maintain long term. In addition, exacerbations of pain and other symptoms related to OA may interfere with the ability to maintain treatments long term.[8]

Most adherence research in OA populations has focused on the knee, particularly investigating exercise and physical activity, which is unsurprising given that the benefits of exercise for improving physical function and pain in those with knee OA have been well established.[9] Adherence to other interventions commonly prescribed to those with lower limb OA, such as braces and weight loss, have not been as extensively researched. There is also a noted paucity of research examining adherence in hand OA populations, highlighting this as an area for future research. Adherence to home exercise interventions for hand OA are commonly not measured in randomized controlled trials (RCTs),[10] making it difficult to determine factors/predictors affecting hand OA adherence and treatment effects of the interventions.

This narrative review outlines the measurement of adherence to core treatments in OA populations, summarizes existing evidence of factors affecting adherence and predictors of adherence, and examines the link between adherence and outcomes. Brief practical recommendations for improving adherence to core treatments in OA populations are provided.

Definition of Adherence

The WHO defines adherence as "the extent to which a person's behaviour such as taking medication, following a diet and/or executing lifestyle changes, corresponds with agreed recommendations from a health care provider."[1] Terms such as compliance, concordance, or adherence have often been used interchangeably; however, it should be noted that these terms have distinct meanings. Compliance is defined as "the act or process of complying to a desire, demand, proposal or regimen or to coercion."[11] In medical settings, compliance suggests that the patient does as instructed by the health care practitioner, without taking into account personal preferences or concerns.[12] In contrast, the WHO definition of adherence requires an active, collaborative relationship between patient and clinician, with greater emphasis on the patient role in deciding to undertake a particular treatment.[12]

Adherence is multifaceted and determined by a range of both internal and external factors. Almost 35 years ago, Meichenbaum and Turk[13] suggested 4 interdependent factors that influenced treatment adherence behavior: knowledge and skills, beliefs, motivation, and action. More recently, the WHO uses a model that describes adherence as being determined by the interplay of 5 dimensions: (1) health system factors (eg, inadequate reimbursement by health insurance plans, lack of knowledge and training for health care providers, short consultations), (2) social/economic (eg, socioeconomic status, level of education, distances from treatment centers), (3) therapy related (eg, immediacy of beneficial effects, duration of treatment, previous treatment failures), (4) condition related (eg, severity of symptoms, level of disability, rate of progression), and (5) patient related (eg, knowledge, attitudes, perceptions, and expectations).[1]

Measurement of adherence

The measurement of adherence to treatments for OA is essential in order to assess the effectiveness of an intervention, to identify patterns of adherence and consequences of adherence, and to evaluate interventions aiming to improve adherence. Accurate measurement of adherence is also fundamental to allow appropriate progression or adjustment of elements of the treatment in response to the actual dose being completed.

Because of the multifaceted nature of core treatments for OA, numerous methods to measure adherence exist. These include self-reported measures such as a treatment diary or retrospective self-rated scale, longer self-reported questionnaires, objective measures such as sensors, and patient interviews. Previous systematic reviews investigating the measurement of adherence to exercise and self-management for musculoskeletal pain conditions have been inconclusive in determining a recommended method of measuring adherence[14–17] (**Table 1**). Our recent systematic review investigating measurement of adherence to unsupervised, conservative treatments for knee OA also concluded that a wide variety of measurement methods, parameters, and cut-off values are currently used.[18]

Despite the range of options to measure adherence, we found that many studies investigating conservative interventions for knee OA do not mention how adherence to the intervention was measured (n = 432/1113, 38.8%).[18] When adherence data were reported, there was wide variation in the format in which this was done. Reporting adherence data should be standardized in clinical trials (**Box 1**) to allow improved comparisons between interventions and correlation with important clinical outcomes, such as pain and function.

The most commonly used method for assessing adherence to core treatments in OA, both in research and clinical practice, is self-report.[15,18,19] Self-report measures such as exercise diaries, logs and self-rated scales are inexpensive and simple to use, hence their popularity. The use of self-reported measures is subject to multiple biases[20] and overestimation.[21] Self-reporting bias, which represents a major issue in most observational studies, can include social desirability and recall bias.[20] Social desirability bias can occur when anonymity and confidentiality cannot be guaranteed at the time of data collection and can be prevented by using valid self-report tools.[1] Recall bias can occur when participants erroneously provide responses and depends on their ability to recall past events. Having shorter recall periods is one method to minimize recall bias.[20] Any measurement tool is seldom perfect; however, in order to provide useful information, a measurement tool should possess acceptable levels of both validity and reliability.[22] In recent systematic reviews investigating adherence measurement methods, most measures used were neither reliable nor valid. In our systematic review, only 10 out of 261 treatments included (3.8%) reported any reliability or validity testing of the measurement instrument used.[18] Most of the instruments were for measuring physical activity, including validated questionnaires such as the Physical Activity Scale for the Elderly (PASE), Community Healthy Activities Model Program for Seniors (CHAMPS), and accelerometers. The lack of reliable and valid measures is in accordance with McLean and colleagues,[15] who found that only 10 out of 110 included articles provided any evidence of measurement/practical properties of the measures used. The authors also noted that the assessment of relevance and comprehensiveness was largely absent and there was no patient involvement in the development of the measures.[15] Bollen and colleagues[17] assessed self-reported adherence measures to rehabilitation programs and found that most measures included did not report any reliability or validity testing of the included measures, and only 2 of 61 measures scored positively for one psychometric property.

Recently, an increasing number of studies have used objective methods to measure adherence. For example, studies evaluating physical activity have used wearable accelerometers or pedometers, and those evaluating online educational programs have assessed the number of hours of online content watched.[18] Combining objective and

Table 1
Systematic reviews investigating adherence measurement

Study	Population	Intervention/s	Main Findings
Bailey et al.,[42] 2018	Adults with MSK pain	Therapeutic exercise	Exercise frequency through self-reported diaries were were most commonly used Most studies did not define "satisfactory adherence"; an 80%–99% completion rate was most frequently used
Bollen et al.,[17] 2014	Adults with a long-term physical condition	Unsupervised, home-based exercise program	There were 61 different adherence measurement methods used in the 58 studies included. These measures included 29 questionnaires, 20 logs, 2 visual analog scales, and 1 tally counter. Only 2 measures scored positively for 1 psychometric property (content validity). Most studies did not report any validity or reliability measures
Duong et al.,[18] 2021	Adults with OA	Unsupervised, conservative interventions	Most studies investigated exercise and measured frequency through a self-reported diary Most studies used 1 measurement method only; however, for education and physical activity interventions, objective measures such as from a wearable accelerometer were also used Most studies did not define "satisfactory adherence"; the most common reported values were 75%–99% Only a small number of studies reported any reliability or validity measures of the tool being used Unable to make formal comparisons between measurement methods because of the large variability in reporting
Hall et al.,[14] 2015	Adults with a chronic MSK condition	Unsupervised self-management component	No names of referenced adherence measurement tools were found; a total of 47 self-invented measures were identified. The main method used was home diaries, and all measured varied in type of information obtained and scoring methods No consistency among adherence measurement tools; the construct is ill-defined
McLean et al.,[15] 2017	Adults with MSK pain	Therapeutic exercise	Seven clearly defined measures of exercise adherence identified No clear recommendation of an adherence measurement because of significant methodological and quality issues

Abbreviation: MSK, musculoskeletal.

Box 1
Clinical and research considerations for measuring adherence

- Method for measuring adherence (eg, self-reported diary/log book, telephone interview, questionnaire, objective measure)

- Which parameters of adherence measurement are you most interested in (eg, frequency, duration, intensity, weight, accuracy/quality, if applicable)?

- Which time points are most relevant?

- Consider the recall period and time to complete being asked of patients (eg, recall bias may be greater if periods are too long; however, too short/frequent and they may present as a time burden to participants)

- Are validity and/or reliability data available for the method?

- If analyzing adherence as an outcome, consider including cutoff values for satisfactory adherence

---

self-reported measures is also becoming more common. Self-reported questionnaires such as the Short Questionnaire to Assess Health Enhancing Physical Activity (SQUASH)[23] or PASE[24] have been validated in multiple populations, including those with OA. The Exercise Adherence Rating Scale (EARS) is a brief questionnaire designed to explicitly measure adherence to home exercise, as well as investigate potential barriers/facilitators to exercise.[25] For dietary weight loss interventions, participants' body weight can be measured in conjunction with a food diary and/or validated self-reported questionnaire. Objective measures in combination with self-reported measures may provide a more accurate representation of an individuals' adherence, and they offer great potential for monitoring of adherence in the future.

In the hand OA population, where exercise is also an important core treatment, adherence has not been extensively measured or investigated. In a Cochrane Review of 7 RCTs investigating the effects of exercise on hand OA, only one study reported how many sessions were attended by participants, and only 3 studies reported adherence to the unsupervised home exercise sessions using a self-reported diary.[10] Common parameters of exercise adherence measurement were frequency,[26,27] duration,[27] and the number of exercises completed.[28] One study further categorized adherence as high if greater than or equal to 75% of group exercises sessions were attended and greater than or equal to 60% of home exercises were completed as recorded by a diary.[28] The use of orthoses is also a common intervention for patients with thumb base OA and is recommended by guidelines.[6] A review published in 2017 investigating orthosis design on thumb OA functional outcomes found that only 5 of the included 14 studies reported adherence measures to the orthoses, all of which were self-reported.[29] Although 3 studies reported the mean number of days or hours the orthosis was worn, there is limited information on how this information was collected, and the articles fail to mention crucial adherence information such as the methods of measurement or recall periods.[30–32] The most common parameter of adherence to orthoses is measures such as the frequency or time worn using self-reported diaries.[33–36] Two studies have reported the frequency of the orthoses worn in a self-reported diary that was checked at subsequent follow-up visits.[34,36] One study further categorized adherence as good if the orthosis was worn 5 to 7 nights a week, fair if worn 3 or 4 nights a week, and absent if worn less than 1 night a week.[34] Other studies had participants self-report the number of hours the splint was worn each day in a diary.[33,35] Another method of adherence measurement was to have participants self-report their frequency of wear on a 5-point scale (no orthoses wear, 1–2 times per month, 1 to 2 times per week, minimum of 4 times per week, or daily) at follow-up.[37] Other studies investigating orthoses in thumb base OA make no mention of measures of adherence.[38–41]

Previous systematic reviews have attempted to quantify values for satisfactory adherence, or a minimum level of adherence to gain benefits from an intervention. A cutoff value of greater than or equal to 75% has been suggested by multiple authors.[18,42] However, given the complex nature of adherence, using a definitive cutoff value may result in loss of important information in the data. Using continuous measures rather than cutoff values allows better comparisons between groups and correlation with patient outcomes, such as pain and function. Currently, evidence is lacking as to whether there is a threshold of adherence to treatments for OA in order for benefits to be seen, from a behavior change perspective. Future research examining this is warranted, and the standardization of adherence measurements will facilitate research in this area.

At present, there is no validated measure of adherence, and developing a tool to measure adherence to core treatments for OA remains a priority. Guidelines for developing clinical measurement tools have been previously established.[22] However, because of the complexity of adherence, developing tools that encompass all aspects of adherence is particularly challenging. Input and collaboration from patients, clinicians, and researchers in the development of future tools should be sought.[43] Adherence measurement tools should be multifaceted to focus on aspects such as frequency/duration of the treatment, as well as encompass a measure of accuracy/quality, which is particularly important for exercise treatments, and are commonly used in clinical practice.[15]

Factors Influencing Adherence

Many theories and models that are designed to explain human behavior and its influences have been proposed. Bandura's Social Cognitive Theory framework provides a model of how people's self-efficacy beliefs operate with goals, outcome expectations, perceived environmental factors, and facilitators in the regulation of human motivation, action, and well-being.[44] In this theory, individual beliefs in self-efficacy can be developed by various sources of influence. These different sources could be mastery of experiences, vicarious experiences through social models (eg, seeing someone with knee OA also exercise), or social persuasion (eg, verbal persuasion/encouragement).[44] In the context of adherence to core treatments for OA, targeting these different sources is a potential mechanism to improve self-efficacy, which may lead to greater adherence. A more recent framework is the Behaviour Change Wheel (BCW) proposed by Michie and colleagues,[45] which synthesizes 19 behavior change theories. At the core of the BCW is a framework coined the COM-B. In the COM-B model, for a behavior to occur, 3 essential conditions must be satisfied: capability, opportunity, and motivation. Capability is defined as the individual's psychological and physical capacity to partake in the activity, which also requires the necessary knowledge and skills; motivation is the processes that energize and direct behavior, such as habitual processes and analytical decision making; and opportunity refers to the external factors that make the behavior possible or prompt it.[45] Opportunity and capability influence motivation, and all 3 components influence behavior.[45] A recent study that used the BCW to develop a text message intervention aiming to improve adherence to a home exercise program for knee OA found that, at 24-week follow-up, self-reported adherence was higher in the text message group, compared with control.[46] These models provide fundamental knowledge and greater insight into how behavior is influenced and should be considered when planning interventions to identify perceived barriers and facilitators to executing and adhering to core OA treatments.

Adherence to OA core treatments is multifaceted and can be influenced by the interplay of intrinsic and/or extrinsic factors, particularly because the treatment generally comprises several components.[47,48] These factors, and their impact on adherence, may vary between individuals, and within an individual over time. Factors affecting exercise behavior have been summarized by Petursdottir and colleagues,[47] who separated intrinsic factors into individual attributes (eg, motivation, self-image, personality, knowledge) or personal experience (eg, symptoms, mental status), and extrinsic factors into social (eg, social support, time, patient-provider relationship) or physical environment (eg, weather, access, transport). Internal, external, and systems-level factors influencing adherence to core OA treatments are illustrated in **Fig. 1**.

Individual factors such as patient preference have been shown to be important influences of adherence to OA treatments in clinical trials. A systematic review found that participants who were randomized to their preferred intervention groups had greater effect sizes for self-reported musculoskeletal disability questionnaires

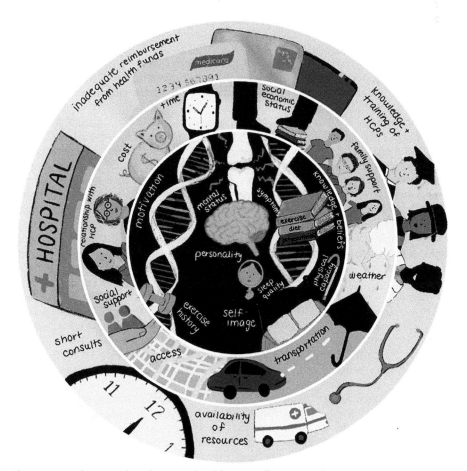

Fig. 1. Internal, external, and systems-level factors influencing adherence to core treatments for osteoarthritis.

compared with those who were indifferent about their treatment allocation at follow-up (ranging from 6 weeks to 24 months).[49] Patient preference was also found to be an important factor influencing adherence to a walking program for knee OA. Patients who had a preference for walking were twice as likely to adhere to a home walking program over 3 months.[50] Other individual factors, such as high level of physical fitness and an absence of emotional involvement, were also important factors linked to the adherence to a walking program in knee OA participants.[50]

The attitudes and beliefs of those living with OA have also been found to influence adherence to core treatments. Participants with knee OA who had poor awareness of treatment options available (besides surgical and pharmacologic treatment), and those that believed that exercise could accelerate joint damage, had low adherence to an exercise program.[51] Conversely, high self-determination was found to be linked to high adherence to strength training at 2-year follow-up in knee OA participants in a qualitative study. Extrinsic factors have also been found to influence adherence. Social factors such as having an opportunity to complete an organized/supervised exercise session and social support from family/friends have been shown to improve exercise adherence.[50,52] Among participants with knee OA undertaking an exercise intervention, those who were supervised by a health practitioner were found to be nearly 3 times more likely to adhere compared with those who were not supervised.[50]

Predictors of Adherence

A limited number of studies have examined predictors of adherence to core treatments in OA populations, and the results have been inconsistent. Adherence to a 12-week home exercise program was investigated in a recent large secondary analysis of 325 participants aged greater than or equal to 45 years with knee OA and meniscus damage. Of the various factors examined, including demographic data, subjective clinical data (eg, symptoms of anxiety, depression, expectations, knee pain, and meniscal tear symptoms), objective data (eg, functional tests, severity of OA on radiographs), and extrinsic factors, low socioeconomic status was the only factor linked to poor adherence.[53] A systematic review found that intention to engage in home-based physical therapies, self-motivation, self-efficacy, previous adherence behavior, and social support were strong predictors of adherence to home-based physical therapies in patients with musculoskeletal conditions.[54] However, the authors noted that, because of the difficulty in measuring home exercise adherence, the predictive ability of these factors is limited.[54] These findings are consistent with the findings from an 8-week study investigating a home exercise program; the authors found that having previous good adherence in weeks 1 to 4 was the strongest predictor of adherence in weeks 5 to 8.[55] In a Web-based education intervention for hip/knee OA, higher age and the presence of comorbidities predicted nonadherence. Adherence was measured as the number of online modules completed over a 9-week period, and participants were considered adherent if they completed greater than or equal to 6 modules. The authors postulate that, since the website was OA focused, older patients with multiple comorbidities may require a more personalized approach.[56]

There is limited evidence on the predictors of adherence to a home program in hand OA populations. In a cohort study with thumb base osteoarthritis, patients with higher baseline levels of pain were more adherent to a 12-week home program consisting of hand exercises, topical antiinflammatory gel, and splint for the base of the thumb.[57] This finding suggests that participants were more likely to adhere to the home program if they were motivated by pain symptoms. To our knowledge, there are no studies in hand OA populations that explicitly aim to measure adherence, highlighting an area for future research. A summary of the predictors of adherence in OA populations is presented in **Table 2**.

When attempting to investigate predictors of adherence to OA, a longer-term RCT model should be used with standardized measurements and reporting of adherence to improve predictive modeling techniques. Information on the duration of the intervention and follow-up periods, recall times, and methods of adherence measurement should be standardized.

Consequences of Poor Adherence

Twenty years ago, Carr[3] proposed that poor adherence was one of the main barriers to achieving and maintaining the benefits of interventions for people with OA. Despite this widely held view, a limited number of studies have evaluated the relationship between adherence and patient outcomes, particularly long term. However, if the short-term benefits of core treatments, and in particular exercise, for OA are used as a guide, the effects of nonadherence long term are likely to be significant. Higher adherence to exercise in the short term has been identified as a predictor of better long-term outcomes among people with hip and/or knee OA.[58] Secondary analysis of an 18-month study investigating a dietary and exercise intervention in obese and overweight participants with knee OA found those with higher adherence had improved physical function at both 6-month and 18-month follow-up, as measured through 6-minute walking distance.[59] Similarly, an RCT comparing a 3-month behavioral graded exercise intervention with usual exercise therapy reported increased adherence was associated with better outcomes of pain, self-reported function, physical performance, and self-perceived effect at 3-month, 15-month, and 60-month follow-up.[60]

Assessing the relationship between adherence and outcomes is further complicated by the absence of a gold standard for adherence measurement. Previous studies have largely relied on self-reported measures, which, as previously discussed, are subject to reporting bias, overestimation, and poor recall. In a small study that used concealed accelerometers placed in ankle cuff weights to measure home exercise adherence among patients with knee OA, no association was found between home exercise adherence and self-reported pain or function at 12-week follow-up.[61] Further exploration of this topic, including standardized measures of adherence, should be addressed.

DISCUSSION
Improving Adherence

Maximizing adherence can greatly dictate the success of the treatment, and the implementation of strategies to improve and maintain adherence is recommended.[58] Adhering to the core treatments for OA long term often requires significant behavior change. Using existing models of behavior change when developing interventions targeting adherence is crucial. The COM-B is one such model, which summarizes the required elements of capability, opportunity, and motivation that are needed for a behavior to take place.[45] Clinicians should carefully examine the barriers and facilitators to treatment adherence before prescribing an intervention. After consideration of patient barriers and facilitators, the prescribed intervention/s should be individualized to consider the patient's abilities and preferences. Regular supervision, such as in a class-based setting and monitoring through telephone/email contact, can also assist in improving self-efficacy and treatment beliefs.[51]

One way to identify sources of behavior is by using motivational interviewing, a technique that can be used to promote behavior change by helping patients realize why

Table 2
Predictors of adherence to osteoarthritis

Population	Study	Intervention	Variables	Findings
Knee OA	Seçkin et al.,[68] 2000	Home exercise program: flexibility, strengthening, endurance, active ROM	Pain	Associated with higher adherence
Knee OA and meniscal tear	Tuakli-Wosornu et al.,[53] 2016	Home exercise program: strengthening	Lower income, no baseline pain with pivoting and twisting	Associated with greater risk of nonadherence to home exercise program
Hip/knee OA	Schoo et al.,[55] 2005	Home exercise program: strengthening and mobility	Previous good adherence, high levels of physical activity, perceptions of physical inactivity	Associated with higher adherence
Hip/knee OA	Bossen et al.,[56] 2013	Web-based education program	Higher age, presence of comorbidities	Associated with less usage
Thumb base OA	Duong et al.,[57] 2021	Home program: topical NSAID, exercises, and splint	Higher baseline pain Lower baseline function	Associated with higher adherence No association

Abbreviations: NSAID, nonsteroidal antiinflammatory drug; ROM, range of movement.

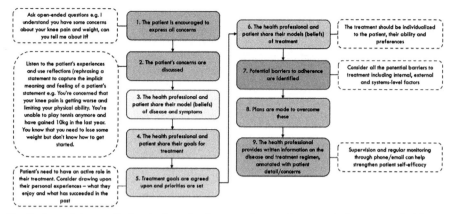

Fig. 2. A model consultation to target adherence to core treatments for osteoarthritis.

and how they might change. Motivational interviewing is based on the use of a guiding style of open-ended questions, which is superior to standard advice giving.[62] The BCW can assist in identifying interventions targets, such as education, training, or incentivization. These general intervention targets can be translated into specific techniques aimed at changing behaviors and encompassing replicable components, coined behavior change techniques. A systematic review and meta-analysis found that booster sessions with a physiotherapist and behavioral graded activity provided moderate quality of evidence to support patient adherence to exercise in hip/knee OA.[63] Behavioral graded exercise uses principles of operant conditioning and self-regulation with booster sessions to improve and maintain adherence[64] and can be implemented for home exercise programs. The aim of behavioral graded approaches is to gradually increase the time spent undertaking the intervention and gradually incorporate it into daily living. A model consultation to improve adherence, based on the work of Carr,[3] is presented in **Fig. 2.** Educational resources relevant to health professionals and patients are provided in **Box 2.**

Sound explanations and educational resources about the benefits of core interventions, such as exercise, physical activity, and weight management, should not be overlooked as part of an OA management plan, because patient beliefs toward exercise can heavily influence their actions. There are numerous opportunities for education, whether they are structured education resources or other forms of individual (unstructured) education.[65] Structured education can be delivered in person during a consultation, in a small group, or as part of a larger multidisciplinary team.[65] Other

---

Box 2
Resources for health professionals and patients

Health professionals
- The British Medical Journal Motivational Interviewing
- Royal Australian College of General Practitioners (RACGP) Motivational Interviewing: facilitating behavior change in the general practice setting

Patients
- MyJointPain: Exercising with osteoarthritis: staying motivated
- The Joint Action Podcast

forms of unstructured educational resources can include books, pamphlets, or internet resources[65] such as podcasts. Podcast platforms have become popular recently and have allowed wider dissemination of OA information.[66] Dissemination of information in a digital format is particularly useful during times of isolation, such as during coronavirus disease 2019 (COVID-19), whereby patients living with OA can receive accessible and credible information. Regardless of the mode of education, the main outcomes are to increase patient knowledge, desirable behaviors (adherence with prescribed intervention/s), self-efficacy, and functional status.[67]

SUMMARY

Adherence to core treatments for OA remains a challenge for researchers, clinicians, and patients. Adherence is influenced by multiple factors, both intrinsic and extrinsic. These factors differ between individuals, and within an individual over time, making predicting adherence difficult and unreliable. Measurement and reporting of adherence are essential. The measurement of adherence should be standardized for various OA interventions, and developing a tool to measure adherence is a priority. Identifying the barriers and enablers to treatments by using existing frameworks such as the Behaviour Change Wheel and implementing behavior change techniques known to improve adherence, such as booster sessions, should be used to assist in improving adherence in clinical trials and practice. All prescribed interventions should include patient education and consider patient barriers, abilities, and preferences to maximize adherence long term.

CLINICS CARE POINTS

- In order to better understand the influence of adherence on clinical outcomes, the first priority is to standardize measures of reporting adherence in clinical trials.
- A standardized reporting guideline for core interventions should be developed and established to enhance the quality and transparency of health and medical research.
- Following the implementation of improved adherence reporting, measurement methods can be further compared (ie, comparing self-reported with objective methods) to develop a tool that provides a valid and reliable measure of adherence for future trials and in clinical practice.
- Exploration of further factors influencing adherence and their behavior over time should be investigated, and whether a minimum threshold of adherence is required to have benefits from the prescribed treatments.

DISCLOSURE

V. Duong is supported by a University of Sydney Postgraduate Award scholarship. D.J. Hunter is supported by a National Health and Medical Research Council (NHMRC) Investigator Fellowship. P.J.A. Nicolson is funded by a Versus Arthritis Foundation Fellowship (grant reference number 22428).

REFERENCES

1. World Health Report. Adherence to long term therapies, evidence for action. Geneva (Switzerland): World Health Organization; 2003.
2. Sabaté E, Organization WH. Adherence to long-term therapies: policy for action: meeting report, 4-5 June 2001. Geneva(Switzerland): World Health Organization; 2001.

3. Carr A. Barriers to the effectiveness of any intervention in OA. Best Pract Res Clin Rheumatol 2001;15(4):645–56.
4. Elshaug AG, Rosenthal MB, Lavis JN, et al. Levers for addressing medical underuse and overuse: achieving high-value health care. Lancet 2017;390(10090): 191–202.
5. McAlindon TE, Bannuru RR, Sullivan M, et al. OARSI guidelines for the non-surgical management of knee osteoarthritis. Osteoarthr Cartil 2014;22(3):363–88.
6. Kolasinski SL, Neogi T, Hochberg MC, et al. 2019 American College of Rheumatology/Arthritis Foundation guideline for the management of osteoarthritis of the hand, hip, and knee. Arthritis Rheumatol 2020;72(2):220–33.
7. Fernandes L, Hagen KB, Bijlsma JW, et al. EULAR recommendations for the non-pharmacological core management of hip and knee osteoarthritis. Ann Rheum Dis 2013;72(7):1125–35.
8. Farr JN, Going SB, Lohman TG, et al. Physical activity levels in patients with early knee osteoarthritis measured by accelerometry. Arthritis Care Res 2008;59(9): 1229–36.
9. Lange AK, Vanwanseele B, Fiatarone singh MA. Strength training for treatment of osteoarthritis of the knee: a systematic review. Arthritis Care Res 2008;59(10): 1488–94.
10. Østerås N, Kjeken I, Smedslund G, et al. Exercise for hand osteoarthritis. Cochrane Database Syst Rev 2017;(1):CD010388.
11. Merriam-webster. Compliance. In Merriam-Webster.com dictionary Retrieved June 28, 2021. Available at: https://wwwmerriam-webstercom/dictionary/compliance. Accessed June 28, 2021.
12. Myers LB, Midence K. Concepts and issues in adherence. Amsterdam (Netherlands): Harwood Academic; 1998.
13. Meichenbaum D, Turk DC. Facilitating treatment adherence: a practitioner's guidebook. New York: Plenum Press; 1987.
14. Hall AM, Kamper SJ, Hernon M, et al. Measurement tools for adherence to non-pharmacologic self-management treatment for chronic musculoskeletal conditions: a systematic review. Arch Phys Med Rehabil 2015;96(3):552–62.
15. McLean S, Holden MA, Potia T, et al. Quality and acceptability of measures of exercise adherence in musculoskeletal settings: a systematic review. Rheumatology 2016;56(3):426–38.
16. Bailey DL, Holden MA, Foster NE, et al. Defining adherence to therapeutic exercise for musculoskeletal pain: a systematic review. Br J Sports Med 2020;54(6): 326–31.
17. Bollen JC, Dean SG, Siegert RJ, et al. A systematic review of measures of self-reported adherence to unsupervised home-based rehabilitation exercise programmes, and their psychometric properties. BMJ open 2014;4(6):e005044.
18. Duong V, Daniel MS, Ferreira ML, et al. Measuring adherence to unsupervised, conservative treatment for knee osteoarthritis: a systematic review. Osteoarthr Cartil Open 2021;3(2):100171.
19. Holden MA, Nicholls EE, Hay EM, et al. Physical therapists' use of therapeutic exercise for patients with clinical knee osteoarthritis in the United Kingdom: in line with current recommendations? Phys Ther 2008;88(10):1109–21.
20. Althubaiti A. Information bias in health research: definition, pitfalls, and adjustment methods. J Multidiscip Healthc 2016;9:211.
21. Nicolson PJ, Hinman RS, Wrigley TV, et al. Self-reported home exercise adherence: a validity and reliability study using concealed accelerometers. J Orthop Sports Phys Ther 2018;48(12):943–50.

22. De Vet HC, Terwee CB, Mokkink LB, et al. Measurement in medicine: a practical guide. Cambridge, UK: Cambridge University Press; 2011.
23. Wendel-Vos GW, Schuit AJ, Saris WH, et al. Reproducibility and relative validity of the short questionnaire to assess health-enhancing physical activity. J Clin Epidemiol 2003;56(12):1163–9.
24. Washburn RA, McAuley E, Katula J, et al. The physical activity scale for the elderly (PASE): evidence for validity. J Clin Epidemiol 1999;52(7):643–51.
25. Meade L, Bearne LM, Godfrey EL. Comprehension and face validity of the Exercise Adherence Rating Scale in patients with persistent musculoskeletal pain. Musculoskelet Care 2018;16(3):409–12.
26. Dziedzic K, Nicholls E, Hill S, et al. Self-management approaches for osteoarthritis in the hand: a 2× 2 factorial randomised trial. Ann Rheum Dis 2015; 74(1):108–18.
27. Hennig T, Hæhre L, Hornburg VT, et al. Effect of home-based hand exercises in women with hand osteoarthritis: a randomised controlled trial. Ann Rheum Dis 2015;74(8):1501–8.
28. Østerås N, Hagen K, Grotle M, et al. Limited effects of exercises in people with hand osteoarthritis: results from a randomized controlled trial. Osteoarthr Cartil 2014;22(9):1224–33.
29. de Almeida PHT, MacDermid J, Pontes TB, et al. Differences in orthotic design for thumb osteoarthritis and its impact on functional outcomes: a scoping review. Prosthet Orthot Int 2017;41(4):323–35.
30. Ahmadi Bani M, Arazpour M, Hutchins SW, et al. A custom-made neoprene thumb carpometacarpal orthosis with thermoplastic stabilization: an orthosis that promotes function and improvement in patients with the first carpometacarpal joint osteoarthritis. Prosthet Orthot Int 2014;38(1):79–82.
31. Bani MA, Arazpour M, Kashani RV, et al. Comparison of custom-made and prefabricated neoprene splinting in patients with the first carpometacarpal joint osteoarthritis. Disabil Rehabil Assistive Technol 2013;8(3):232–7.
32. Bani MA, Arazpour M, Kashani RV, et al. The effect of custom-made splints in patients with the first carpometacarpal joint osteoarthritis. Prosthet Orthot Int 2013; 37(2):139–44.
33. Sillem H, Backman CL, Miller WC, et al. Comparison of two carpometacarpal stabilizing splints for individuals with thumb osteoarthritis. J Hand Ther 2011;24(3): 216–26.
34. Rannou F, Dimet J, Boutron I, et al. Splint for base-of-thumb osteoarthritis: a randomized trial. Ann Intern Med 2009;150(10):661–9.
35. Maddali-Bongi S, Del Rosso A, Galluccio F, et al. Is an intervention with a custom-made splint and an educational program useful on pain in patients with trapeziometacarpal joint osteoarthritis in a daily clinical setting? Int J Rheum Dis 2016; 19(8):773–80.
36. Deveza LA, Robbins SR, Duong V, et al. Efficacy of a combination of conservative therapies vs an education comparator on clinical outcomes in thumb base osteoarthritis: a randomized clinical trial. JAMA Intern Med 2021;181(4):429–38.
37. Hermann M, Nilsen T, Eriksen CS, et al. Effects of a soft prefabricated thumb orthosis in carpometacarpal osteoarthritis. Scand J Occup Ther 2014;21(1):31–9.
38. Wajon A, Ada L. No difference between two splint and exercise regimens for people with osteoarthritis of the thumb: a randomised controlled trial. Aust J Physiother 2005;51(4):245–9.

39. Boustedt C, Nordenskiöld U, Nilsson ÅL. Effects of a hand-joint protection programme with an addition of splinting and exercise. Clin Rheumatol 2009;28(7): 793–9.
40. Arazpour M, Soflaei M, Ahmadi Bani M, et al. The effect of thumb splinting on thenar muscles atrophy, pain, and function in subjects with thumb carpometacarpal joint osteoarthritis. Prosthet Orthot Int 2017;41(4):379–86.
41. Tsehaie J, Spekreijse KR, Wouters RM, et al. Predicting outcome after hand orthosis and hand therapy for thumb carpometacarpal osteoarthritis: a prospective study. Arch Phys Med Rehabil 2019;100(5):844–50.
42. Bailey DL, Holden MA, Foster NE, et al. Defining adherence to therapeutic exercise for musculoskeletal pain: a systematic review. Br J Sports Med 2018;54(6): 326–31.
43. Staniszewska S, Haywood KL, Brett J, et al. Patient and public involvement in patient-reported outcome measures. Patient 2012;5(2):79–87.
44. Bandura A. Health promotion from the perspective of social cognitive theory. Psychol Health 1998;13(4):623–49.
45. Michie S, Van Stralen MM, West R. The behaviour change wheel: a new method for characterising and designing behaviour change interventions. Implementation Sci 2011;6(1):1–12.
46. Bennell K, Nelligan RK, Schwartz S, et al. Behavior change text messages for home exercise adherence in knee osteoarthritis: randomized trial. J Med Internet Res 2020;22(9):e21749.
47. Petursdottir U, Arnadottir SA, Halldorsdottir S. Facilitators and barriers to exercising among people with osteoarthritis: a phenomenological study. Phys Ther 2010;90(7):1014–25.
48. Marks R. Knee osteoarthritis and exercise adherence: a review. Curr Aging Sci 2012;5(1):72–83.
49. Group PCR. Patients' preferences within randomised trials: systematic review and patient level meta-analysis. BMJ 2008;337:a1864.
50. Loew L, Brosseau L, Kenny GP, et al. Factors influencing adherence among older people with osteoarthritis. Clin Rheumatol 2016;35(9):2283–91.
51. Hurley MV, Walsh N, Bhavnani V, et al. Health beliefs before and after participation on an exercised-based rehabilitation programme for chronic knee pain: doing is believing. BMC Musculoskelet Disord 2010;11(1):1–12.
52. Damush TM, Perkins SM, Mikesky AE, et al. Motivational factors influencing older adults diagnosed with knee osteoarthritis to join and maintain an exercise program. J Aging Phys Activity 2005;13(1):45–60.
53. Tuakli-Wosornu YA, Selzer F, Losina E, et al. Predictors of exercise adherence in patients with meniscal tear and osteoarthritis. Arch Phys Med Rehabil 2016; 97(11):1945–52.
54. Essery R, Geraghty AW, Kirby S, et al. Predictors of adherence to home-based physical therapies: a systematic review. Disabil Rehabil 2017;39(6):519–34.
55. Schoo AM, Morris ME, Bui QM. Predictors of home exercise adherence in older people with osteoarthritis. Physiother Can 2005;57(3):179–87.
56. Bossen D, Buskermolen M, Veenhof C, et al. Adherence to a web-based physical activity intervention for patients with knee and/or hip osteoarthritis: a mixed method study. J Med Internet Res 2013;15(10):e223.
57. Duong V, Nicolson PJ, Robbins SR, et al. High baseline pain is associated with treatment adherence in persons diagnosed with thumb base osteoarthritis: an observational study. J Hand Ther 2021. https://doi.org/10.1016/j.jht.2021.04.024.

58. Roddy E, Zhang W, Doherty M, et al. Evidence-based recommendations for the role of exercise in the management of osteoarthritis of the hip or knee—the MOVE consensus. Rheumatology 2004;44(1):67–73.

59. Van Gool CH, Penninx BW, Kempen GI, et al. Effects of exercise adherence on physical function among overweight older adults with knee osteoarthritis. Arthritis Care Res 2005;53(1):24–32.

60. Pisters MF, Veenhof C, Schellevis FG, et al. Exercise adherence improving long-term patient outcome in patients with osteoarthritis of the hip and/or knee. Arthritis Care Res 2010;62(8):1087–94.

61. Nicolson PJ, Hinman RS, Wrigley TV, et al. Effects of covertly measured home exercise adherence on patient outcomes among older adults with chronic knee pain. J Orthop Sports Phys Ther 2019;49(7):548–56.

62. Rubak S, Sandbæk A, Lauritzen T, et al. Motivational interviewing: a systematic review and meta-analysis. Br J Gen Pract 2005;55(513):305–12.

63. Nicolson PJ, Bennell KL, Dobson FL, et al. Interventions to increase adherence to therapeutic exercise in older adults with low back pain and/or hip/knee osteoarthritis: a systematic review and meta-analysis. Br J Sports Med 2017;51(10): 791–9.

64. Pisters MF, Veenhof C, de Bakker DH, et al. Behavioural graded activity results in better exercise adherence and more physical activity than usual care in people with osteoarthritis: a cluster-randomised trial. J Physiother 2010;56(1):41–7.

65. Schrieber L, Colley M. Patient education. Best Pract Res Clin Rheumatol 2004; 18(4):465–76.

66. Mobasheri A, Costello KE. Podcasting: an innovative tool for enhanced osteoarthritis education and research dissemination. Osteoarthr Cartil Open 2020;3(1): 100130.

67. Daltroy LH. Doctor-patient communication in rheumatological disorders. Baillières Clin Rheumatol 1993;7(2):221–39.

68. Seçkin Ü, Gündüz S, Borman P, et al. Evaluation of the compliance to exercise therapy in patients with knee osteoarthritis. J Back Musculoskelet Rehabil 2000;14(3):133–7.

A Framework to Guide the Development of Health Care Professional Education and Training in Best Evidence Osteoarthritis Care

Sarah Kobayashi, PhD, BLAS[a,1,*], Kelli Allen, PhD[b,2],
Kim Bennell, PhD[c,3], Jocelyn L. Bowden, BHMSc, BSc(Hon), PhD[a,1],
Andrew M. Briggs, PhD, BSc(PT)Hons[d,10],
Annette Burgess, PhD, MMedEd, MEd, MBioethics, MBT[e,4],
Rana S. Hinman, PhD, BPhysio (Hons)[c,3], Melanie Holden, PhD[f,5],
Nina Østerås, PhD[g,6], May Arna Godaker Risberg, PhD[h,7],
Saurab Sharma, PhD[i,j,8], Martin van der Esch, PhD[k,9],
Jillian P. Eyles, PhD, BAppSc(Phty)[a,1]

[a] Kolling Institute of Medical Research, Faculty of Medicine and Health, University of Sydney, Sydney, Australia; [b] Thurston Arthritis Research Center, University of North Carolina, Chapel Hill, NC, USA; [c] Centre for Health, Exercise and Sports Medicine, University of Melbourne, Australia; [d] Curtin School of Allied Health, Faculty of Health Sciences, Curtin University, Perth, Australia; [e] Sydney Medical School, Faculty of Medicine and Health, University of Sydney, Sydney, Australia; [f] Primary Care Centre Versus Arthritis, School of Medicine, Keele University, Keele, Staffordshire, United Kingdom; [g] Division of Rheumatology and Research, Diakonhjemmet Hospital, Oslo, Norway; [h] Norwegian School Sport Sciences, Oslo, Norway; [i] Centre for Pain IMPACT, Neuroscience Research Australia (NeuRA), Sydney, Australia; [j] University of New South Wales, Sydney, Australia; [k] Amsterdam University of Applied Sciences, Faculty of Health, Reade, Centre for Rehabilitation and Rheumatology, Amsterdam, the Netherlands

[1] Level 10 Kolling Building 10 Westbourne Street, St Leonards, NSW 2064, AUSTRALIA
[2] Thurston Arthritis Research Center The University of North Carolina at Chapel Hill 3300 Thurston Bldg., CB# 7280 Chapel Hill, NC 27599-7280, UNITED STATES OF AMERICA
[3] Centre for Health, Exercise & Sports Medicine, The University of Melbourne, Alan Gilbert Building, 161 Barry Street, Carlton, Victoria 3053 AUSTALIA
[4] Rm 208E, Edward Ford Building A27, The University of Sydney, NSW 2006, AUSTRALIA
[5] Primary Care Centre Versus Arthritis, School of Medicine, Keele University, Staffordshire ST5 5BG, UNITED KINGDOM
[6] Division of Rheumatology and Research, Diakonhjemmet Hospital, Postboks 23 Vinderen, 0319 Oslo, NORWAY
[7] Norwegian School Sport Sciences, Postboks 4014 Ullevål stadion, 0806 Oslo, Norway
[8] Centre for Pain IMPACT, Neuroscience Research Australia (NeuRA), PO Box 1165 Randwick, NSW 2031, AUSTRALIA
[9] Amsterdam University of Applied Sciences, Faculty of Health, Reade, Centre for Rehabilitation and Rheumatology, Nicolaes Tulphuis (NTH), Tafelbergweg 51, 1105 BD Amsterdam, NETHERLANDS
[10] Curtin School of Allied Health, Curtin University, GPO Box U1987, Perth, WA 6845, AUSTRALIA
* Level 10 Kolling Building 10 Westbourne Street, St Leonards, NSW 2064, Australia
E-mail address: sarah.kobayashi@sydney.edu.au

Clin Geriatr Med 38 (2022) 361–384
https://doi.org/10.1016/j.cger.2021.11.008
0749-0690/22/© 2021 Elsevier Inc. All rights reserved.

geriatric.theclinics.com

KEYWORDS

- Osteoarthritis • Health care professionals • Education • Training
- Professional development • Students

KEY POINTS

- There is currently no education and training available for health care professionals (HCPs) to support them in best evidence osteoarthritis (OA) care that is interdisciplinary and addresses core capabilities.
- Knowledge and skill gaps are barriers for HCPs to deliver best evidence OA care.
- Addressing system-level, clinician-level, and patient-level barriers, and collaborating with key stakeholders are critical when designing education and training, especially in low- and middle-income countries and low-resourced settings.
- An evidence-informed framework to guide development and evaluation of education and training for delivery of evidence-based OA care includes overarching principles for education and training, core capabilities for the delivery of OA care, theories of learning and preferences for delivery, and evaluation of education and training.

INTRODUCTION

Osteoarthritis (OA) is a leading cause of pain and disability worldwide, affecting 500 million people[1] and recognized by the World Health Organization as a condition that limits daily functioning in older people as they age.[2] Current clinical practice guidelines strongly recommend education on how to manage OA, exercise, and weight control as core components of care[3–5] (**Fig. 1**). However, the widespread adoption of core OA care into clinical practice has been poor, especially compared with lower tier care such as referral for surgery.[6] The implementation of core OA care is complex, and barriers arise at multiple levels; from point of care, to service delivery and system-level factors, and social determinants of health such as education level and socioeconomic status.[7,8] It is well-recognized that implementation of core OA care is limited by gaps in the knowledge and skills of health care professionals (HCPs).[8–11] This presents an opportunity to improve OA care through evidence-informed training and education of HCPs.[12]

There is currently no coordinated, common curricula across multiple disciplines that reflect best evidence OA care for HCPs or students.[13] The International Association for the Study of Pain has developed an "Interprofessional Pain Curriculum Outline" and encourages all interprofessional medical programs to embed this curriculum into pain education and training.[14] However, this curriculum is not disease-specific. Given the substantial prevalence and burden of OA,[15] specific attention to best evidence OA care in the chronic disease management curriculum is justified.

This article presents an evidence-informed framework that can be used to guide the development and evaluation of education and training to support HCPs and students in the delivery of evidence-based OA care. The framework includes the following 4 key components:

- Overarching principles for education and training of HCPs;
- Core capabilities for the delivery of best evidence OA care;
- Theories of learning and preferences for delivery;
- Evaluation of education and training for HCPs.

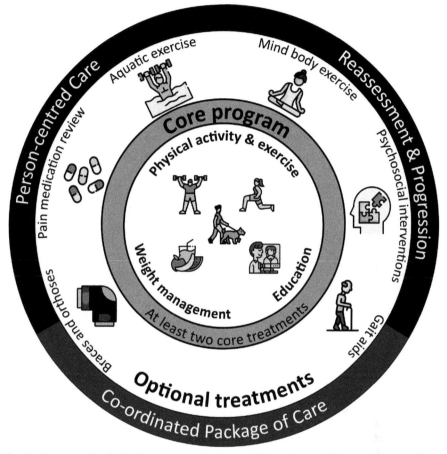

Fig. 1. Core aspects of OA Management Programs. (*From* Eyles JP, Hunter DJ, Bennell KL, et al. Priorities for the effective implementation of osteoarthritis management programs: an OARSI international consensus exercise. Osteoarthritis Cartilage. 2019;27(9):1270–1279. https://doi.org/10.1016/j.joca.2019.05.015; with permission.)

DISCUSSION

Overarching Principles for Education and Training of HCPs

The Global Independent Commission into Education of Health Professionals for the 21st century made broad recommendations for reforms to HCP's education and training.[16] The 5 recommendations that are most relevant to developing education and training programs for HCPs are summarized in the following subsections.

Take a competency/capability-driven approach that allows for adaptations to local contexts

Professional competence has been defined as "*the habitual and judicious use of communication, knowledge, technical skills, clinical reasoning, emotions, values, and reflection in daily practice for the benefit of the individual and community being served.*"[17] Professional capability goes even further, referring to the capacity of individuals to adapt to change, generate new knowledge, and improve their performance.[18] Ideally, a set of capabilities should be identified to define what HCPs need to know and be able to do.

Support interprofessional education that cuts across generic competencies and enhances collaborative relationships across different health care professions
Interprofessional education refers to when two-or-more professions learn with, from and about each other to improve collaborative working and the quality of care.[19] Interprofessional education is important in developing a workforce that practices collaboratively,[20] especially in low-resourced settings[21] and has been associated with improvements in HCP behavior, service organization, and quality of care.[22]

Harness tools and innovations made available through information technology to enable enhanced collaboration through connectivity and distance learning
Internet-based Learning (eLearning) has proliferated in health care education in recent years. There is emerging evidence to support the efficacy and acceptability of eLearning in OA care.[23] Lack of time and financial support are known barriers to HCPs participating in professional development activities,[24] particularly in low-income and middle-income countries (LMICs),[25] both barriers which may be overcome by eLearning modalities.[26] The COVID-19 pandemic has given rise to new technologies, systems, and processes,[27] which are likely to stimulate the development of new innovations such as artificial intelligence for eLearning.[28]

Draw on global knowledge, experience, and share educational resources while adapting them for local contexts
Communities of practice (COPs) refer to groups of people who share dialogue around common topics, which can lead to the development and sharing of knowledge and educational materials to support their work. A current example of a virtual COP in OA care is the "Joint Effort Initiative" (JEI; https://oarsi.org/discussion-group-joint-effort-initiative), which operates under the auspices of the Osteoarthritis Research Society International (OARSI), outlined in **Box 1**.

Strengthen the availability of educational resources through investment in their development and providing access to low-resourced settings
Sharing international educational resources allows for greater efficiencies and economies of scale. Although the benefits of sharing resources are clear, barriers to this include confusion around issues such as intellectual property, copyright, and lack of technical support and user-friendly technologies, which need to be overcome.[29–31] There are barriers to open access publishing, including (i) academics prioritizing perceived journal reputation over making the paper freely available; (ii) inadequate funding for article publication charges, particularly for academics in LMICs[32]; and

---

Box 1
The Joint Effort Initiative: a community of practice

The "Joint Effort Initiative" (JEI) is an international collaboration and virtual community of practice. Comprising 100+ researchers (22 countries and 6 continents), clinicians, consumers, and consumer organizations, the JEI is concerned with the implementation of evidence-based, cost-effective, osteoarthritis care through osteoarthritis management programs. The mission of the JEI is to investigate the best osteoarthritis management program models to use, develop long-term strategies for effective implementation of these programs in different socioeconomic and cultural environments, and identify research priorities to facilitate best evidence care internationally. Priorities for the work of the JEI were established in 2018 through an international survey and consensus study,[5] and the development of the core capabilities framework was finalized in 2019.[35]

Table 1
Domain and capabilities for high-value OA care

Capabilities

DOMAIN A: Person-Centered Approaches

1. Communication—The healthcare professional can do the following within their role and scope of practice	Apply a critical self-awareness of their own values.
	Recognize and practice two-way communication.
	Modify conversations to avoid jargon and negative descriptors.
	Respond to communication and information needs of individuals.
	Involve individuals and their carers in their management and respond to their questions and concerns.
	Direct individuals to sources of high-quality information and support.
	Communicate with other HCPs to facilitate timely and integrated care.
	When possible, draw on the expertise of other HCPs from the interdisciplinary team.
2. Person-centered care	Recognize individuals as experts in their own care and demonstrate sensitivity to their background, needs, and experiences.
	Explore the impact of the individuals' symptoms on their life, including relationships, social roles, and participation.
	Demonstrate an awareness of the burden of treatment (time & money) during care planning.
	Progress care recognizing that symptoms such as pain may not improve dramatically, but other aspects such as quality of life or participation may improve over time.
	Empower individuals to set priorities and goals, explain all management options, their risks, and benefits to support their decision-making.

DOMAIN B: Assessment, Investigation, & Diagnosis

3. History-taking—The health care professional can do the following within their role and scope of practice	Listen to individuals, asking questions to elicit additional information to optimize the efficiency and effectiveness of the subjective examination.
	Gather and synthesize information on symptoms, past history, comorbidities, and other determinants of health.
	Assess an individuals' preferences when determining goals & priorities with them.
	Assess the impact of an individuals' OA symptoms on their quality of life, impairments, limitations in activity, and participation.
	Ask individuals about previous treatments and their level of effectiveness.

(continued on next page)

Table 1 (continued)	
Capabilities	
	Record the information accurately adhering to local protocols and professional requirements.
4. Physical assessment—The health care professional can do the following within their role and scope of practice	Obtain individuals' consent to physical examination, respect privacy and dignity while adhering to infection control protocols.
	Adapt practice to suit the needs of individuals, including cultural, religious factors, and other factors such as cognitive impairment.
	Perform relevant observational and functional assessments to identify and characterize impairments
	Record assessment information accurately adhering to local protocols and professional requirements.
5. Investigations and diagnosis—The health care professional can do the following within their role and scope of practice	Understand that the diagnosis of OA is based on clinical symptoms and radiological imaging is unnecessary for diagnosis.
	Assess the important features of the clinical assessment recognizing the wide variety of presentations in OA.
	Identify serious pathologies and make appropriate onward referrals.
	Identify risk factors for the rapid progression of OA.
	Recognize scenarios where early referral and diagnosis may impact long-term outcomes.
	Recognize how OA can interact with comorbidities.
	Describe OA using accurate and nonthreatening language.
DOMAIN C: Management, Interventions, & Prevention	
6. Interventions and care planning—The health care professional can do the following within their role and scope of practice	Develop management plans in partnership with individuals, accounting for their preferences and needs, within the services available.
	Recognize where different types of pain may require different management, eg, neuropathic pain.
	Include accessible pain management options in an individuals' management plan.
	Ensure an individuals' management plan considers all management options, their underlying evidence, risks, and benefits.
	Provide advice on nonpharmacologic and pharmacologic pain management options.
	Review and adjust management plans regularly according to an individuals' symptoms and treatment tolerability.

(continued on next page)

Table 1
(continued)

Capabilities

7. Prevention and lifestyle interventions—The health care professional can do the following within their role and scope of practice	Provide advice on increasing physical activity, refer to services as needed and explain the effects of inactivity. Provide advice on the effects of overweight and obesity on OA and where relevant, promote weight management and refer to services as needed. Support positive changes in lifestyle that may lead to improved health. Use behavior change techniques that support self-management.
8. Self-management and behavior change—The health care professional can do the following within their role and scope of practice	Explain the role of self-management strategies and lifestyle changes in pain management. Support self-management and lifestyle changes using behavior change techniques that aim to achieve an individuals' goals. Assist individuals to understand the consequences of their actions/inactions on their health and achievement of their goals. Support and encourage individuals to ask questions and discuss their concerns and priorities. Identify risk factors for persistent OA symptoms.
9. Rehabilitative interventions—The health care professional can do the following within their role and scope of practice	Explain the role of common rehabilitative interventions and the evidence to support their use. Provide advice on the benefits and risks, pros and cons of using different rehabilitative interventions. Provide advice on pain management, including graded activity, pacing, and direct individuals to self-management resources Recognize that individuals living with additional challenges, such as mental health issues and comorbidities, may need additional support during treatment. Work with individuals to explore the suitability of rehabilitative options, including referral to community-based programs. Refer individuals on to rehabilitation specialists when indicated
10. Pharmacotherapy—The health care professional can do the following within their role and scope of practice	Understand the role of medications and the evidence available for their effectiveness. Refer on for advice on medications when needed.

(continued on next page)

Table 1 (continued)	
Capabilities	
11. Surgical interventions—The health care professional can do the following within their role and scope of practice	Understand the role and evidence for the use of surgical interventions (arthroscopy and arthroplasty) for OA. Provide advice on the benefits, risks, advantages, disadvantages, and limitations of surgical procedures in the context of nonsurgical options Refer for surgical opinion when nonsurgical management is not providing sufficient symptomatic management.
12. Referrals and collaborative working—The health care professional can do the following within their role and scope of practice	Work within their role access specialist advice when needed. Communicate effectively with, and draw on the expertise of interdisciplinary colleagues to optimize an individuals' integrated care. Contribute to interdisciplinary service development and continuing education. Take part in the interdisciplinary team with an understanding of team dynamics. Refer individuals to other HCPs when appropriate.
DOMAIN D: Service & Professional Development	
13. Evidence-based practice and service development—The health care professional can do the following within their role and scope of practice	Identify and apply clinical practice guidelines appropriate to context Use data collection and evaluation to monitor service level outcomes, eg, quality of OA care, pain, and function outcomes. Engage in quality improvement, evaluation, and research as appropriate. Engage individuals and carers in providing feedback for quality improvement. Report service deficiencies that have the potential to affect an individual's care to relevant clinical service managers. Take part in relevant continued professional development opportunities. Take part in reflective practice and clinical supervision as part of professional development, to inform service development and quality improvement

Adapted from Hinman RS, Allen KD, Bennell KL, et al. Development of a core capability framework for qualified health professionals to optimize care for people with osteoarthritis: an OARSI initiative. Osteoarthritis Cartilage. 2020;28(2):154–166. https://doi.org/10.1016/j.joca.2019.12.001; with permission

(iii) high prevalence of predatory journals making authors especially in LMICs susceptible.[33,34]

Core Capabilities for the Delivery of Best Evidence OA Care

The JEI adapted a generic, skills-based capability framework for HCPs of any discipline providing care for people with OA, using a Delphi Panel to achieve expert

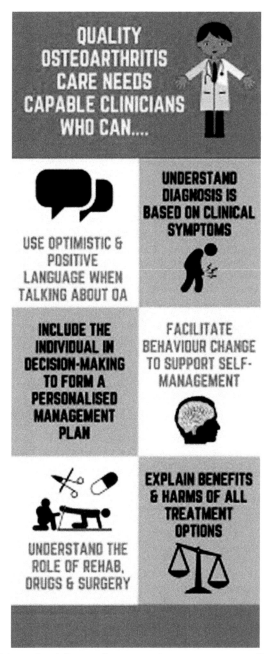

Fig. 2. Core capabilities for delivery of OA care. (*From* Hinman RS, Allen KD, Bennell KL, et al. Development of a core capability framework for qualified health professionals to optimise care for people with osteoarthritis: an OARSI initiative. Osteoarthritis Cartilage. 2020;28(2):154–166. https://doi.org/10.1016/j.joca.2019.12.001; with permission.)

Box 2
Key theories for educators in continuing professional education

1. **Cognitive load theory:** states that working memory has limitations, which impacts a learner's cognitive processing. Learning can be enhanced by managing different types of cognitive load.

Implementation: Educators can apply cognitive load theory to their courses by ensuring that content is digestible and relevant. Infographics, figures, or graphs could be helpful in illustrating content while minimizing intrinsic and extraneous cognitive load. Educators may also use several examples to help learners make sense of the content, such as through case studies. In education contexts where learners are acquiring a new skill or behavior, continued practice can help with easing cognitive load ("automatic processing").

2. **Constructivism:** views learning as being socially constructed, involving a process that builds new knowledge that is founded on an individual's previous understanding and experience. The educator encourages and promotes the learner to explore, discuss, and question their knowledge of the content (often through dialogue with the educator), by considering how it fits/does not fit into their own constructed framework.

Implementation: Depending on the format, constructivist methods can be applied to deepen the learner's understanding of concepts. Educators who adopt a constructivist's approach may engage in a discourse with their learners to understand the learner's preconceptions/pre-existing knowledge base. Identifying barriers to core skills and competencies may also be useful in identifying the learner's pre-existing knowledge base. The educators can then tailor the education or training to help the learner create either a new framework or alter their current framework to accommodate new concepts. This can be achieved by questioning and challenging the learner's current perspective or encouraging them to explain the rationale for their understanding (active discovery).

3. **Analogical transfer:** occurs "when a solution to a problem is used or transferred to solve a new and analogous problem in another situation."[39] This can only occur if the "deep structure" of 2 problems is equivalent.

Implementation: Educators can facilitate analogical transfer by developing a framework for a concept's deep structure that is common across multiple problems with different surface structures. By providing examples, sometimes in the form of stories or metaphors, learners can recognize situations or problems where analogical transfer can occur.

Adapted from Weidman J, Baker K. The Cognitive Science of Learning: Concepts and Strategies for the Educator and Learner. Anesth Analg. 2015;121(6):1586–1599. https://doi.org/10.1213/ANE.0000000000000890; with permission

---

consensus.[35] The resulting framework outlines a core set of capabilities to ensure that any HCPs managing a person with OA is able to implement evidence-based care. The final framework comprised 70 specific capabilities across 13 broad areas, mapped to 4 domains (**Table 1**), which can be used as a learning content framework for the development of education and training initiatives (**Fig. 2**).

Theories and Styles of Learning, and Preferences for Delivery

Learning theories

Learning theories provide education developers and designers the "strategies, tactics, and techniques" to optimize learning.[36] The main paradigms in adult learning are cognitivism, behaviorism, humanism, social learning (or social cognitive theory), and constructivism.[37] Despite the breadth of literature on learning theory for higher education, there is little focus on adult learning theory in continuing professional education (CPE).[38] Weidman and Baker (2015)[39] outlined key principles and theories of learning in CPE in medicine (cognitive load theory, constructivism, and analogical transfer).[39]

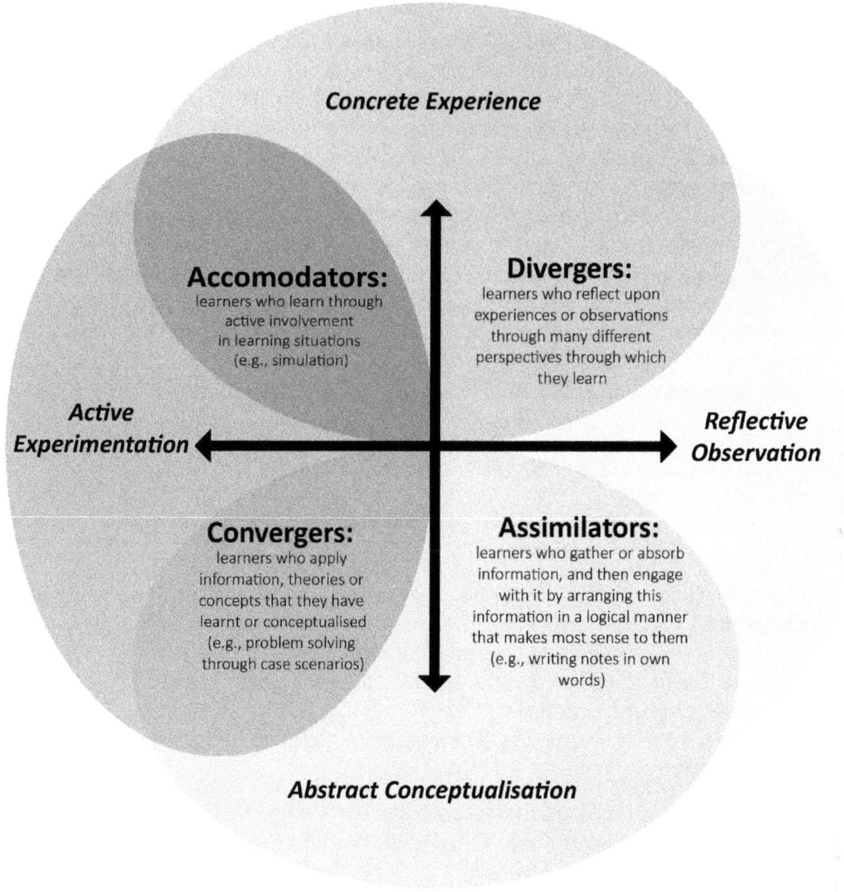

Fig. 3. Learning styles according to Kolb's Experiential Learning Theory. (KOLB, DAVID A, EXPERIENTIAL LEARNING: EXPERIENCE AS THE SOURCE OF LEARNING AND DEVELOPMENT, 2nd edition, ©2015. Reprinted by permission of Pearson Education, Inc.)

These theories and tips for their implementation are summarized in **Box 2** to guide the development of education and training for HCPs.

Understanding learning styles of HCPs

To further understand how HCPs engage with education and training, it is important to recognize the influence of learning styles. The literature surrounding learning styles for HCPs adopts Kolb's experiential learning theory, which is grounded on the idea that learning is a process, and that process is informed by experience.[40,41] Although learners may use different modes of learning, Kolb identified that learners can be categorized into 4 learning styles: convergers, accommodators, assimilators, and divergers (**Fig. 3**). Convergers and assimilators are the most popular learning styles for HCPs overall[42–45]; however, there is no "one-size-fits-all" approach,[42] and it is likely that learners will identify with several learning styles.[42–45]

Learning preferences

Despite an increase in online-based education and a rapid transformation from face-to-face modalities to eLearning options,[46] most HCPs prefer to engage and consume face-to-face education and training.[47–53] HCPs also prefer programs where there are opportunities for peer discussion and to apply new knowledge and skills in a practical setting.[48,54] A randomized trial comparing a face-to-face workshop with an eLearning workshop found that although learning outcomes were similar, physiotherapists were more satisfied with the face-to-face workshop.[55] To address this preference for face-to-face learning, eLearning should be interactive, stimulate reflection, and enable practice of new skills.[46] This could be achieved through creative use of discussion boards, audio-visual resources to demonstrate implementation of new skills in a clinical situation, and case scenarios to emulate face-to-face programs.[12,46,56] Emerging artificial intelligence programs may also have a role in simulating "real-life" case scenarios to engage HCPs.[57] A blended approach to education and training should be considered, where HCPs can asynchronously acquire knowledge, and then apply their new knowledge to practical situations while also exchanging ideas with peers and receiving feedback from instructors.[46,53]

Development of education and training: barriers, engaging with key stakeholders, and understanding context
Barriers to engaging with education and training. The most common barriers to HCPs completing CPE and training are:

- Lack of time,[46,47,50,54,58] other work/non–work-related priorities take precedence[49,58];
- Cost of courses, particularly face-to-face workshops[47,50];
- Access to education and training (both face-to-face and eLearning), especially those in remote/rural practices[49,50,58,59];
- Lack of interest in the topic,[54] perceived lack of relevance to practice.[49,58]

Although lack of time and motivation are still reported as common barriers to HCP participation, eLearning allows more flexibility with time, location, and choice of learning content.[46,60] However, there are specific barriers to eLearning, namely limited or no Internet access and digital literacy.[46,48] A systematic review recommended that workplaces provide dedicated time and space for online-based CPE, where opportunities are provided to practice skills learned online.[46,61]

Engaging with key stakeholders. Involving key stakeholders at decisive stages in the development of education and training programs can enhance uptake and engagement by HCPs. Key stakeholders may include:

1. clinical champions at different career levels, from diverse settings;
2. researchers who are content experts and/or skilled in implementation;
3. experts in educational design; and
4. professional societies and consumer groups.[62],

Engaging with these stakeholders during development and before implementation will ensure the education and training is more likely to be:

1. Relevant and necessary to the target HCP group;
2. Engaging for the target HCP group;
3. Linked with workforce capability plans and models of service delivery;
4. Consistent with professional development requirements of professional societies and/or accrediting organizations.

A recent survey of general practitioners, general practice nurses, and pharmacists in Scotland identified that meeting CPE requirements for registration was a powerful motivator for completion of education and training.[63] Involving professional societies, key stakeholders, and ensuring that HCPs are recognized for CPE could be used to enhance engagement with, and the sustainability of education and training programs.[63]

Importance of cultural and socioeconomic context. It is critical to consider the cultural and socioeconomic context in which the HCPs practice when designing education and training. Recently, there has been an increased focus on implementing models of care for musculoskeletal pain in LMICs to reduce the global burden of disability.[64,65] A strategy to build system capacity to deliver high-value musculoskeletal care in these countries is to ensure that there are enough trained and competent HCPs to provide this care.[66,67] A recently published systematic review highlighted an increase in education programs for nurses in LMICs from 2007 to 2017, particularly in Asia.[68] The authors highlighted the importance of context and culture in administering training programs, especially in rural settings. They identified several strategies to navigate the challenges of adapting educational materials to different cultural contexts including:

- Language translation and cross-cultural adaptations;
- Identifying and navigating local barriers to education;
- Identifying and using local cultural learning preferences;
- Collaborating with local administrators and professional societies to develop culturally acceptable education and training and seek their endorsement;
- Recognizing the limitations of infrastructure for community groups, including access to Internet, computers, and space to complete education and training.[68]

Other strategies may also include:

- Raising awareness of the high prevalence and burden of OA to advocate for the implementation of OA management programs[69];
- Ensuring that local guidelines are in accordance with international guidelines;
- Identifying and challenging existing attitudes or beliefs of HCPs in these contexts[70]; and
- Understanding differences in health care services in different countries and cultural contexts, and ensuring that educational materials are responsive to these differences.

It is important to recognize the specific contexts and needs of indigenous and ethnic minority communities. Many of these communities reside in rural and remote areas, where there is reduced health care infrastructure and limited access to information and technology services.[71,72] In addition, cultural beliefs about health care may impact how it is delivered, and diverge from Western beliefs about what constitutes high-value care.[71,73] Working in partnership with HCPs and leaders from these communities is critical to the successful implementation of sustainable education and training for HCPs. It is also important to understand and acknowledge the indigenous experience with OA and ensure that "cultural security" is embedded in their care, whereby "cultural rights, values, beliefs, knowledge systems, and expectations" are considered and included in the delivery of care.[74]

Evaluation of Education and Training for HCPs

Creating education and training content is costly, and HCPs are required to commit valuable time and money to participate fully in education and training initiatives. Therefore, it is important to evaluate the quality and efficacy of education and training to

Table 2
Framework for the evaluation of education and training based on the Kirkpatrick Evaluation Model and Implementation Outcomes

i. Reaction: Degree to Which the Education and/or Training was Favourable, Engaging, and Relevant to Their Work.

Construct	Outcome Measure	Related Implementation Outcomes
Satisfaction	HCP satisfaction can be measured using Likert or VAS/NRS customized to a specific learning activity and context	**Acceptability**—The perception that a given educational activity or resource is agreeable to HCPs,[77] can be measured using customized questions with Likert scales, or explored using qualitative methods such as interviews or focus groups,[23] or the *Acceptability of Intervention Measure*.[78]
Barriers	Factors that affect HCPs engaging with educational resources and implementing recommended care can be assessed using survey questions, semistructured interviews, or focus groups.	**Appropriateness**—The perceived fit, relevance, or compatibility of given educational resource of activity for a particular setting, audience, problem, or stakeholder,[77] it can be measured using customized questions with Likert scales or explored using qualitative methods such as interviews or focus groups,[23] or the *Intervention Appropriateness Measure*.[78]
Learning analytics	When using online resources, learning analytics can measure HCPs engagement with learning activities (eg, number of sites visited, time spent with each learning item).[57]	**Feasibility**—The extent to which an educational activity or resource can be used successfully within a particular setting,[77] it can be measured using customized questions with Likert scales the *Feasibility of Intervention Measure*.[78]
Usability	Assessment of how easily a resource is used by intended audiences is important when delivered via technology. The System Usability Scale assesses the usability of interface technologies and can be applied to different types of technology.[79]	

ii. Learning: Degree to Which HCPs Acquire the Knowledge, Skills, Attitudes, and Confidence Based on Their Interactions With the Education and/or Training.

Construct	Outcome measurement	Related implementation outcomes
Knowledge	The extent of knowledge gained from educational resources is often measured using custom-developed knowledge tests. For example, Peter et al. (2015) developed a knowledge questionnaire based on OA clinical practice	**Adoption/uptake**—Actions that indicate the intention to initiate an educational activity or use a resource,[77] usually expressed as a proportion of HCPs who engaged with a learning activity/educational resource (eg, attended a workshop) compared with the total number of people who

Skills

guidelines that they implemented in a randomized trial.[80]

Assessments of specific clinical skills of HCPs can be conducted through audio/video recordings of clinical encounters and scoring the encounters against specific criteria using trained assessors. For example, Elwyn et al. (2016) assessed shared decision-making between physiotherapists and people with OA using audio recordings and the Observing Patient Involvement in Decision Making (OPTION) instrument. A surrogate for assessing skills during clinical practice is measuring how HCPs respond to a clinical case (vignette).[81]

Confidence in knowledge and/or skills

The level of confidence that HCPs have in knowing "what" to do and "how" to do it can be measured using a customized questionnaire with Likert scales or VAS/NRS. Briggs et al. (2019) adapted a questionnaire to measure confidence in knowledge and skills of health professionals delivering OA care.[9]

Attitudes to aspects of recommended care

were eligible/invited.

Fidelity—The degree to which an educational resource or activity was implemented as was intended,[77] often reported in terms of adherence, dose, and quality of the intervention delivered.

Attitudes toward aspects of recommended care can be measured by rating agreement (on Likert scales) with statements regarding recommended, or nonrecommended management. For example, Moseng et al. (2019) asked HCPs to rate their agreement with statements about recommended treatments for OA before and after an education and training workshop.[82] Individual or focus group interviews can also be helpful for the assessment of attitudes to recommended care.[23,83]

iii. Behavior: the Degree to Which HCPs Apply What They Learned During Education and Training When They are Back at Work

Construct	Outcome measurement	Related implementation outcomes
Process outcomes	Outcomes that indicate that HCPs have followed recommended care can be recorded as a simple yes/no variable. For example, referrals rates to HCPs or services have been used in several previous randomized trials.[84,85] Quality Indicators represent an important standard of care for a particular condition and describe the process elements of care that should occur.[86] Two large implementation trials assessed patient-reported quality indicators for OA care[85,87]	**Factors that influence changes in clinical behaviors**—Education and training resources aim to change specific behaviors of HCPs. The theoretic domain framework provides a set of domains to help explain behavior change.[88,89] The Implementation Behavior Questionnaire was developed to identify factors influencing the behaviors of HCPs to enable assessment of efficacy and to assist with the design of implementation strategies.[90]

iv. Results: the Impact that the Education and Training Has Had on Broader Organizational Goals and Objectives

Construct	Outcome measurement	Related implementation outcomes
Patient-reported outcomes	Recommended patient-reported outcomes for OA include measurement of pain using an NRS or VAS, and function with a questionnaire such as the Knee injury and Osteoarthritis Outcome Score or Western Ontario and McMaster Universities Osteoarthritis Index as has been used in previous randomized controlled trials[87,91]	**Cost**—refers to the cost impact of an implementation effort.[77] This can be achieved through simple costing of treatments. The cost-effectiveness of a model OA consultation to support self-management compared with usual care was assessed through incremental cost-utility analysis using the EuroQoL-5D questionnaire.[92] **Penetration**—indicates the integration of an educational activity or resource within a service setting and its subsystems.[77] **Sustainability**—is the extent to which educational activities, resources, and innovation are maintained within an ongoing service setting, including stable operation over time.[77]
Rates of joint replacement surgery	The rate of joint replacement surgery within a population can be an informative outcome where the goals of the education and/or training are to increase access to joint replacement surgery or reduce unnecessary surgeries.	
Equity of access to OA care	Differences in access to and outcomes of OA care across groups with different socioeconomic, geographic, and racial/ethnic characteristics.[93]	

Abbreviations: NRS, numeric rating scale; OA, osteoarthritis; VAS, visual analog scale.

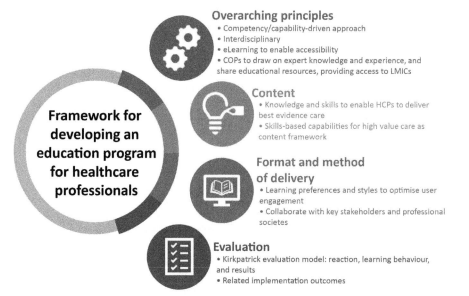

Overarching principles
- Competency/capability-driven approach
- Interdisciplinary
- eLearning to enable accessibility
- COPs to draw on expert knowledge and experience, and share educational resources, providing access to LMICs

Content
- Knowledge and skills to enable HCPs to deliver best evidence care
- Skills-based capabilities for high value care as content framework

Format and method of delivery
- Learning preferences and styles to optimise user engagement
- Collaborate with key stakeholders and professional societes

Evaluation
- Kirkpatrick evaluation model: reaction, learning behaviour, and results
- Related implementation outcomes

Framework for developing an education program for healthcare professionals

Fig. 4. Framework to guide clinicians in developing education and training for HCPs.

ensure it meets the needs of learners and is successful at achieving its intended aims. The Kirkpatrick Evaluation Model[75] is well-accepted for the evaluation of education and training. It has 4 levels:

1. Reaction: the degree to which HCPs find the education and training favorable, engaging, and relevant;
2. Learning: the degree to which HCPs acquire the knowledge, skills, attitude, confidence, and commitment through the education and training;
3. Behavior: the degree to which HCPs apply what they learned during education and training; and
4. Results: the impact that the education and training has had on broader organizational goals and objectives.

Despite its popularity, this simple model has been criticized for not adequately accounting for contextual factors.[75] Implementation outcomes can be considered alongside the evaluation domains of the Kirkpatrick Evaluation Model to enrich the evaluation of education and training programs. Implementation outcomes arise from implementation research, which can be broadly defined as the study of carrying research evidence into practice.[76] The Kirkpatrick Model is outlined in **Table 2**, with relevant outcomes at each level, and related implementation outcomes that can be used as a framework for evaluation.

SUMMARY

This article presents a framework to guide the development and evaluation of education and training for HCPs in the delivery of best evidence OA care (**Fig. 4**). It is important to consider the barriers for the implementation of core components of OA care, including system-based, clinician-based, and patient-based barriers when designing education and training for HCPs by engaging with key stakeholders. This is even more critical when designing education and training for low-resourced settings where HCPs may not have access to the infrastructure or the facilities to deliver care in the same way that it is recommended in high-resourced settings. Developing education and training materials that are culturally appropriate to local contexts, particularly in LMICs or non-western cultures should be a priority.

At present, there is no generally available education and training to support HCPs in best evidence OA care that is interdisciplinary in nature and that addresses the core capabilities of OA care. Work is currently being undertaken to address this through a project led by members of the JEI, and based around this framework, to develop, evaluate and implement an interdisciplinary eLearning program for any HCP delivering care for OA.

CLINICS CARE POINTS

- Key overarching principles for HCP education and training are as follows: (1) ensuring that education is competency/capability-driven; (2) interdisciplinary; (3) uses innovation and technology (eLearning); (4) draws on expert knowledge and experience; and (5) is inclusive and accessible for LMICs and low-resourced settings.

- There is no "one-size-fits-all" learning style for HCPs. Engaging with all learning styles needs to be considered when designing education and training.

- A blended approach to education and training (eLearning and synchronous workshops) may be effective for HCPs learning new knowledge and skills for best evidence OA care.

- Meeting CPD requirements may be a key motivator to engage HCPs in education and training.

- Engaging with professional societies, community members, and HCPs in LMICs and low-resourced settings is crucial for the successful implementation of education and training in these contexts.

- Education and training should be available in multiple languages to meet the needs of clinicians of diverse cultural and language skills.

- The Kirkpatrick Evaluation Model is a well-accepted framework for evaluating professional education and training.

DISCLOSURE

R.S. Hinman is supported by a National Health & Medical Research Council Senior Research Fellowship (#1154217). All other authors have nothing to disclose.

REFERENCES

1. Global Burden of Disease Collaborative Network. Global burden of disease study 2019 (GBD 2019) results. http://ghdx.healthdata.org/gbd-results-tool. [Accessed 2 September 2021].
2. World Health Organization. World report on ageing and health. Geneva: World Health Organization; 2015.
3. Kolasinski SL, Neogi T, Hochberg MC, et al. 2019 American College of Rheumatology/Arthritis Foundation guideline for the management of osteoarthritis of the hand, hip, and knee. Arthritis Care Res (2010) 2020;72(2):149–62.
4. Bannuru RR, Osani MC, Vaysbrot EE, et al. OARSI guidelines for the non-surgical management of knee, hip, and polyarticular osteoarthritis. Osteoarthritis Cartilage 2019;27(11):1578–89.

5. Eyles JP, Hunter DJ, Bennell KL, et al. Priorities for the effective implementation of osteoarthritis management programs: an OARSI international consensus exercise. Osteoarthritis Cartilage 2019;27(9):1270–9.

6. Hagen KB, Smedslund G, Østerås N, et al. Quality of community-based osteoarthritis care: a systematic review and meta-analysis. Arthritis Care Res 2016; 68(10):1443–52.

7. Ackerman IN, Livingston JA, Osborne RH. Personal perspectives on enablers and barriers to accessing care for hip and knee osteoarthritis. Phys Ther 2016; 96(1):26–36.

8. Briggs AM, Houlding E, Hinman RS, et al. Health professionals and students encounter multi-level barriers to implementing high-value osteoarthritis care: a multi-national study. Osteoarthritis Cartilage 2019;27(5):788–804.

9. Briggs AM, Hinman RS, Darlow B, et al. Confidence and attitudes toward osteoarthritis care among the current and emerging health workforce: a Multinational interprofessional study. ACR Open Rheumatol 2019;1(4):219–35.

10. Egerton T, Diamond LE, Buchbinder R, et al. A systematic review and evidence synthesis of qualitative studies to identify primary care clinicians' barriers and enablers to the management of osteoarthritis. Osteoarthritis Cartilage 2017;25(5): 625–38.

11. Selten EMH, Vriezekolk JE, Nijhof MW, et al. Barriers impeding the use of non-pharmacological, non-surgical care in hip and knee osteoarthritis: the views of general practitioners, physical therapists, and medical specialists. J 2017; 23(8):405–10.

12. Chehade MJ, Gill TK, Kopansky-Giles D, et al. Building multidisciplinary health workforce capacity to support the implementation of integrated, people-centred Models of Care for musculoskeletal health. Best Pract Res Clin Rheumatol 2016;30(3):559–84.

13. Sharma M, Murphy R, Doody GA. Do we need a core curriculum for medical students? A scoping review. BMJ open 2019;9(8):e027369.

14. International association for the study of pain. IASP interprofessional pain curriculum outline. https://www.iasp-pain.org/education/curricula/iasp-interprofessional-pain-curriculum-outline/.

15. Vos T, Abajobir A, Abate K, et al. Global, regional, and national incidence, prevalence, and years lived with disability for 328 diseases and injuries for 195 countries, 1990-2016: a systematic analysis for the Global Burden of Disease Study 2016. Lancet 2017;390(10100):1211–59.

16. Frenk J, Chen L, Bhutta ZA, et al. Health professionals for a new century: transforming education to strengthen health systems in an interdependent world. Lancet 2010;376(9756):1923–58.

17. Epstein RM, Hundert EM. Defining and assessing professional competence. JAMA 2002;287(2):226–35.

18. Fraser SW, Greenhalgh T. Coping with complexity: educating for capability. BMJ (Clinical Research Ed) 2001;323(7316):799–803.

19. Barr H, Koppel I, Reeves S, et al. Effective interprofessional education: argument, assumption and evidence. Oxford: Blackwell; 2005.

20. Brack P, Shields N. Short duration clinically-based interprofessional shadowing and patient review activities may have a role in preparing health professional students to practice collaboratively: a systematic literature review. J Interprof Care 2019;33(5):446–55.

21. World Health Organization. Framework for action on interprofessional education & collaborative practice. Geneva, Switzerland: World Health Organization; 2010.

22. Hammick M, Freeth D, Koppel I, et al. A best evidence systematic review of inter-professional education: BEME Guide no. 9. Med Teach 2007;29(8):735–51.

23. Jones SE, Campbell PK, Kimp AJ, et al. Evaluation of a novel e-learning program for physiotherapists to manage knee osteoarthritis via telehealth: qualitative study nested in the PEAK (physiotherapy exercise and physical activity for knee osteoarthritis) randomized controlled trial. J Med Internet Res 2021;23(4):e25872.

24. Haywood H, Pain H, Ryan S, et al. Continuing professional development: issues raised by nurses and allied health professionals working in musculoskeletal settings. Musculoskelet Care 2013;11(3):136–44.

25. Feldacker C, Pintye J, Jacob S, et al. Continuing professional development for medical, nursing, and midwifery cadres in Malawi, Tanzania and South Africa: a qualitative evaluation. PLoS One 2017;12(10):e0186074.

26. Barton CJ, Ezzat AM, Bell EC, et al. Knowledge, confidence and learning needs of physiotherapists treating persistent knee pain in Australia and Canada: a mixed-methods study. Physiother Theor Pract 2021;1–13.

27. Zuo L, Miller Juve A. Transitioning to a new era: future directions for staff development during COVID-19. Med Educ 2021;55(1):104–7.

28. Arora A. Disrupting clinical education: using artificial intelligence to create training material. Clin Teach 2020;17(4):357–9.

29. Maloney S, Moss A, Keating J, et al. Sharing teaching and learning resources: perceptions of a university's faculty members. Med Educ 2013;47(8):811–9.

30. Rolfe V. Open educational resources: staff attitudes and awareness. Res Learn Technology 2012;20(1):1–13.

31. Regmi K, Jones L. A systematic review of the factors - enablers and barriers - affecting e-learning in health sciences education. BMC Med Educ 2020;20(1):91.

32. Iyandemye J, Thomas MP. Low income countries have the highest percentages of open access publication: a systematic computational analysis of the biomedical literature. PLoS One 2019;14(7):e0220229.

33. Greussing E, Kuballa S, Taddicken M, et al. Drivers and obstacles of open access publishing. A qualitative investigation of individual and Institutional factors. Front Commun 2020;5(90).

34. Severin A, Strinzel M, Egger M, et al. Characteristics of scholars who review for predatory and legitimate journals: linkage study of Cabells Scholarly Analytics and Publons data. BMJ Open 2021;11(7):e050270.

35. Hinman RS, Allen KD, Bennell KL, et al. Development of a core capability framework for qualified health professionals to optimise care for people with osteoarthritis: an OARSI initiative. Osteoarthritis Cartilage 2019;28(2):154–66.

36. Ertmer PA, Newby TJ. Behaviorism, cognitivism, constructivism: comparing critical features from an instructional design perspective. Perform improvement Q 2013;26(2):43–71.

37. Marquardt M, Waddill D. The power of learning in action learning: a conceptual analysis of how the five schools of adult learning theories are incorporated within the practice of action learning. Action Learn Res Pract 2004;1(2):185–202.

38. Wittnebel L. Business as usual? A review of continuing professional education and adult learning. J Adult Cont Educ 2012;18(2):80–8.

39. Weidman J, Baker K. The cognitive science of learning: concepts and strategies for the educator and learner. Anesth Analgesia 2015;121(6):1586–99.

40. Kolb DA. Experiential learning: experience as the source of learning and development. New Jersey, United States of America: Pearson FT Press; 2014.

41. Manolis C, Burns DJ, Assudani R, et al. Assessing experiential learning styles: a methodological reconstruction and validation of the Kolb Learning Style Inventory. Learn Individual Diff 2013;23:44–52.

42. Stander J, Grimmer K, Brink Y. Training programmes to improve evidence uptake and utilisation by physiotherapists: a systematic scoping review. BMC Med Educ 2018;18(1):1–12.

43. Smith A. Learning styles of registered nurses enrolled in an online nursing program. J Prof Nurs 2010;26(1):49–53.

44. Rassin M, Kurzweil Y, Maoz Y. Identification of the learning styles and "on-the-job" learning methods implemented by nurses for promoting their professional knowledge and skills. Int J Nurs Educ Scholarship 2015;12(1):75–81.

45. Jack MC, Kenkare SB, Saville BR, et al. Improving education under work-hour restrictions: comparing learning and teaching preferences of faculty, residents, and students. J Surg Education 2010;67(5):290–6.

46. Lawn S, Zhi X, Morello A. An integrative review of e-learning in the delivery of self-management support training for health professionals. BMC Med Educ 2017; 17(1):183.

47. Barton CJ, Ezzat AM, Bell EC, et al. Knowledge, confidence and learning needs of physiotherapists treating persistent knee pain in Australia and Canada: a mixed-methods study. Physiother Theor Pract 2021;1–13.

48. Micallef R, Kayyali R. A systematic review of models used and preferences for continuing education and continuing professional development of pharmacists. Pharmacy 2019;7(4):154.

49. Goodyear-Smith F, Whitehorn M, McCormick R. Experiences and preferences of general practitioners regarding continuing medical education : a qualitative study. New Zealand Med J 2003;116(1172):10p.

50. Maher B, O'Neill R, Faruqui A, et al. Survey of Irish general practitioners' preferences for continuing professional development. Educ Prim Care 2018;29(1): 13–21.

51. Muñoz-Castro FJ, Valverde-Gambero E, Herrera-Usagre M. Predictors of health professionals' satisfaction with continuing education: a cross-sectional study. Revista Lat Am Enfermagem 2020;28:e3315.

52. Jeong D, Presseau J, ElChamaa R, et al. Barriers and facilitators to self-directed learning in continuing professional development for physicians in Canada: a scoping review. Acad Med 2018;93(8):1245–54.

53. Jones SE, Campbell PK, Kimp AJ, et al. Evaluation of a novel e-learning program for physiotherapists to manage knee osteoarthritis via telehealth: qualitative study nested in the PEAK (physiotherapy exercise and physical activity for knee osteoarthritis) randomized controlled trial. J Med Internet Res 2021;23(4):e25872.

54. Xing W, Ao L, Xiao H, et al. Chinese nurses' preferences for and attitudes about e-learning in continuing education: a correlational study. J Contin Educ Nurs 2020;51(2):87–96.

55. Richmond H, Hall AM, Hansen Z, et al. Using mixed methods evaluation to assess the feasibility of online clinical training in evidence based interventions: a case study of cognitive behavioural treatment for low back pain. BMC Med Educ 2016;16:163.

56. Cook DA, Levinson AJ, Garside S, et al. Instructional design variations in internet-based learning for health professions education: a systematic review and meta-analysis. Acad Med 2010;85(5):909–22.

57. Chan AK, Botelho MG, Lam OL. Use of learning analytics data in health care-related educational disciplines: systematic review. J Med Int Res 2019;21(2): e11241.
58. French HP, Dowds J. An overview of continuing professional development in physiotherapy. Physiotherapy 2008;94(3):190–7.
59. Macaden L, Washington M, Smith A, et al. Continuing professional development: needs, facilitators and barriers of registered nurses in India in rural and remote settings: findings from a cross sectional survey. Open J Nurs 2017;7(8).
60. Carroll C, Booth A, Papaioannou D, et al. UK health-care professionals' experience of on-line learning techniques: a systematic review of qualitative data. J Contin Educ Health Prof 2009;29(4):235–41.
61. Campbell C, Lockyer J. Categorising and enhancing the impacts of continuing professional development to improve performance and health outcomes. Med Educ 2019;53(11):1066–9.
62. Sinclair PM, Levett-Jones T, Morris A, et al. High engagement, high quality: a guiding framework for developing empirically informed asynchronous e-learning programs for health professional educators. Nurs Health Sci 2017;19(1):126–37.
63. Cunningham DE, Alexander A, Luty S, et al. CPD preferences and activities of general practitioners, registered pharmacy staff and general practice nurses in NHS Scotland – a questionnaire survey. Education Prim Care 2019;30(4):220–9.
64. Briggs AM, Chan M, Slater H. Models of Care for musculoskeletal health: moving towards meaningful implementation and evaluation across conditions and care settings. Best Pract Res Clin Rheumatol 2016;30(3):359–74.
65. Briggs AM, Shiffman J, Shawar YR, et al. Global health policy in the 21st century: challenges and opportunities to arrest the global disability burden from musculoskeletal health conditions. Best Pract Res Clin Rheumatol 2020;34(5):101549.
66. Sharma S, Blyth FM, Mishra SR, et al. Health system strengthening is needed to respond to the burden of pain in low- and middle-income countries and to support healthy ageing. J Glob Health 2019;9(2):020317.
67. Lim KK, Chan M, Navarra S, et al. Development and implementation of Models of Care for musculoskeletal conditions in middle-income and low-income Asian countries. Best Pract Res Clin Rheumatol 2016;30(3):398–419.
68. Azad A, Min J-G, Syed S, et al. Continued nursing education in low-income and middle-income countries: a narrative synthesis. BMJ Glob Health 2020;5(2): e001981.
69. Woolf ADBMF, Brooks PFFF, Åkesson KMDP, et al. Prevention of musculoskeletal conditions in the developing world. Best Pract Res Clin Rheumatol 2008;22(4): 759–72.
70. Arshad A, Rashid R. A pilot study of the primary care management of knee osteoarthritis in the Northern States of Malaysia. IIUM Med J Malaysia 2008;7(2).
71. Vindigni D, Parkinson L, Blunden S, et al. Aboriginal health in Aboriginal hands: development, delivery and evaluation of a training programme for Aboriginal health workers to promote the musculoskeletal health of Indigenous people living in a rural community 2004;4(4):281.
72. Vindigni D, Griffen D, Perkins J, et al. Prevalence of musculoskeletal conditions, associated pain and disability and the barriers to managing these conditions in a rural. Aust Aboriginal Community 2004;4(3):230.
73. World Health Organization. The health of indigenous peoples. Geneva, Switzerland: World Health Organization; 1999.

74. O'Brien P, Bunzli S, Lin I, et al. Tackling the burden of osteoarthritis as a health care opportunity in indigenous communities—a call to action. J Clin Med 2020; 9(8):2393.
75. Bates R. A critical analysis of evaluation practice: the Kirkpatrick model and the principle of beneficence. Eval Program Plann 2004;27(3):341–7.
76. Peters DH, Adam T, Alonge O, et al. Implementation research: what it is and how to do it. BMJ (Clinical Research Ed) 2013;347:f6753.
77. Proctor E, Silmere H, Raghavan R, et al. Outcomes for implementation research: conceptual distinctions, measurement challenges, and research Agenda. Adm Policy Ment Health Ment Health Serv Res 2011;38(2):65–76.
78. Weiner BJ, Lewis CC, Stanick C, et al. Psychometric assessment of three newly developed implementation outcome measures. Implement Sci 2017;12(1):108.
79. Bangor A, Kortum PT, Miller JT. An empirical evaluation of the system usability scale. Int J Human Computer Interaction 2008;24(6):574–94.
80. Peter W, van der Wees PJ, Verhoef J, et al. Effectiveness of an interactive post-graduate educational intervention with patient participation on the adherence to a physiotherapy guideline for hip and knee osteoarthritis: a randomised controlled trial. Disabil Rehabil 2015;37(3):274–82.
81. Evans SC, Roberts MC, Keeley JW, et al. Vignette methodologies for studying clinicians' decision-making: validity, utility, and application in ICD-11 field studies. Int J Clin Health Psychol 2015;15(2):160–70.
82. Moseng T, Dagfinrud H, Osteras N. Implementing international osteoarthritis guidelines in primary care: uptake and fidelity among health professionals and patients. Osteoarthritis Cartilage 2019;27(8):1138–47.
83. Lawford BJ, Delany C, Bennell KL, et al. "I was really pleasantly surprised": first-hand experience with telephone-delivered exercise therapy shifts physiotherapists' perceptions of such a service for knee osteoarthritis. A qualitative study. Arthritis Care Res (Hoboken) 2019;71(4):545–57.
84. Allen KD, Yancy WS Jr, Bosworth HB, et al. A combined patient and provider intervention for management of osteoarthritis in veterans: a randomized clinical trial [with consumer summary]. Ann Intern Med 2016;164(2):73–83.
85. Osteras N, Moseng T, van Bodegom-Vos L, et al. Implementing a structured model for osteoarthritis care in primary healthcare: a stepped-wedge cluster-randomised trial. PLoS Med 2019;16(10):e1002949.
86. Osteras N, Garratt A, Grotle M, et al. Patient-reported quality of care for osteoarthritis: development and testing of the osteoarthritis quality indicator questionnaire. Arthritis Care Res 2013;65(7):1043–51.
87. Dziedzic KS, Healey EL, Porcheret M, et al. Implementing core NICE guidelines for osteoarthritis in primary care with a model consultation (MOSAICS): a cluster randomised controlled trial. Osteoarthritis Cartilage 2018;26(1):43–53.
88. Cane J, O'Connor D, Michie S. Validation of the theoretical domains framework for use in behaviour change and implementation research. Implement Sci 2012;7:37.
89. Michie S, Johnston M, Abraham C, et al. Making psychological theory useful for implementing evidence based practice: a consensus approach. Qual Saf Health Care 2005;14(1):26–33.
90. Huijg JM, Gebhardt WA, Dusseldorp E, et al. Measuring determinants of implementation behavior: psychometric properties of a questionnaire based on the theoretical domains framework. Implement Sci 2014;9:33.
91. Allen KD, Oddone EZ, Coffman CJ, et al. Patient, provider, and combined interventions for managing osteoarthritis in primary care: a cluster randomized trial. Ann Intern Med 2017;166(6):401–11.

92. Oppong R, Jowett S, Lewis M, et al. Cost-effectiveness of a model consultation to support self-management in patients with osteoarthritis. Rheumatology (Oxford) 2018;57(6):1056–63.

93. Callahan LF, Cleveland RJ, Allen KD, et al. Racial/ethnic, socioeconomic, and geographic disparities in the epidemiology of knee and hip osteoarthritis. Rheum Dis Clin North Am 2021;47(1):1–20.

Surgery for Osteoarthritis

Total Joint Arthroplasty, Realistic Expectations of Rehabilitation and Surgical Outcomes: A Narrative Review

Kaka Martina, RN, BN, GradDip (Clinical Teaching)[a,b,c,d,*],
David J. Hunter, MBBS, MSc (Clin Epi), M SpMed, PhD, FRACP (Rheum)[a,b,e],
Lucy J. Salmon, BAppSci (Physio), PhD[d,f,1],
Justin P. Roe, MBBS, FRACS[d,g,1],
Michelle M. Dowsey, BHealthSci (Nursing), MEpi, PhD[h,2]

KEYWORDS

• Arthroplasty • Expectation • Rehabilitation • Inpatient • Surgery • THA • TKA

KEY POINTS

• The increase in demand for TJA will require a sustainable health care expenditure budget with an appropriate health care workforce and resource allocation, while concurrently optimizing the quality of care.

• A better understanding of realistic patient expectations will assist surgeons and clinicians to better modify care and accommodate patients' needs, to meet the important concept of patient-centered care.

• Both in public and private sectors, rehabilitation services are integrated into postoperative care after TJA; however, there are inconsistencies in what is believed to be the benchmark for a rehabilitation setting, level of care, and duration after TJA.

• Assessing outcomes of TJA go beyond what was conventionally determined by prosthesis survivorship or surgeon-based clinical and radiological assessments, to a patient-centered approach inclusive of patient-reported outcomes.

[a] Rheumatology Department, Royal North Shore Hospital, Sydney, New South Wales, Australia; [b] Institute of Bone and Joint Research, Kolling Institute, University of Sydney, Sydney, New South Wales, Australia; [c] Mater Hospital Sydney, Sydney, New South Wales, Australia; [d] North Sydney Orthopedic and Sports Medicine Center, Sydney, New South Wales; [e] Kolling Institute, Level 10, 10 Westbourne Street, St Leonards, New South Wales 2064, Australia; [f] University of Notre Dame, Sydney, New South Wales, Australia; [g] University of New South Wales, Sydney, New South Wales, Australia; [h] Department of Surgery, University of Melbourne, St Vincent's Hospital, Melbourne, Victoria, Australia
[1] Present address: Suite G.02, 3 Gillies Street, Wollstonecraft, NSW 2065, Australia.
[2] Present address: Level 2, Clinical Sciences Building, 29 Regent Street, Fitzroy, VIC 3010, Australia
* Corresponding author. Suite G.02, 3 Gillies Street, Wollstonecraft, New South Wales 2065, Australia.
E-mail address: kmartina@nsosmc.com.au

Clin Geriatr Med 38 (2022) 385–396
https://doi.org/10.1016/j.cger.2021.11.009
0749-0690/22/© 2021 Elsevier Inc. All rights reserved.

geriatric.theclinics.com

INTRODUCTION

Osteoarthritis (OA) is a chronic joint disease that is associated with a substantial and increasing individual, socioeconomic, and health burden.[1] OA is the single leading cause of disability worldwide in older adults because of its disabling impact on joints and the primary symptom of pain.[2-4] With an aging population, the continual growth of obesity and increasing sports-related injuries,[5] the prevalence of OA is becoming more common, with more than 500 million people affected by this disease globally.[6]

Although OA is an irreversible condition, interventions do exist that lessen or effectively manage symptoms.[7,8] Conservative treatment is promoted as the first-line treatment for OA,[9] and involves interventions that target modifiable risk factors, such as obesity, joint malalignment, or muscle weakness.[10] The aim of these interventions is to increase physical functionality by minimizing the effects of pain and how it negatively impacts an individual's quality of life (QoL).[9,11] This may include weight management, physical therapy, and activity modification.[9,11,12] In addition, pharmacologic treatment modalities are regularly integrated into conservative management in various forms, from oral regimes to more targeted treatments, such as intra-articular injections.[8] When all appropriate nonsurgical treatments have been attempted for a reasonable period and are no longer sufficiently effective, only then should surgical treatment be considered.

The referral to see an orthopedic specialist is generally completed by a primary care physician. This referral should be based on a pattern of deterioration in overall physical functioning or mobility, combined with poor health-related QoL.[9,13] The frequency of elective surgery for OA is increasing, despite well-documented reports that it does not always lead to desirable outcomes.[14] This reflects the increasing burden of end-stage OA. The most frequently performed surgical treatment for individuals with end-stage OA, especially of the hip and knee, is total joint arthroplasty (TJA).[15,16] Globally, the incidence of TJA is predicted to grow.[5] Between 2000 and 2014, the estimated annual incidence of THA and TKA in the United States increased by 105% (from 56.80 to 116.26 per 100,000 population) and 119% (from 97.37 to 213.28 per 100,000 population), respectively.[17] Multiple studies have projected significant growth in future THA and TKA procedure volumes in the United States for the next few decades.[17-19] In Australia, the age-standardized rate of TJA with OA as the primary diagnosis increased by 27% for TKA (from 144 to 183 per 100,000 population) and 33% (from 85 to 113 per 100,000 population) for THA, from 2008 to 2009 to 2017 to 2018.[12] The continuous increase in demand for TJA will require a sustainable health care expenditure budget with an appropriate health care workforce and resource allocation, while concurrently optimizing the quality of care.[5]

TJA: WHAT, WHY, WHO, AND WHEN

TJA, a gold standard treatment for end-stage OA,[20] involves removing and substituting the arthritic part of the joint with a prosthesis, which imitates the movement of a normal healthy joint. TJA should ideally be offered to individuals who have exhausted sufficient conservative interventions, where activities of daily living are affected and QoL is declining.[20,21] The effectiveness of TJA to treat end-stage OA is well-documented in the literature.[22] Up until 2019, the Australian Orthopedic Association National Joint Replacement Registry (AOANJRR) recorded OA as the primary diagnosis in 98% of knee replacement and 88% of hip replacement surgeries performed in Australia since data collection commenced in 1999.[23]

TJA is a resource-intensive procedure that can lead to serious risks and adverse events.[21,24,25] A significant proportion (~50%) of the direct health care cost of OA derives from the cost of this surgery.[5,26,27]With the continuous growth of TJA per-formed worldwide, selecting suitable candidates for surgery and optimizing after-care algorithms become vital to consider.

Although an orthopedic surgeon can indicate the need for surgery based on clinical and radiographic assessments, decision-making for TJA should always be shared and patient-centered, weighing up the personal risks and benefits. The indication for TJA becomes challenging when orthopedic surgeons are presented with individuals who fall outside the "ideal candidate", such as those who are younger or much older, or who are obese, or have other pre-existing health comorbidities.[25,28,29] **Table 1** refers to some common criteria to consider in recommending a referral for TJA.

Before recommending surgery, it is critical for surgeons to determine a patient's un-derstanding of what the surgery involves, particularly on the pattern and length of re-covery, and ascertain the ultimate goal of surgery from the patient's perspective.[30–33] The process needs to be collaborative where both parties jointly discuss all aspects of the surgery while incorporating the patient's needs and preferences[34]. This "partner-ship" model of patient-clinician communication is preferable to a paternalistic approach, whereby decisions are heavily weighted by surgical opinion, independent of individual patients' needs and choices.[34–36] The shared-decision making process is beneficial to improve patient knowledge, reduce the risk of inaccurate patient per-ceptions of the treatment and outcomes, which will diminish any decisional conflict between a clinician and patient.[36] This process will empower patients to make informed decisions, and establish realistic expectations of their rehabilitation journey and surgery outcomes.

REALISTIC EXPECTATIONS: REHABILITATION AFTER TJA

In the "ideal" clinical care for TJA, surgeons and hospital staff involved spend a considerable amount of time with surgery candidates, explaining not only the risks and benefits of surgery, but also the extent and length of the recovery effort required to reach a specific outcome or goal.[37] This is aimed to facilitate patients setting realistic anticipations of what events are expected in the perioperative period, and what can result from surgery itself.[38] However, whether or not patients' and surgeons' expectations are aligned despite the efforts mentioned earlier re-mains debatable.[38,39]

Table 1
Surgical indications and contraindications for THA and TKA

Indications	Contraindications
Significant pain with no adequate pain relief	Active sepsis or existing infection in the joint
Progressive physical function loss or disability due to pain, swelling or deformity	Other ongoing remote source of infection
Deteriorated quality of life	Poorly controlled pre-existing mental and/or physical health comorbidities*
Significant radiographic changes (Kellgren-Lawrence grade 3 or 4)	Obesity/morbidly obese**
Failed conservative therapy	

Note * and ** Relative contraindications
** The recommended 'ideal' Body Mass Index (BMI) for best outcomes following TJA is BMI ≥ 20 and ≤ 30 kg/m^2
Data from the Royal Australian College of General Practitioners. Guideline for the management of knee and hip osteoarthritis. 2nd edn. East Melbourne, Vic: RACGP, 2018

Postacute rehabilitation service is a controversial topic in relation to after-hospital care following TJA. In current clinical practice, after a THA or TKA, patients are typically either transferred to an inpatient rehabilitation (IPR) facility as another hospital admission, or discharged directly home. Discharge directly home can occur with or without an outpatient-based physiotherapy program. Outpatient-based physiotherapy may be delivered via day hospital-based therapy, private clinic physiotherapy, or through a physiotherapy-in-the-home program, where patients are treated in their own home and/or provided exercise guidance via teleconference.[40,41] Both in public and private sectors, rehabilitation services are integrated into the postoperative care for TJA.[42] However, there is a high variance both nationally and internationally in what is believed to be the benchmark for postacute rehabilitation setting, level of care, and duration after TJA.[43–49]

Multiple studies have highlighted that after-hospital discharge to IPR versus home after THA and TKA does not lead to better functional and patient-reported outcomes, and is associated with increased risks of postdischarge complications and unexpected readmission.[44,46,50] In Australia, the uptake of IPR from individual hospitals across the states/territories varies greatly from 4% to 64%.[42,48] A report in 2018 highlighted that the use of IPR service after THA and TKA in the United States reached a median of 26% (range, 3.1%–58%), with the rest of this population either being referred to a "skilled nursing facility" or home-based rehabilitation service, with or without supervision of a physiotherapist.[42] However, the recent initiation to rule out TJA from "Medicare Inpatient Only List -list of procedures which are covered under Medicare, only when the treatment takes place in an inpatient setting-," in the United States, has driven surgeons to offer same-day discharge TJA.[51] Although the potential candidate selection may be more restricted for day surgery TJA, this trend has become increasingly common in the United States, and research has demonstrated this as a feasible option to address the mounting health care cost.[51]

In Australia, most THAs and TKAs are performed in the private sector; in 2020, 71% of TKA and 60% of THA were undertaken in private hospitals across the country.[23] The uptake for referral to an IPR facility following elective THA and TKA in privately insured patients is 33% and 56%, respectively, compared with only 4% of THA and 8% of TKA patients who are publicly insured, in Australia.[46] Hence, insurance status is a significant aspect that influences patient's decision in relation to TJA-related expenses and medical care, particularly in the private sector. Previous research has suggested the views of privately insured patients on the effectiveness of IPR as a service of choice following acute hospital care, are strongly influenced by their own and close social environment.[52–54] It is not uncommon that a patient who was transferred to an extended IPR facility after their previous TJA surgery will choose the same option again with their subsequent TJA in the future, regardless of a clinical indication for this medical care. A sense of self-entitlement to the costly medical treatment and/or service, such as IPR, is also driven by the accumulated expensive premium paid to the private insurance provider by the patient, rather than driven by evidence for its benefit.[52–54]

The inconsistency in utilization of IPR after TJA proposes either underuse or overuse of this service[49] globally, nationally, regionally, or even locally from center-to-center. The cost of IPR is significantly higher compared with other home-based rehabilitation service; hence its referral should be judicious and based on clinical necessity, not personal preference.[55] Although studies have been conducted to address the effectiveness of IPR versus home discharge on surgical outcomes, and predictors of appropriate postacute discharge destinations after TJA, further research is warranted to standardize the best clinical practice for rehabilitation care after TJA.

REHABILITATION AFTER THA AND TKA: CURRENT CLINICAL PRACTICE

A major focus of current research in TJA is directed to advancing the technical aspects of TJA surgery, and enhancing the recovery clinical pathway.[21,56,57] This is aimed to address the mounting health care cost related to TJA, which threatens the long-term sustainability of a high-quality standard care with the demands for TJA projected to rise rapidly.[5]

After it was first introduced in 1997, rapid recovery, commonly referred as "enhanced recovery after surgery (ERAS)," has evolved in orthopedic surgery, particularly in THA and TKA.[56,58] Aligned with its term, ERAS, is an accelerated recovery program that consists of evidence-based interventions. The purpose of ERAS is to shorten acute hospital length of stay (LoS) without increasing the risk of postoperative complications and readmission, improve satisfaction with surgery outcomes, and maximize health care cost savings.[56,58,59] ERAS advocates preoperative institutional-based education sessions/classes, which covers critical aspects of the surgery and its recovery journey, such as "prehabilitation," acute hospital stay, and early discharge planning.[58] This adopts the concept of informed decision-making and realistic expectation of the rehabilitation journey to create a smooth recovery and transition to early discharge home after the acute hospital stay. ERAS programs promote both early discharge planning and early return to patient's "normal" day-to-day activities.[60,61] When compared with the use of an extended IPR facility, home discharge has been increasingly promoted as a superior choice, when it is safe and suitable, where patients are able to manage their rehabilitation at home, either with or without supervision from an outpatient physiotherapist.[48,49,62,63]

Although the benefits offered by ERAS are promising, currently there is no standardized program that can be offered to everyone independent of the individual's circumstances. In today's arthroplasty practice, ERAS components are "practiced" reasonably well, but are reliant on effectiveness of the multidisciplinary team involved in the patient care and institutional and/or clinician standard clinical practice. With its multimodal approach, ERAS programs have been shown to be effective in reducing the acute LoS after TJA, which directly correlates with effective resource utilization and efficiency in health care cost.[61,64] However, although ERAS has been positively associated with increasing rates of home discharge after TJA, the evidence of this is sparse because of the high variance in today's arthroplasty clinical practice.

In light of the current COVID-19 pandemic, recent published literature has emphasized that both patients and clinicians are more likely to be enthused with the indication of early discharge directly home when it is clinically safe and possible to do so, to reduce the risk of contracting the SARS-CoV-2 virus in the clinical setting such as hospital facility.[64,65] In a recent study, an observed reduction of referral to an IPR facility after elective THA and TKA was observed, particularly in the private sector, as a direct result of the COVID-19 pandemic in Melbourne, Victoria, which was a place of significant COVID-19 outbreak.[65] However, further research is needed in the postpandemic environment, to determine if the perceived reduction in the use of IPR is sustained.

REALISTIC EXPECTATIONS: OUTCOMES OF THE SURGERY

Studies have determined positive associations between preoperative patient expectations and subsequent satisfaction with surgery outcomes.[30–32,66] A better understanding of realistic patient expectations will assist surgeons and clinicians to better modify care and accommodate patients' needs, to meet the important concept of patient-centered care.[31] However, the practice variation of delivery of patient-centered care in TJA is concerning, particularly when a customary surgeon-patient relationship is still observed, where decision-making processes seem to be guided more by surgeons than shared with the patients.[33]

Research has demonstrated that discussing and adjusting the expectations to align with a more accurate outlook of the advantages and limitations of TJA can have a positive impact on satisfaction with surgery.[67,68] Patient-reported satisfaction with surgery outcomes is reliant on the fulfillment of their preoperative expectations after surgery. Despite the well-documented favorable result of TJA, studies have reported that 7% to 15% of THA and 11% to 22% of TKA patients were still dissatisfied with their surgery outcomes at 1 year after surgery.[69,70] This is primarily caused by unfulfilled expectations in certain aspects of the anticipated surgery outcomes, with "kneeling" and "squatting" in TKA, and ability to "bend down" in THA, being the most commonly reported issues.[70] Patient expectations of pain relief, psychological well-being, and restoration of functional ability are the most frequently reported determinants to self-reported satisfaction after surgery.[71–73] The discrepancy between patient and surgeon perceptions of their satisfaction to surgical outcomes is commonly seen, with patients typically reporting greater dissatisfaction compared with surgeons.[74,75]

Patients tend to set high expectations in terms of pain relief and their ability to return to the "normal" activities within a certain timeframe, which can differ from person-to-person.[76,77] It is not uncommon that patients expect to be completely pain-free and off opioid-based medications within weeks of surgery, when research has shown that it can take up to 6 months to a year after THA and TKA for the operative joint to feel "normal again."[78,79] Despite technically successful surgery, it has been shown that 1 in 5 TKA patients experience chronic pain after the surgery,[80] compared with 1 in 10 THA patients.[81] Opioid use after TJA is a multifactorial issue, which can be dependent on an individual's other underlying clinical condition, such as OA, in another part of body. However, studies have shown that preoperative opioid use is a significant predictor of ongoing opioid use after TJA surgery.[82,83] This highlights the importance of discussing the probability of persisting pain or incomplete functional recovery after surgery in the preoperative period to avoid unfulfilled expectations of anticipated surgery outcomes.[71]

Surgery outcomes for TJA go beyond what is conventionally determined by prosthesis survivorship or surgeon-based clinical and radiological assessments.[27] The trend to use patient-reported outcome measures (PROMS) has been increasing as a method to assess patients' self-reported opinion on the effectiveness or impact of a disease/disorder and/or medical care to treat it.[27,84,85] PROMS generally consist of validated surveys completed by patients to establish their insights on an individual's health status, disease-specific symptoms severity, level of impairment and disability, and other health dimensions specific to the patients, that at times only the patient can determine.[86] Thus, PROMS offers vital insights to evaluate the effectiveness of medical care or treatment outcomes, such as TJA. However, the collection of PROMS data is time-consuming, and is therefore potentially a costly exercise.[87]

SUMMARY

Understanding the suitability of patients for surgical treatment of OA, such as TJA, is vital, not only to maximize the efficacy of the procedure itself, but also its efficiency in terms of health care resource allocation. With the advancements of surgical technique, technology, and overall improvement in orthopedic-specific clinical practice, rapid recovery protocols, such as ERAS, have been increasingly promoted as a way out to address the ever-growing OA-related health expenditure from the cost of TJA surgery. Considering that the use of IPR service takes a significant proportion of health care costs related to TJA, further research to address the inappropriate utilization of IPR is warranted. There is a need to gain a greater understanding of factors influencing the choice of certain TJA-related medical care after surgery, which are applicable in both private and public sectors. Finally, it is evident that setting predetermined expectations before surgery based on a more realistic outlook of the rehabilitation or recovery involved and the likely outcomes of surgery will result in greater patient satisfaction.

CLINICS CARE POINTS

- 17. *Sloan and colleagues (2018)*

Using data from the US National Inpatient Sample on over 116 million all hospital discharges from 2000 to 2014, the simulated annual growth of total hip and knee arthroplasty was predicted to grow by 71% (to 635,000 procedures) and 85% (to 1.26 million procedures) respectively, by the year 2030.

- 44. *Naylor and colleagues (2019)*

This study of 610 total knee arthroplasty and 690 total hip arthroplasty patients in a total of 19 private and public hospitals in Australia, determined that insurance status is the strongest predictor to facility-based rehabilitation program in "most" total knee arthroplasty and "some" total hip arthroplasty patients.

- 50. *Naylor and colleagues (2021)*

This prognostic study of 520 total hip and knee arthroplasty patients in the public sector found "physical impairment" and "health factors'"as the determinant of care for inpatient rehabilitation service after surgery.

- 65. *Wallis and colleagues (2020)*

This study of 222 total hip and knee replacement patients was the first to indicate the direct result of COVID-19 pandemic on reduction in inpatient rehabilitation after elective total hip and knee arthroplasties in private sector in Australia.

- 67. *Conner-Spady et al (2020)*

This study of 556 total hip and knee arthroplasty patients demonstrated that patient expectations of surgery outcomes need to be discussed before surgery and should be appropriate, to anticipate potential unfulfilled expectations that can have a significant impact on patient satisfaction after surgery.

ACKNOWLEDGMENTS

D.J.H. is supported by an NHMRC Investigator Grant Leadership 2 (#1194737). MMD is supported by a University of Melbourne Dame Kate Campbell Fellowship.

DISCLOSURE

K. Martina and L.J. Salmon have nothing to disclose. D.J. Hunter provides consulting advice on scientific advisory boards for Pfizer, Lilly, TLCBio, Novartis, Tissuegene, Biobone. JPR holds shares in 360MEDCARE, has done consulting work for Smith and Nephew Surgical, and Johnson & Johnson Depuy, and receives institutional support from 360MEDCARE and Smith and Nephew Surgical. M.M. Dowsey reports grants from Medacta International, grants from National Health and Medical Research Council, grants from Australian Research Council, personal fees from Pfizer, grants from HCF Research Foundation, grants from the Australian Orthopaedic Association, outside the submitted work.

REFERENCES

1. Litwic A, Edwards MH, Dennison EM, et al. Epidemiology and burden of osteoarthritis. Br Med Bull 2013;105:185–99.
2. Neogi T. The epidemiology and impact of pain in osteoarthritis. Osteoarthritis and cartilage 2013;21(9):1145–53.
3. Fransen M, Bridgett L, March L, et al. The epidemiology of osteoarthritis in Asia. Int J Rheum Dis 2011;14(2):113–21.
4. Hunter DJ, Bierma-Zeinstra S. Osteoarthritis. Lancet. 2019;393(10182):1745–59.
5. Ackerman IN, Bohensky MA, Zomer E, et al. The projected burden of primary total knee and hip replacement for osteoarthritis in Australia to the year 2030. BMC Musculoskelet Disord 2019;20(1):90.
6. Hunter DJ, March L, Chew M. Osteoarthritis in 2020 and beyond: a lancet commission. Lancet 2020;396(10264):1711–2.
7. Bennell KL, Hunter DJ, Hinman RS. Management of osteoarthritis of the knee. BMJ 2012;345:e4934.
8. Abramoff B, Caldera FE. Osteoarthritis: pathology, diagnosis, and treatment options. Med Clin North Am 2020;104(2):293–311.
9. The Royal Australian College of General, Practitioners. Guideline for the management of knee and hip osteoarthritis. 2018.
10. Hunter DJ. Focusing osteoarthritis management on modifiable risk factors and future therapeutic prospects. Ther Adv Musculoskelet Dis 2009;1(1):35–47.
11. Meneses SR, Goode AP, Nelson AE, et al. Clinical algorithms to aid osteoarthritis guideline dissemination. Osteoarthritis Cartilage 2016;24(9):1487–99.
12. Australian institute of health, and welfare. Osteoarthritis. 2020. Available at: https://www.aihw.gov.au/reports/chronic-musculoskeletal-conditions/osteoarthritis. Accessed August 26 2020.
13. Waugh EJ, Badley EM, Borkhoff CM, et al. Primary care physicians' perceptions about and confidence in deciding which patients to refer for total joint arthroplasty of the hip and knee. Osteoarthritis Cartilage 2016;24(3):451–7.
14. Selten EM, Vriezekolk JE, Geenen R, et al. Reasons for treatment choices in knee and hip osteoarthritis: a qualitative study. Arthritis Care Res (Hoboken) 2016; 68(9):1260–7.
15. Sinusas K. Osteoarthritis: diagnosis and treatment. Am Fam Physician 2012; 85(1):49–56.
16. Registry AOANJR. Hip, Knee & Shoulder Arthoplasty 2019 Annual Report. In. Adelaide2019.
17. Sloan M, Premkumar A, Sheth NP. Projected volume of primary total joint arthroplasty in the U.S., 2014 to 2030. J Bone Joint Surg Am 2018;100(17):1455–60.
18. Singh JA, Yu S, Chen L, et al. Rates of total joint replacement in the United States: future projections to 2020-2040 using the national inpatient Sample. J Rheumatol 2019;46(9):1134–40.
19. Kurtz SM, Ong KL, Lau E, et al. Impact of the economic downturn on total joint replacement demand in the United States: updated projections to 2021. J Bone Joint Surg Am 2014;96(8):624–30.
20. Choong ALC, Shadbolt C, Dowsey MM, et al. Sex-based differences in the outcomes of total hip and knee arthroplasty: a narrative review. ANZ J Surg 2021; 91(4):553–7.

21. de l'Escalopier N, Anract P, Biau D. Surgical treatments for osteoarthritis. Ann Phys Rehabil Med 2016;59(3):227–33.
22. Skou ST, Roos EM, Laursen MB, et al. A randomized, controlled trial of total knee replacement. N Engl J Med 2015;373(17):1597–606.
23. Registry AOANJR. Demographics of hip, knee & shoulder arthroplasty. Adelaide: AOANJRR; 2020.
24. Hügle T, Geurts J, Nüesch C, et al. Aging and osteoarthritis: an inevitable encounter? J Aging Res 2012;2012:950192.
25. Dowsey MM, Kilgour ML, Santamaria NM, et al. Clinical pathways in hip and knee arthroplasty: a prospective randomised controlled study. Med J Aust 1999; 170(2):59–62.
26. Dieppe P, Brandt KD. What is important in treating osteoarthritis? Whom should we treat and how should we treat them? Rheum Dis Clin North Am 2003;29(4): 687–716.
27. Lau RL, Gandhi R, Mahomed S, et al. Patient satisfaction after total knee and hip arthroplasty. Clin Geriatr Med 2012;28(3):349–65.
28. Sherman WF, Patel AH, Kale NN, et al. Surgeon decision-making for individuals with obesity when indicating total joint arthroplasty. J Arthroplasty 2021;36(8): 2708–2715 e2701.
29. Jauregui JJ, Boylan MR, Kapadia BH, et al. Total joint arthroplasty in nonagenarians: what are the risks? J Arthroplasty 2015;30(12):2102–2105 e2101.
30. Dyck BA, Zywiel MG, Mahomed A, et al. Associations between patient expectations of joint arthroplasty surgery and pre- and post-operative clinical status. Expert Rev Med Devices 2014;11(4):403–15.
31. Padilla JA, Feng JE, Anoushiravani AA, et al. Modifying patient expectations can enhance total hip arthroplasty postoperative satisfaction. J Arthroplasty 2019; 34(7S):S209–14.
32. Haanstra TM, van den Berg T, Ostelo RW, et al. Systematic review: do patient expectations influence treatment outcomes in total knee and total hip arthroplasty? Health Qual Life Outcomes 2012;10:152.
33. Wiering B, de Boer D, Delnoij D. Meeting patient expectations: patient expectations and recovery after hip or knee surgery. Musculoskelet Surg 2018;102(3): 231–40.
34. Edusei E, Anoushiravani AA, Slover J. Modern clinical decision-making in total joint arthroplasty. Ann Joint 2017;2(6).
35. Barlow T, Griffin D, Barlow D, et al. Patients' decision making in total knee arthroplasty: a systematic review of qualitative research. Bone Joint Res 2015;4(10): 163–9.
36. Hoffmann TC, Del Mar CB. Shared decision making: what do clinicians need to know and why should they bother? Med J Aust 2014;201(9):513–4.
37. Dieppe P, Lim K, Lohmander S. Who should have knee joint replacement surgery for osteoarthritis? Int J Rheum Dis 2011;14(2):175–80.
38. Ghomrawi HM, Franco Ferrando N, Mandl LA, et al. How often are patient and surgeon recovery expectations for total joint arthroplasty aligned? Results of a pilot study. HSS J 2011;7(3):229–34.
39. Scott CE, Bugler KE, Clement ND, et al. Patient expectations of arthroplasty of the hip and knee. J Bone Joint Surg Br 2012;94(7):974–81.
40. Halawi MJ, Vovos TJ, Green CL, et al. Patient expectation is the most important predictor of discharge destination after primary total joint arthroplasty. J Arthroplasty 2015;30(4):539–42.

41. Sharareh B, Le NB, Hoang MT, et al. Factors determining discharge destination for patients undergoing total joint arthroplasty. J Arthroplasty 2014;29(7): 1355–1358 e1351.

42. Surgeons RACo. Rehabilitation pathways following hip and knee arthroplasty. North Adelaide: Royal Australasian College of Surgeons; 2018.

43. Ponnusamy KE, Naseer Z, El Dafrawy MH, et al. Post-discharge care duration, Charges, and outcomes Among Medicare patients after primary total hip and knee arthroplasty. J bone Jt Surg 2017;99(11):e55. American volume U6 - ctx_ver=Z3988-2004&ctx_enc=info%3Aofi%2Fenc%3AUTF-8&rfr_id=info%3As id%2Fsummonserialssolutionscom&rft_val_fmt=info%3Aofi%2Ffmt%3Akev%3A mtx%3Ajournal&rftgenre=article&rftatitle=Post-Discharge+Care+Duration%2C+ Charges%2C+and+Outcomes+Among+Medicare+Patients+After+Primary+ Total+Hip+and+Knee+Arthroplasty&rftjtitle=Journal+of+bone+and+joint+ surgery+American+volume&rftau=Ponnusamy%2C+Karthikeyan+E&rftau=''' Naseer%2C+Zan&rftau=El+Dafrawy%2C+Mostafa+H&rftau=Okafor%2C+ Louis&rftdate=2017-06-07&rfteissn=1535-1386&rftvolume=99&rftissue=11 &rftspage=e55&rft_id=info%3Apmid%2F28590385&rft_id=info%3Apmid%2F2 8590385&rftexternalDocID=28590385&paramdict=en-US U7 - Journal Article.

44. Fu MC, Samuel AM, Sculco PK, et al. Discharge to inpatient Facilities after total hip arthroplasty is associated with increased Postdischarge Morbidity. J Arthroplasty 2017;32(9S):S144–149 e141.

45. Heligman JL. The effect of a discharge Disposition algorithm on patient outcomes and satisfaction. Orthop Nurs 2021;40(3):125–33.

46. Naylor JM, Hart A, Harris IA, et al. Variation in rehabilitation setting after uncomplicated total knee or hip arthroplasty: a call for evidence-based guidelines. BMC Musculoskelet Disord 2019;20(1):214.

47. Westby MD. Rehabilitation and total joint arthroplasty. Clin Geriatr Med 2012; 28(3):489–508.

48. Hutchinson AG, Gooden B, Lyons MC, et al. Inpatient rehabilitation did not positively affect 6-month patient-reported outcomes after hip or knee arthroplasty. ANZ J Surg 2018;88(10):1056–60.

49. Buhagiar MA, Naylor JM, Harris IA, et al. Effect of inpatient rehabilitation vs a Monitored home-based program on mobility in patients with total knee arthroplasty: the HIHO Randomized clinical Trial. JAMA 2017;317(10):1037–46.

50. Padgett DE, Christ AB, Joseph AD, et al. Discharge to inpatient Rehab does not result in improved functional outcomes following primary total knee arthroplasty. J Arthroplasty 2018;33(6):1663–7.

51. Scully RD, Kappa JE, Melvin JS. Outpatient"-Same-calendar-day discharge hip and knee arthroplasty. J Am Acad Orthop Surg 2020;28(20):e900–9.

52. Naylor JM, Frost S, Farrugia M, et al. Patient factors associated with referral to inpatient rehabilitation following knee or hip arthroplasty in a public sector cohort: a prognostic factor study. J Eval Clin Pract 2021;27(4):809–16.

53. Buhagiar MA, Naylor JM, Simpson G, et al. Understanding consumer and clinician preferences and decision making for rehabilitation following arthroplasty in the private sector. BMC Health Serv Res 2017;17(1):415.

54. Schilling C, Keating C, Barker A, et al. Predictors of inpatient rehabilitation after total knee replacement: an analysis of private hospital claims data. Med J Aust 2018;209(5):222–7.

55. Naylor JM, Hart A, Mittal R, et al. The value of inpatient rehabilitation after uncomplicated knee arthroplasty: a propensity score analysis. Med J Aust 2017;207(6): 250–5.

56. Kaye AD, Urman RD, Cornett EM, et al. Enhanced recovery pathways in orthopedic surgery. J Anaesthesiol Clin Pharmacol 2019;35(Suppl 1):S35–9.
57. Sattler L, Hing W, Vertullo C. Changes to rehabilitation after total knee replacement. Aust J Gen Pract 2020;49(9):587–91.
58. Soffin EM, YaDeau JT. Enhanced recovery after surgery for primary hip and knee arthroplasty: a review of the evidence. Br J Anaesth 2016;117(suppl 3). iii62-iii72.
59. Deng QF, Gu HY, Peng WY, et al. Impact of enhanced recovery after surgery on postoperative recovery after joint arthroplasty: results from a systematic review and meta-analysis. Postgrad Med J 2018;94(1118):678–93.
60. Wainwright TW, Gill M, McDonald DA, et al. Consensus statement for perioperative care in total hip replacement and total knee replacement surgery: enhanced Recovery after Surgery (ERAS((R))) Society recommendations. Acta Orthop 2020;91(1):3–19.
61. Stowers MD, Manuopangai L, Hill AG, et al. Enhanced Recovery after Surgery in elective hip and knee arthroplasty reduces length of hospital stay. ANZ J Surg 2016;86(6):475–9.
62. DeMik DE, Carender CN, Glass NA, et al. Home discharge has increased after total hip arthroplasty, however rates vary between large Databases. J Arthroplasty 2021;36(2):586–592 e581.
63. DeMik DE, Carender CN, Glass NA, et al. More patients are being discharged home after total knee arthroplasty, however rates vary between large Databases. J Arthroplasty 2021;36(1):173–9.
64. Wainwright TW. Enhanced recovery after surgery (ERAS) for hip and knee replacement-why and how it should Be Implemented following the COVID-19 pandemic. Medicina (Kaunas) 2021;57(1).
65. Wallis JA, Young K, Zayontz S, et al. Utilisation of inpatient rehabilitation following elective total knee or hip replacements in private hospital setting declined during the COVID-19 pandemic. Intern Med J 2021;51(3):446–7.
66. Waljee J, McGlinn EP, Sears ED, et al. Patient expectations and patient-reported outcomes in surgery: a systematic review. Surgery 2014;155(5):799–808.
67. Husain A, Lee GC. Establishing realistic patient expectations following total knee arthroplasty. J Am Acad Orthop Surg 2015;23(12):707–13.
68. Kastner A, Ng Kuet, Leong VSC, Petzke F, et al. The virtue of optimistic realism - expectation fulfillment predicts patient-rated global effectiveness of total hip arthroplasty. BMC Musculoskelet Disord 2021;22(1):180.
69. Conner-Spady BL, Bohm E, Loucks L, et al. Patient expectations and satisfaction 6 and 12 months following total hip and knee replacement. Qual Life Res 2020; 29(3):705–19.
70. Tilbury C, Haanstra TM, Leichtenberg CS, et al. Unfulfilled expectations after total hip and knee arthroplasty surgery: there is a need for better Preoperative patient Information and education. J Arthroplasty 2016;31(10):2139–45.
71. Halawi MJ, Jongbloed W, Baron S, et al. Patient dissatisfaction after primary total joint arthroplasty: the patient Perspective. J Arthroplasty 2019;34(6):1093–6.
72. Kahlenberg CA, Nwachukwu BU, McLawhorn AS, et al. Patient satisfaction after total knee replacement: a systematic review. HSS J 2018;14(2):192–201.
73. Anakwe RE, Jenkins PJ, Moran M. Predicting dissatisfaction after total hip arthroplasty: a study of 850 patients. J Arthroplasty 2011;26(2):209–13.
74. Harris IA, Harris AM, Naylor JM, et al. Discordance between patient and surgeon satisfaction after total joint arthroplasty. J Arthroplasty 2013;28(5):722–7.
75. Janse AJ, Gemke RJ, Uiterwaal CS, et al. Quality of life: patients and doctors don't always agree: a meta-analysis. J Clin Epidemiol 2004;57(7):653–61.

76. Lespasio MJ, Guarino AJ, Sodhi N, et al. Pain management associated with total joint arthroplasty: a primer. Perm J 2019;23.

77. Mahomed NN, Liang MH, Cook EF, et al. The importance of patient expectations in predicting functional outcomes after total joint arthroplasty. J Rheumatol 2002; 29(6):1273–9.

78. Carlson VR, Post ZD, Orozco FR, et al. When does the knee feel normal again: a Cross-Sectional study assessing the Forgotten joint score in patients after total knee arthroplasty. J Arthroplasty 2018;33(3):700–3.

79. Beswick AD, Wylde V, Gooberman-Hill R, et al. What proportion of patients report long-term pain after total hip or knee replacement for osteoarthritis? A systematic review of prospective studies in unselected patients. BMJ Open 2012;2(1): e000435.

80. Wylde V, Beswick A, Bruce J, et al. Chronic pain after total knee arthroplasty. EFORT Open Rev 2018;3(8):461–70.

81. Wylde V, Sayers A, Lenguerrand E, et al. Preoperative widespread pain sensitization and chronic pain after hip and knee replacement: a cohort analysis. Pain 2015;156(1):47–54.

82. Naylor JM, Pavlovic N, Farrugia M, et al. Associations between pre-surgical daily opioid use and short-term outcomes following knee or hip arthroplasty: a prospective, exploratory cohort study. BMC Musculoskelet Disord 2020;21(1):398.

83. Kim SC, Choudhry N, Franklin JM, et al. Patterns and predictors of persistent opioid use following hip or knee arthroplasty. Osteoarthritis Cartilage 2017; 25(9):1399–406.

84. Williams K, Sansoni J, Morris D, et al. Patient-reported outcome measures: literature review. Sydney: ACSQHC; 2016.

85. Kyte DG, Calvert M, van der Wees PJ, et al. An introduction to patient-reported outcome measures (PROMs) in physiotherapy. Physiotherapy 2015;101(2): 119–25.

86. Heath EL, Ackerman IN, Cashman K, et al. Patient-reported outcomes after hip and knee arthroplasty : results from a large national registry. Bone Jt Open 2021;2(6):422–32.

87. Weldring T, Smith SMS. Patient-reported outcomes (PROs) and patient-reported outcome measures (PROMs). Health Serv Insights 2013;6:61–8.

Prospects of Disease-Modifying Osteoarthritis Drugs

Win Min Oo, MD, PhD[a,b,*]

KEYWORDS

- Osteoarthritis • DMOADs • Disease-modifying drugs
- Intra-articular therapy: endotype

KEY POINTS

- Despite the massive disease burden of osteoarthritis (OA), there is an immense unmet need owing to the absence of approved disease-modifying osteoarthritis drugs and only modest efficacy of current therapies.
- By virtue of lessons learned from failed clinical trials and insights gained through molecular and imaging research, some promising agents are progressing to late-stage clinical trials.
- International consensus on phenotype classification, appropriate selection criteria, and trial design for each specific targeted therapy, the innovation of drug delivery system, target validation, and linkage with the disease in preclinical research should be the focus.

INTRODUCTION

Osteoarthritis (OA) is the most prevalent arthritis with an estimated global prevalence in 2020 of 22.9% (95% confidence interval [CI], 19.8%-26.1%) in persons over 40 years of age (correspondingly 654.1 million individuals globally).[1] The disease burden impacts on OA patients are substantial in terms of pain, functional limitations, and quality of life, resulting in the 15th highest cause of years lived with disability worldwide. In addition, direct and indirect costs of OA range from 1% to 2.5% of the gross national product across most countries.[2]

Despite the massive disease burden in OA populations, there are currently no disease-modifying osteoarthritis drugs (DMOADs) approved by regulatory bodies.[3]

Funding: No funding is acquired for this work.
Conflicts of Interest: Dr WMO has no conflict of interest.
[a] Department of Physical Medicine and Rehabilitation, Mandalay General Hospital, University of Medicine, Mandalay, Mandalay, Myanmar; [b] Rheumatology Department, Royal North Shore Hospital, Institute of Bone and Joint Research, Kolling Institute, The University of Sydney, Sydney, Australia
* Department of Physical Medicine and Rehabilitation, Mandalay General Hospital, University of Medicine, Mandalay, Mandalay, Myanmar.
E-mail addresses: wioo3335@uni.sydney.edu.au; drwinminoopmr@gmail.com

The current pharmacologic or nonpharmacologic management has revealed only modest efficacy at best,[4] and there are often safety concerns for the long-term use of commonly used analgesics in elderly patients who usually have comorbid diseases.[3] More than half of the patients with moderate and severe OA reported unsatisfactory pain relief,[5] suggesting an immense unmet need in the current therapies. Therefore, finding innovative, effective DMOAD therapies for OA patients is exquisitely urgent, given the global increase of the elderly population and prevalence of obesity.[6]

A DMOAD can be defined as a pharmaceutical agent that will delay or reverse the progression of the structural damage of the joint, thereby leading to clinical translation of improvement in symptoms, manifested either by pain reduction or by benefits in physical function.[7] So far, there is no effective DMOAD approved by the regulatory bodies.

This narrative review focuses on the DMOAD candidates currently undergoing or having completed the active phase 2 and 3 clinical trials within the last 5 years (**Fig. 1**) related to 3 main molecular endotypes: (1) inflammation-driven endotype, (2) bone-driven endotype, (3) cartilage-driven endotype. Although the assignment of a specific drug on account of its predominant activity was made only to 1 specific endotype, some drugs may have broader endotype effects, and where present, these are duly described. The electronic and manual searches were conducted on the https://clinicaltrials.gov/ site for detecting the phase 2/3 clinical trials, which are either active or have been completed within the last 5 years (**Table 1**). Moreover, the PubMed and Embase via Ovid trials from the inception to August 31, 2021 were used for electronic database searches for publications of these phase 2/3 clinical trials with the following MESH or keywords: osteoarthritis OR osteoarthrosis AND disease-modifying osteoarthritis drugs/OR DMOAD/OR structure modification. Then, the current challenges and potential research opportunities are discussed by using the PICO (population, intervention, control, and outcomes) approach commonly applied to formulate a research question in evidence-based medicine (**Fig. 2**).

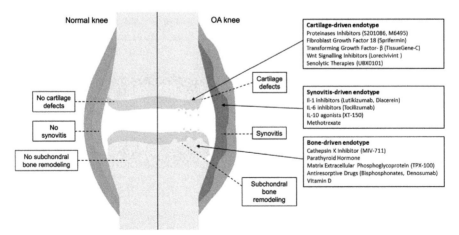

Fig. 1. Active drugs related to the 3 main OA endotypes (phase 2 and 3 RCT). (*Adapted from* Oo WM, Little C, Duong V, Hunter DJ. The Development of Disease-Modifying Therapies for Osteoarthritis (DMOADs): The Evidence to Date. Drug Des Devel Ther. 2021;15:2921–2945. Published 2021 Jul 6. https://doi.org/10.2147/DDDT.S295224; with permission from Dove Medical Press)

Table 1
Summary of disease-modifying osteoarthritis drugs clinical trials that are active or finished within 5 y in osteoarthritis (phase 2 and 3)

Targeted Endotype	Drug Class	Name of Investigational Drug	Route	OA Site	Active Trial IDs/Estimated Completion Date	Completed Trial IDs/Completed Date
Inflammation	Anti-IL-1	Lutikizumab (ABT-981)	SC	Hand		NCT02087904 (Dec 2016) NCT02384538 (July 2016)
	Anti-IL-6	Diacerein	Oral	Knee		NCT02688400 (Dec 2019)
		Tocilizumab	IV	Hand		NCT02477059 (Feb 2019)
	DNA plasmid with IL10 transgene	XT-150	IA	Knee	NCT04124042 (Feb 2022)	
	DMARD	Methotrexate	Oral	Knee	NCT03815448 (Dec 2022)	ISRCTN77854383 (2018)
Subchondral bone	Cathepsin K inhibitors	MIV-711	Oral	Knee		NCT02705625 (May 2017) NCT03037489 (Nov 2017)
	Parathyroid hormone	Teriparatide	SC	Knee	NCT03072147 (Oct 2022)	NCT01925261 (Sept 2016) NCT02837900 (Aug 2017)
	Matrix extracellular phosphoglycoprotein	TPX-100	IA	Knee		
	Anti-resorptives	Zoledronic acid	IV	Hip	NCT04303026 (Mar 2022)	
		Denosumab	SC	Hand	NCT02771860 (May 2021)	
		Vitamin D	Oral	Knee	NCT04739592 (Jul 2024)	
Cartilage	ADAMTS-5 inhibitors	GLPG1972/s201086	Oral	Knee		NCT03595618 (Jul 2020)
	Fibroblast growth factor	Sprifermin (AS902330)	IA	Knee		NCT01919164 (May 2019)
	Gene therapy	TissueGene-C	IA	Knee	NCT03291470 (Sept 2021) NCT03203330 (Oct 2024)	
	Wnt/β-catenin signaling pathway inhibitors	Lorecivivint	IA	Knee	NCT03928184 (Aug 2021) NCT03727022 (Sept 2021) NCT04385303 (Sept 2021) NCT03706521 (Dec 2021) NCT04520607 (Sept 2022)	NCT02536833 (April 2017) NCT03122860 (April 2018)
		SM04690				
	Senolytic agents	UBX0101	IA	Knee		NCT04129944 (Aug 2020) NCT04349956 (Nov 2020)

Abbreviations: IV, intravenous; SC, subcutaneous.

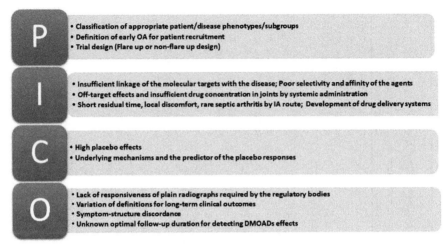

P
- Classification of appropriate patient/disease phenotypes/subgroups
- Definition of early OA for patient recruitment
- Trial design (Flare up or non-flare up design)

I
- Insufficient linkage of the molecular targets with the disease; Poor selectivity and affinity of the agents
- Off-target effects and insufficient drug concentration in joints by systemic administration
- Short residual time, local discomfort, rare septic arthritis by IA route; Development of drug delivery systems

C
- High placebo effects
- Underlying mechanisms and the predictor of the placebo responses

O
- Lack of responsiveness of plain radiographs required by the regulatory bodies
- Variation of definitions for long-term clinical outcomes
- Symptom-structure discordance
- Unknown optimal follow-up duration for detecting DMOADs effects

Fig. 2. Barriers to be overcome in the context of the PICO approach.

OSTEOARTHRITIS SUBTYPES: PHENOTYPES AND ENDOTYPES

Because of marked heterogeneity in clinical and structural manifestations and the complexity of the pathobiological mechanism of the OA disease process, targeting a particular subtype of the OA population would be meaningful for a target therapy in drug development.[8] Broadly, OA disease can be divided into either a phenotype based on observable traits (ie, similar clinically observable characteristics, such as etiologic factors, risk factors), or an endotype that possesses a distinct pathophysiologic mechanism via cellular, molecular, and biomechanical signaling pathways.[9] As a note, a given clinical OA phenotype may reveal overlapping molecular endotypes at some stages of the disease process.[7] From the perspective of drug development, there seems to be a consensus on the presence of 3 endotypes, namely synovitis-driven endotype, bone-driven endotype, and cartilage-driven endotype.

SYNOVITIS-DRIVEN ENDOTYPE

The synovium in OA patients undergoes infiltration of mononuclear cells,[10] synovial hypertrophy, and generation of inflammatory cytokines, such as tumor necrosis factor-alpha (TNF-α), interleukin-1β (IL-1β), and IL-6,[11] leading to the synovitis evidenced by the histologic studies[12] and imaging modalities.[13] As synovitis may be associated with pain and radiographic progression,[14] investigating the anti-inflammatory agents is a promising approach for a subset of the OA population with predominant inflammation (**Tables 2 and 3**).

INTERLEUKIN-1 INHIBITORS

IL-1 can induce the production of proteinases[15] in chondrocytes and synoviocytes, leading to cartilage destruction, and it also inhibits the generation of proteoglycan and collagen type II.[16] Therefore, inhibition of the IL-1 pathway can be considered a promising target.[17] Phase 2/3 clinical trials for 2 investigational drugs that can inhibit IL-1 pathway have finished recently.

Table 2
Published results of phase 2/3 clinical trials related to the symptomatic efficacy of pharmaceutical agents in synovitis-driven endotype

Authors/Ref.	ClinialTrials. gov Identifier	OA Site	Dosage, Route of Interventions	N	Follow-Up Duration	Efficacy in Symptomatic Modification		Phase of Development
						Pain (0–50) (WOMAC if not Denoted Otherwise)	Function (0–170) (WOMAC if not Denoted Otherwise)	
Lutikizumab (ABT-981)								
Fleischmann et al,[19] 2019	NCT02087904	Knee	Placebo	85	16 wk	−8.1 (−10.44, −5.79)	−29.1 (−36.46, −21.82)	Phase 2
			Lutikizumab 25 mg SC q2w	89		−10.3 (−12.58, −8.08)	−31.4 (−38.53, −24.34)	
			Lutikizumab 100 mg SC q2w	87		−11.7 (−14.17, −9.26)*	−36.3 (−43.99, −28.53)	
			Lutikizumab 200 mg SC q2w	89		−11.9 (−14.11, −9.66)*	−32.6 (−39.61, −25.52)	
Kloppenburg et al,[20] 2019	NCT02384538	Hand	Placebo	67	16 wk	−10.7 (−15.4 to −6.0)	−17.2 (−24.9 to −9.4)	Phase 2
			Lutikizumab 200 mg SC q2w	64		−9.2 (−13.8 to −4.6) AUSCAN pain range 0–50	−14.6 (−22.1 to −7.1) AUSCAN function ranges 0—90	
Diacerein								
Pelletier et al,[22] 2020	NCT02688400	Knee	Diacerein 50 mg OD for 1 mo and then BD	140	6 mo	−11.1 (0.9)	−27.2 (39.0)	Phase 2
			Celecoxib 200 mg OD	148		−11.8 (0.9)	−29.3 (39.8)	
Tocilizumab								
Richette et al,[28] 2021	NCT02477059	Hand	Placebo	41	6 wk	−9.9 (SD 20.1)	0.2 ± 0.6	Phase 3
			Tocilizumab 8 mg/kg IV at weeks 0 and 4	42		−7.9 (SD 19.4) VAS pain range 0–100	−0.04 ± 0.6 FIHOA (0—30)	

(continued on next page)

Table 2
(continued)

Authors/Ref.	ClinialTrials. gov Identifier	OA Site	Dosage, Route of Interventions	N	Follow-Up Duration	Efficacy in Symptomatic Modification		Phase of Development
						Pain (0–50) (WOMAC if not Denoted Otherwise)	Function (0–170) (WOMAC if not Denoted Otherwise)	
Methotrexate								
Kingsbury et al,[33] 2019	ISRCTN77854383	Knee	Placebo 10 mg to 25 mg over 8 wk and then maintenance at 25 mg	68 66	6 mo	−0.83 (−1.55, −0.10) (mean difference, NRS pain)	−5.01 (−8.74, −1.29)	Phase 3

Abbreviations: AUSCAN, the Australian Canadian Osteoarthritis Hand Index; BD, ; FIHOA, Functional Index for Hand Osteoarthritis; NRS, numerical rating scale; OD, ; SD, standard deviation.

Table 3
Published results of phase 2/3 clinical trials related to the structural efficacy of pharmaceutical agents in synovitis-driven endotype

Authors/Ref.	ClinialTrials.gov Identifier	OA Site	Dosage, Route of Interventions	N	Follow-Up Duration (wk)	Efficacy in Structural Modification		Phase of Development
						Plain Radiographs	MRI	
Lutikizumab (ABT-981)								
Fleischmann et al,[19] 2019	NCT02087904	Knee	Placebo Lutikizumab 25 mg SC every 2 wk Lutikizumab 100 mg SC every 2 wk Lutikizumab 200 mg SC every 2 wk	85 89 87 89	26 wk for MRI synovitis 52 wk for radiographs	No significant difference in medal or lateral JSN except for Lutikizumab 25 mg	No significant difference in synovial thickness, synovial fluid volume, and WORMS semiquantitative synovitis/effusion volume	Phase 2
Kloppenburg et al,[20] 2019	NCT02384538	Hand	Placebo Lutikizumab 200 mg SC q2w	67 64	26 wk	No significant changes in JSN	No significant changes in HOAMRIS MRI scores	Phase 2
Methotrexate								
Kingsbury et al,[33] 2019	ISRCTN77854383	Knee	Placebo 10 mg to 25 mg over 8 wk and then maintenance at 25 mg	68 66	6 mo	NA	14.89 (−18.19, 47.96) (mean difference, mm³)	Phase 3

Abbreviations: HOAMRIS, Hand Osteoarthritis Magnetic Resonance Imaging Scoring System; NA, nonavailable; WORMS, .

Lutikizumab (ABT-981)

Lutikizumab is a novel human dual-variable domain immunoglobulin, which demonstrated simultaneous blockage of both IL-1a and IL-1b in a mouse OA model.[18] In a phase 2 study in 347 patients with knee OA with MRI- or ultrasound-detected synovitis, Lutikizumab showed limited reduction in the Western Ontario and McMaster Universities Osteoarthritis Index (WOMAC) pain score at week 16 and no significant improvement in structural endpoints, such as MRI synovitis, at 26 weeks and joint space narrowing (JSN) on radiographs at week 52.[19] A preplanned subgroup analysis showed that Lutikizumab 100 mg had statistically significant improvement in pain among patients with K/L grade 3 knee OA, suggesting that more advanced disease may be more responsive from IL-1 blockage. Lutikizumab had more adverse events: injection site reactions (25.2% vs 15.3%) and neutropenia (27.5% vs 2.4%), compared with the placebo. In another phase 2 study evaluating its efficacy in erosive hand OA with ≥3 tender and/or swollen hand joints (n = 132), Lutikizumab demonstrated no symptomatic or structural benefits assessed with multiple imaging scoring systems,[20] in agreement with the previous study in knee OA.

Diacerein

Diacerein acts by suppressing the IL-1b system and related downstream pathways. In mice, diacerein (5.0–25.0 mg/kg) also inhibits IL-1β in a dose-dependent manner and reduces TNF-α–induced nociception.[21] Recently, in an international, multicenter, double-blind randomized clinical trial (RCT) (NCT02688400), the efficacy and safety of administering diacerein 50 mg once per day for 1 month and twice daily thereafter (n = 140), or celecoxib 200 mg once per day for 6 months (n = 148), were compared in moderate and severe knee OA. A similar treatment effect on WOMAC pain and function was detected, starting at 2 months' follow-up and maintained for the entire duration of the study. However, the study did not include the outcomes measures for structural modification. In the diacerein group, gastrointestinal side effects (diarrhea) were more common (10.2% vs 3.7%), and 1 patient had symptoms suggestive of possible hepatitis.[22] The EMA's Pharmacovigilance Risk Assessment Committee recommended restrictions of its use to limit risks of severe diarrhea and hepatotoxicity in 2014.[23] In a recent meta-analysis investigating the adverse effects of OA medications, compared with placebo, diacerein was significantly related to gastrointestinal disorders (odds ratio [OR], 2.53; 95% CI, 1.43–4.46) and renal disorders (OR, 3.16; 95% CI, 1.93–5.15) even when concomitant OA medications were not allowed.[24]

ANTI-INTERLEUKIN-6 INHIBITORS

IL-6 played a direct role in regulating chondrocyte function and cartilage metabolism and seems to have a differential effect on OA pathophysiology depending on the signal via the classic (protective) or transsignaling (inflammatory and catabolic) pathway.[25] In the destabilization of the medial meniscus (DMM) mouse model, neutralizing antibody of the IL-6 receptor reduced osteophyte formation, cartilage lesions, and synovitis.[26]

Tocilizumab

Tocilizumab, an IL-6 antagonist, leads to cartilage preservation in a mouse model of ischemic osteonecrosis.[27] However, in a recent phase 3 clinical trial (n = 83), which evaluated the efficacy of tocilizumab in refractory hand OA with at least 3 painful joints, there was no significant benefits in pain and function.[28] This might suggest that removing IL-6 signaling alone in the short term is not sufficient for pain reduction in human OA. As a note, tocilizumab causes inhibition of all IL-6 signaling pathways, including classic and trans-signaling.[25]

INTERLEUKIN-10 AGONISTS

IL-10 is a potent anti-inflammatory cytokine, which can suppress the generation of key proinflammatory cytokines, such as TNF-α, IL-1β, and IL-6, as well as reduce matrix metallopeptidases (MMPs) expression.[29]

XT-150

IL-10 protein possesses a short half-life in vivo and poor permeation into articular capsule upon systemic administration. Therefore, XT-150 was developed using plasmid DNA-based therapy for the generation of a long-acting human IL-10 variant.[30] XT150 administered into canine OA joints showed an increase in intra-articular (IA) IL-10 levels, showed improved pain, and is well tolerated.[31] Currently, a phase 2 clinical trial is ongoing for knee OA (NCT04124042).

METHOTREXATE

Methotrexate (MTX) is a traditional disease-modifying antirheumatic drug used in a variety of inflammatory rheumatic and autoimmune disorders.[32] In the phase 3 PRO-MOTE trial published as a 2019 OARSI conference abstract (n = 134), oral MTX showed significant improvement in knee pain and function at 6-month follow-up but not at 9 and 12 months with no change in synovial volume on contrast-enhanced MRI at 6 months.[33] Currently, a phase 3 study is active for symptomatic knee OA patients with effusion-synovitis grade of $\geq$2 (NCT03815448).

BONE-DRIVEN ENDOTYPE

Microstructural changes in subchondral bone are attributed to an uncoupled remodeling process owing to the spontaneous activation (in early-stage OA) or inactivation (in late-stage OA) of osteoclastic bone resorption activity.[34] An acidic microenvironment created by bone-resorbing osteoclasts via secreting H+ produced bone pain in animal models of bone metastasis.[35] During aberrant subchondral bone remodeling, Netrin-1 produced by osteoclasts can induce sensory innervation and genesis of OA pain by acting through its receptor DCC (deleted in colorectal cancer).[36] The agents acting through subchondral bone remodeling have reached late clinical trials (**Tables 4 and 5**).

CATHEPSIN K INHIBITOR

Cathepsin K is a lysosomal cysteine protease present in activated osteoclasts for degrading collagen and other matrix proteins during bone resorption.[37] Moreover, it is also involved in cartilage matrix degradation, and OA as a milder cartilage degradation occurred in cathepsin K–deficient mice after anterior cruciate ligament transection (ACLT) when compared with wild-type controls.[38]

MIV-711 is a potent selective cathepsin K inhibitor that revealed reduced subchondral bone loss and cartilage damage in ACLT-induced rabbit OA and partial-medial meniscectomy-induced dog OA.[39] In a 26-week phase 2 human trial in knee OA (n = 244), significant reductions in bone and cartilage OA progression were detected with no improvement in pain. The active treatment groups had 5 cardiovascular events, and skin disorders were more common in the active groups (100 mg/d: 7.3%; 200 mg/d: 12.2%; placebo: 2.5%).[40]

Table 4
Published results of phase 2/3 clinical trials related to the symptomatic efficacy of pharmaceutical agents in bone-driven endotype

Authors/Ref.	ClinialTrials.gov Identifier	OA Site	Dosage, Route of Interventions	N	Follow-up Duration (wk)	Efficacy in Symptomatic Modification		Phase of Development
						Pain (0–50) (WOMAC if not Denoted Otherwise)	Function (0–170) (WOMAC if not Denoted Otherwise)	
Cathepsin K inhibitors								
Conaghan et al,[40] 2020	NCT02705625 NCT03037489	Knee	Placebo MIV-711, 100 mg/d MIV-711, 200 mg/d	80 82 82	26 wk	−1.4 (−1.9 to −0.8) −1.7 (−2.3 to −1.2) −1.5 (−2.0 to −0.9) NRS (0–10)	NA	Phase 2
Matrix extracellular phosphoglycoprotein								
McGuire et al,[45] 2018	—	Knee	Placebo TPX-100 IA 200 mg 4 weekly injections	93 93	12 mo	— Significant WOMAC scores (no numerical data)	— Significant WOMAC scores (no numerical data)	Phase 2
Antiresorptives								
Frediani et al,[56] 2020	—	Knee	Clodronate IM 200 mg/d for 15 d and then q1w for next 2.5 mo Clodronate IM 200 mg/d for 15 d and then q1w for next 11.5 mo	37 37	12 mo	50.3 ± 31.9 (SD) 15.6 ± 9.8 (SD)* (VAS = 0–100)	24.0 ± 11.9 13.5 ± 5.7*	NA
Cai et al,[58] 2020	ACTRN12613000039785	Knee	Placebo saline IV zoledronic acid IV 5 mg baseline and 12 mo	110 113	24 mo	−16.8 (−22.0 to −11.6) −11.5 (−16.9 to −6.2) (VAS)	NA	Phase 3

MacFarlane et al,[60] 2020	NCT01351805	Knee	Placebo Cholecalciferol oral 2000 IU/d	630 591	4 y	34.6 ± 0.9 (SE) 32.7 ± 0.9	34.6 (0.9) (SE) 34.1 (1.0)	NA
Tu et al,[62] 2021	NCT01176344	Knee	Placebo Cholecalciferol oral 50,000 IU (1.25 mg) per month	204 209	2 y	Change from baseline 1.30 (0.51, 2.09) −0.03 (−0.80, 0.74)* (MFPDI range 0–34)	NA	Phase 3

Abbreviations: IM, intramuscular; IU, international units; MFPDI, Manchester Foot Pain and Disability Index scores; NRS; numerical rating scale, SE, .

Table 5
Published results of phase 2/3 clinical trials related to the structural efficacy of pharmaceutical agents in bone-driven endotype

Authors/ Ref.	ClinialTrials.gov Identifier	OA Site	N	Follow-Up Duration (wk)	Efficacy in Structural Modification — Plain Radiographs	Efficacy in Structural Modification — MRI	Phase of Development
Cathepsin K inhibitors							
Conaghan et al,[40] 2020	NCT02705625 NCT03037489	Knee	80 82 82	26 wk	NA	23.3 (15.7–30.9) 7.9 (0.5–15.3)** 8.6 (1.1–16.1)** (bone area, mm^2) −0.066 (−0.119 to −0.013) 0.011 (−0.042–0.063)* −0.022 (−0.074–0.031) (cartilage thickness, mm)	Phase 2
Matrix extracellular phosphoglycoprotein							
McGuire et al,[45] 2018	—	Knee	93 93	12 mo	NA	No significance in cartilage thickness/volume on quantitative MRI (no numerical data)	Phase 2
McGuire et al,[46] 2020	—	Knee	78 78	12 mo	NA	Significant decrease in pathologic bone shape change in the femur (no numerical data) >	Phase 2
Antiresorptives							
Frediani et al,[56] 2020	—	Knee	37 37	12 mo	NA	5.9 ± 4.9 1.1 ± 0.8* (BML)	NA

Dosage, Route of Interventions:
- Conaghan et al,[40] 2020: Placebo; MIV-711, 100 mg/d; MIV-711, 200 mg/d
- McGuire et al,[45] 2018: Placebo; TPX-100 IA 200 mg 4 weekly injections
- McGuire et al,[46] 2020: Placebo; TPX-100 IA 200 mg 4 weekly injections
- Frediani et al,[56] 2020: Clodronate IM 200 mg/d for 15 d and then q1w for next 2.5 mo; Clodronate IM 200 mg/d for 15 d and then q1w for next 11.5 mo

Cai et al,[58] 2020	ACTRN12613000039785	Knee	Placebo saline IV zoledronic acid IV 5 mg baseline and 12 mo	110 113	24 mo	NA	NA	-919 (-1004 to -835) -878 (-963 to -793) (cartilage volume mm^3) -6 (-75–63) -33 (-104–39) (BML mm^2)	Phase 3
Perry et al,[61] 2021	—	Knee	Placebo Cholecalciferol oral 800 IU/d	26 24	24 mo	NA	NA	Change from baseline 61.5 (-1085.6–1208.6) 155.4 (-1097.3–1408.0) (synovial volume mm^3) -193.4 (-2845.7–2459.0) -506.9 (-3395.6–2381.9) (subchondral BML volume mm^3)	NA

Abbreviation: IV, intravenous.

PARATHYROID HORMONE

Recombinant human parathyroid hormone, teriparatide, possesses a bone anabolic effect in the subchondral plate via acting on the osteoblasts. It increased proteoglycan content and inhibited cartilage degeneration in a mouse model of injury-induced knee OA.[41] It can reduce pain by ameliorating temporomandibular joint OA changes in aging mice,[42] decreasing chondrocyte apoptosis via autophagy-related proteins,[43] prostaglandin E2 production, and sensory innervation of subchondral bone in DMM mice.[44] A phase 2 clinical trial in knee OA is currently ongoing (NCT03072147).

MATRIX EXTRACELLULAR PHOSPHOGLYCOPROTEIN

TPX-100 is a matrix extracellular phosphoglycoprotein derivative having a novel 23-amino-acid peptide.[45] IA injections of TPX-100 stimulate articular cartilage proliferation in goats and reduced joint damage in rats. In a phase 2 study involving 93 patients with bilateral patellofemoral OA, 4 weekly injections of 200 mg TPX-100 demonstrated a significant difference in pain when ascending and descending stairs at 12 months but no structural benefits on quantitative MRI,[45] perhaps because of the small sample size. Another 2020 OARSI conference abstract described a reduction in pathologic bone shape change in the femur and stabilization in tibiofemoral cartilage.[46]

ANTIRESORPTIVE DRUGS: BISPHOSPHONATES AND DENOSUMAB

Research has established an association of OA developments and symptoms with bone marrow lesions (BML) on MRI,[47,48] an altered signal pattern related to increased vascularization, bone marrow necrosis, fibrosis, and less mineralized bone.[49] Histochemical analysis of BMLs revealed an abundance of matrix metalloproteinases, TNF-α, and substance P, which might induce pain receptor stimulation.[50] Therefore, antiresorptive agents seem to be a promising therapy because of their implications in pathogenesis and clinical manifestations in OA.

However, in both preclinical and clinical studies, inconsistent results are reported, which is reflected by significant heterogeneity across the studies in the systematic reviews.[51,52] In the latest reviews, bisphosphonates showed neither symptomatic relief nor improved radiographic progression in knee OA.[53,54] However, there may be some benefits in certain subgroups with early OA and high bone-turnover rates.[51,53] An individual patient data meta-analysis examining the effects of bisphosphonates in certain knee OA subgroups is still ongoing.[55]

In a small sample (n = 74), administration of intramuscular clodronate 200 mg daily for 15 days (higher dose than used in osteoporosis) and then once weekly for the next 11.5 months improved BML and pain in knee OA[56] compared with a shorter maintenance regimen (2.5 months).[56] In a propensity-matched retrospective cohort analysis of the Osteoarthritis Initiative in female participants (n = 346), bisphosphonate exposure showed a significant protective effect (51% relative reduction) against 2-year radiographic progression in nonoverweight patients (body mass index <25 kg/m^2) with early radiographic OA.[57]

Recently, in the 2-year Zoledronic Acid for Osteoarthritis Knee Pain (ZAP2) study conducted in 223 knee OA patients with significant knee pain and MRI-detected BMLs, twice yearly administration of 5 mg zoledronic acid (the most potent of all bisphosphonates) did not significantly improve knee pain, cartilage volume loss, or BML size. Although the clinical trial was designed and sufficiently powered for detecting disease-modifying effects on BMLs in the bone-driven subgroup, the more sensitive MRI-detected cartilage volume was measured as the primary outcome, and the follow-up is quite long (2 years).[58] On the exploratory subgroup analysis of the ZAP2 study, there was a greater symptomatic but not structure-modifying benefit in patients without radiographic JSN (n = 44) than those with JSN grade 1 to 2 (-13.5 vs 9.9 on a visual analogue scale [VAS] score).[58] The zoledronic acid group had more knee replacements (9%) compared with the placebo group (2%) over 2 years. Currently, there are 2 clinical trials examining the effects of zoledronic acid in hip OA (NCT04303026) and of denosumab in hand OA (NCT02771860).

VITAMIN D

Vitamin D stimulates proteoglycan synthesis in mature chondrocytes and reduces the production of inflammatory cytokine by activating AMPK/mTOR signaling.[59] In a VITAL (Vitamin D and Omega-3) Trial, which included a subset of patients with chronic knee pain (1,39), vitamin D supplementation neither reduces knee pain nor improves function at 4-year follow-up.[60] Vitamin D supplementation in patients with symptomatic knee OA showed no significant difference in MRI-detected synovial tissue volume and subchondral BML volume at 2-year follow-up (n = 50).[61] A recent post hoc study in patients with knee OA showed that foot pain scores remained unchanged in the vitamin D group (-0.03 [-0.80, 0.74]) (n = 209) over 2 years while worsening in the placebo group (1.30 [0.51, 2.09]) (n = 204).[62] A recent meta-analysis reported that it had symptomatic benefits but no structure-modifying effect in knee OA.[63] A small phase 4 clinical trial is ongoing (NCT04739592).

CARTILAGE-DRIVEN ENDOTYPE

Cartilage failure to maintain homeostasis between synthesis and degradation of extracellular matrix components is a major contributor to OA pathogenesis, leading to cartilage softening, fibrillation and fissuring of the superficial cartilage layers, and diminished cartilage thickness.[64] **Tables 6 and 7** show the DMOAD candidates for this endotype.

PROTEINASE INHIBITORS

Articular cartilage is formed by chondrocytes, which are embedded in an ECM that has an abundance of type II collagen fibrils and aggrecan. Collagenases, such as matrix metalloproteinases (MMPs), and aggrecanase, such as a disintegrin and metalloproteinases, with thrombospondin motifs (ADAMTSs) belong to the family of zinc endopeptidases and are responsible for degradation of triple-helical type II collagen fibrils (collagenolysis) and aggrecan, the major proteoglycan in articular cartilage.[65] As broad-spectrum MMP inhibitors with strong Zn^{2+} chelating properties, such as PG-116800, showed poor selectivity and caused adverse effects, such as musculoskeletal triad (arthralgia, myalgia, tendinitis), also known as the musculoskeletal syndrome (MSS), and gastrointestinal disorders perhaps owing to a nonselective inhibition of other metalloproteinases or a combined inhibition of a series of critical MMPs, further development has been terminated.[66]

Preclinical studies revealed overwhelming data on a potential role of MMP-13 in OA pathogenesis, and MMP 13 has been a potential target.[67] Because of the unusual presence of the large hydrophobic S1' pocket of MMP-13, non-zinc-binding MMP-13 inhibitors with higher potency and superior selectivity profiles by occupying themselves deeper in the S1' pocket have been developed to avoid MSS, but have not reached the phase 2 clinical trials owing to poor solubility, biodistribution, permeability, metabolic stability, or bioavailability.[68]

Table 6
Published results of phase 2/3 clinical trials related to the symptomatic efficacy of pharmaceutical agents in cartilage-driven endotype

Authors/Ref.	ClinialTrials.gov Identifier	OA Site	Dosage, Route of Interventions	N	Follow-Up Duration (wk)	Efficacy in Symptomatic Modification		Phase of Development
						Pain (0–50) (WOMAC if not Denoted Otherwise)	Function (0–170) (WOMAC if not Denoted Otherwise)	
Proteinases inhibitors								
Galapagos and Servier,[71] 2020	NCT03595618	Knee	Placebo S201086/GLPG1972 low dose S201086/GLPG1972 medium dose S201086/GLPG1972 high dose (no numerical report)	932 (total)	52 wk	No significance (no numerical report)	No significance (no numerical report)	Phase 2
Fibroblast growth factor-18								
Lohmander et al,[80] 2014	NCT01033994	Knee	Placebo Sprifermin IA 10 μg 3 once weekly Sprifermin IA 30 μg 3 once weekly Sprifermin IA 100 μg 3 once weekly	42 21 42 63	12 mo	−5.56 (4.17) −4.10 (5.11) −3.54 (3.67) −2.87 (4.76)* (mean change from baseline, SD)	−17.02 (13.56) −15.76 (13.72) −12.12 (12.06) −11.28 (15.30)* (mean change from baseline, SD)	Phase 1b
Hochberg et al,[83] 2019	NCT01919164	Knee	Placebo Sprifermin IA 30 μg 3 once weekly q6 mo Sprifermin IA 30 μg 3 once weekly q12 mo Sprifermin IA 100 μg 3 once weekly q6 mo Sprifermin IA 100 μg 3 once weekly q12 mo	108 111 110 110 110	24 mo	NA 2.58 (−3.47, 8.64) 1.29 (−4.53, 7.10) −0.06 (−5.76, 5.65) 3.65 (−1.99, 9.28) (difference with placebo; total WOMAC score)	No numerical data for individual WOMAC scores	Phase 2

Study	NCT	Joint	Intervention	N	Duration	Outcome 1	Outcome 2	Phase
Eckstein et al,[86] 2021	NCT01919164	Knee	Placebo Sprifermin IA 30 μg 3 once weekly q12 mo Sprifermin IA 30 μg 3 once weekly q6 mo Sprifermin IA 100 μg 3 once weekly q12 mo Sprifermin IA 100 μg 3 once weekly q6 mo	108 110 111 110 110	60 mo	−22.38 (22.19) −24.41 (22.48) −20.38 (22.49) −24.94 (19.95) −24.00 (22.38) (change from baseline, VAS pain score)	−17.03 (24.15) −18.74 (21.87) −18.55 (23.76) −18.82 (21.62) −18.56 (23.60) (change from baseline at 5 y)	Phase 2
Gene therapy								
Lee et al,[94] 2020	NCT01221441	Knee	Placebo IA (2 mL normal saline 0.9%) TissueGene-C IA	35 67	12 mo	Significant improvement in VAS pain	Significant improvement in IKDC scores	Phase 2
Kim et al,[95] 2018	—	Knee	Placebo IA (2 mL normal saline 0.9%) TissueGene-C IA	81 78	12 mo	−10 −25*** (change from baseline, VAS pain score)	NA	Phase 3
Wnt/β-catenin signaling pathway inhibitors								
Yazici et al,[103] 2020	NCT02536833	Knee	Placebo Lorecivivint (SM04690) 0.03 mg Lorecivivint (SM04690) 0.07 mg Lorecivivint (SM04690) 0.23 mg	114 112 117 109	13 wk	−22.1 ± 2.1 −23.3 ± 2.2 −23.5 ± 2.1 −23.5 ± 2.1 (mean ± SD change from baseline)	NA	Phase 2
Yazici et al,[104] 2021	NCT03122860	Knee	Dry needle Placebo Lorecivivint (SM04690) 0.03 mg Lorecivivint (SM04690) 0.07 mg Lorecivivint (SM04690) 0.15 mg Lorecivivint (SM04690) 0.23 mg	117 116 116 115 115 116	24 wk	NA 6.2 (1.0) 6.2 (1.1)* 6.1 (1.1) 6.1 (1.0) 6.1 (1.0)* (mean ± SD change from baseline, NRS pain)	NA 59.2 (9.8) 59.0 (10.9) 58.1 (11.2) 57.7 (11.1) 57.3 (11.4)* (mean ± SD change from baseline)	Phase 2b

(continued on next page)

Table 6
(continued)

Authors/Ref.	ClinialTrials.gov Identifier	OA Site	Dosage, Route of Interventions	N	Follow-Up Duration (wk)	Efficacy in Symptomatic Modification		Phase of Development
						Pain (0–50) (WOMAC if not Denoted Otherwise)	Function (0–170) (WOMAC if not Denoted Otherwise)	
Senolytic agents								
UNITY Biotechnology,[110] 2021	NCT04129944	Knee	Placebo	46	12 wk	−1.017	NA	Phase 2
			UBX0101 IA 0.5 mg	45		−0.924		
			UBX0101 IA 2.0 mg mg	46		−1.052		
			UBX0101 IA 4.0 mg mg	46		−1.019 (mean change from baseline)		

Abbreviations: IKDC, international knee documentation committee scores; NRS, numerical rating scale.

Table 7
Published results of phase 2/3 clinical trials related to the structural efficacy of pharmaceutical agents in cartilage-driven endotype

Authors/Ref.	ClinialTrials.gov Identifier	OA Site	Dosage, Route of Interventions	N	Follow-up Duration (wk)	Efficacy in Structural Modification		Phase of Development
						Plain Radiographs	MRI	
Proteinases Inhibitors								
Galapagos and Servier,[71] 2020	NCT03595618	Knee	Placebo	932 (total)	52 wk	NA	−0.116 (0.27)	Phase 2
			S201086/GLPG1972 low dose				−0.068 (0.20), −0.097 (0.27)	
			S201086/GLPG1972 medium dose				0.085 (0.22) change in cartilage thickness (in mm [SD])	
			S201086/GLPG1972 high dose (no numerical report)					
Fibroblast growth factor-18								
Lohmander et al,[80] 2014	NCT01033994	Knee	Placebo	42	12 mo	−0.02 (0.90)	−0.11 (−0.20, −0.02)	Phase 1b
			Sprifermin IA10 μg 3 once weekly	21		0.05 (1.00)	0.02 (−0.18, 0.23)	
			Sprifermin IA 30 μg 3 once weekly	42		0.03 (0.72)	−0.11 (−0.18, −0.03)	
			Sprifermin IA 100 μg 3 once weekly	63		−0.04 (0.90) (mean change, MFTC JSW, mm)	−0.03 (−0.11, 0.04) (mean change, cMFTC cartilage thickness, mm)	
						−0.18 (0.74)	−0.03 (−0.04, 0.01)	
						−0.02 (0.86)	0.00 (−0.08, 0.08)	
						1.0 (0.73)	−0.01 (−0.02, 0.01)	
						0.34 (0.90)* (mean change, LFTC JSW, mm)	0.01 (0.00, 0.03)* (mean change, TFTC cartilage thickness, mm)	

(continued on next page)

Table 7
(continued)

Authors/Ref.	ClinialTrials.gov Identifier	OA Site	Dosage, Route of Interventions	N	Follow-up Duration (wk)	Efficacy in Structural Modification		Phase of Development
						Plain Radiographs	MRI	
			Proteinases Inhibitors					
Hochberg et al,[83] 2019	NCT01919164	Knee	Placebo	108	24 mo	NA	−0.02(−0.04, −0.01)	Phase 2
			Sprifermin IA 30 µg 3 once weekly q12 mo	110		0.08 mm (−0.08, 0.25)	0.00 (−0.02, 0.02)	
			Sprifermin IA 30 µg 3 once weekly q6 mo	111		0.04 mm (−0.13, 0.20)	−0.01(−0.03, 0.00)	
			Sprifermin IA 100 µg 3 once weekly q12 mo	110		0.26 mm (0.12, 0.40)**	0.03 (0.01, 0.04)	
			Sprifermin IA 100 µg 3 once weekly q6 mo	110		0.26 mm (0.12, 0.41)** (difference vs placebo, LFTC JSW, mm)	0.02 (0.00, 0.03)*** (mean change, TFTC cartilage thickness, mm)	
Eckstein et al,[86] 2021	NCT01919164	Knee	Placebo	108	60 mo	−0.38 (0.72); mean (SD)	—	Phase 2
			Sprifermin IA 30 µg 3 once weekly q12 mo	110		−0.47 (1.02)	—	
			Sprifermin IA 30 µg 3 once weekly q6 mo	111		−0.31 (0.75)	—*	
			Sprifermin IA 100 µg 3 once weekly q12 mo	110		−0.27 (0.75)	No numerical data reported for TFTC cartilage thickness	
			Sprifermin IA 100 µg 3 once weekly q6 mo	110		−0.16 (0.77) Change from baseline at 5 y; MFTC JSW, mm −0.13 (0.65) −0.05 (0.60) −0.03 (0.69) 0.03 (0.88) 0.02 (0.76) Change from baseline at 5 y; LFTC JSW, mm		

Gene therapy

Study	Trial	Joint	Intervention	N	Duration		Outcomes	Phase
Guermazi et al,[91] 2017	NCT01221441	Knee	Placebo IA (2 mL normal saline 0.9%) TissueGene-C IA	29 57	12 mo	—	47.9% 34.6% Progression of cartilage morphology in any subregion 21.1% 9.6% Any worsening in Hoffa-synovitis/ effusion-synovitis combined 60.6% 66.2% (any BML progression) 32.4% 31.6% any meniscal damage progression	Phase 2
Lee et al,[94] 2020	NCT01221441	Knee	Placebo IA (2 mL normal saline 0.9%) TissueGene-C IA	35 67	12 mo	—	47.9% 34.6% Progression of cartilage morphology in any subregion 21.1% 9.6% Any worsening in Hoffa-synovitis/ effusion-synovitis combined	Phase 2

(continued on next page)

Table 7
(continued)

Authors/Ref.	CliniaTrials.gov Identifier	OA Site	Dosage, Route of Interventions	N	Follow-up Duration (wk)	Efficacy in Structural Modification		Phase of Development
						Plain Radiographs	MRI	
			Proteinases Inhibitors					
Kim et al,[95] 2018	—	Knee	Placebo IA (2 mL normal saline 0.9%) TissueGene-C IA	81 78	12 mo	Not significant (JSW)	No significant change in any of WORMS subscore	Phase 3
Wnt/ß-catenin signaling pathway inhibitors								
Yazici et al,[103] 2020	NCT02536833	Knee	Placebo IA Lorecivivint (SM04690) IA 0.03 mg Lorecivivint (SM04690) IA 0.07 mg Lorecivivint (SM04690) IA 0.23 mg	114 112 117 109	26 wk	−0.20 mm −0.07 mm −0.11 mm −0.02 mm* (mean ± SD change from baseline, medial JSW)	NA	Phase 2
Yazici et al,[104] 2021	NCT03122860	Knee	Dry needle IA Placebo IA Lorecivivint (SM04690) IA 0.03 mg Lorecivivint (SM04690) IA 0.07 mg Lorecivivint (SM04690) IA 0.15 mg Lorecivivint (SM04690) IA 0.23 mg	117 116 116 115 115 116	24 wk	NA 3.44 (1.31) 3.30 (1.26) 3.16 (1.10) 3.26 (1.24) 3.27 (1.08) (mean ± SD change from baseline, medial JSW)	NA	Phase 2

Abbreviations: cMFTC, central medial femorotibial compartment; LFTC, lateral femorotibial compartment; TFTC, total femorotibial compartment.

ADAMTS-5 has been a target for OA therapy, as it is the most potent aggrecanase in vitro (30-fold more potent than ADAMTS-4) and ADAMTS-5 ablation or inhibition prevents joint damage in mice and human chondrocytes.[69] S201086/GLPG1972 is orally administered and a potent active site inhibitor of ADAMTS5[69] with an 8-fold selectivity over ADAMTS-4 in preclinical studies.[70] In a phase 2 study (Roccella study) including 932 knee OA patients, no significant difference was found between the active treatment arms (all 3 different dose levels) and placebo arm in both quantitative MRI cartilage thickness and clinical outcomes,[71] although the study was optimally designed by applying 2 radiologically based selection criteria for structural severity in the cartilage damage (ie, the combined Kellgren/Lawrence [KL] 2 or 3 and OARSI medial JSN 1 or 2 grading).[72] Phase 1 studies for an ADAMTS5 nanobody (M6495) were recently completed (NCT03583346, NCT03224702).

A major problem in the application of small molecules for directly targeting protease activity is the high degree of conservation in the sequence and structure of the active site, leading to unintended cross-inactivation of multiple metalloproteinases. This can result in possible short- and long-term side effects with systemic administration of the drug.[73] As an example, blocking the aggrecan degradation may be desired in the articular cartilage[74] but simultaneously may cause undesirable effects in tendons and the aorta, where aggrecan accumulation in tendons resulted in decreased mechanical properties,[75] and aggrecan and versican accumulation in thoracic aortic aneurysms can lead to aortic dissection and rupture.[76]

FIBROBLAST GROWTH FACTOR-18

Sprifermin is a recombinant human fibroblast growth factor-18 (FGF-18), which is a 19.83-kDa protein derived from the *Escherichia coli* expression system.[77] It induces the proliferation of chondrocytes and promotes hyaline extracellular matrix synthesis in preclinical models.[78] In 2007, a first-in-human trial (NCT00911469) for IA sprifermin administration was commenced in 73 end-stage knee OA patients who were scheduled for knee replacement within the next 6 months and showed positive effects on histologic cartilage parameters with no major safety issues over 24 weeks.[79] In the second proof-of-concept phase 1b trial (NCT01033994) conducted in 2008, a significant dose-dependent response in the sprifermin groups was detected in the secondary structural outcomes, such as radiographic JSW, and MRI-detected total and lateral tibiofemoral cartilage thickness over 12 months (n = 168).[80] The sprifermin also improved WOMAC pain score from baseline, but there was no significant difference, compared with the placebo group. The post hoc analyses of the same studies showed the structure-protective effects on cartilage damage and BMLs at 12-month follow-up.[81,82]

In the third phase 2 dose-ranging clinical trial (FGF18 Osteoarthritis Randomized Trial with Administration of Repeated Doses [FORWARD] study) (NCT01919164), there was a statistically significant dose-dependent improvement, but of uncertain clinical importance, in total tibiofemoral cartilage thickness in patients administered with a dose of 100 μg sprifermin every 6 and 12 months, but not with the dose of 30 μg at 2 years (n = 549). No symptomatic improvement is revealed in the active groups, compared with the placebo saline injection.[83] An exploratory analysis of the same study for 3-year follow-up (n = 442) revealed similar results. These findings were published in the *Journal of the American Medical Association* in 2019. In the post hoc analysis, a "subgroup at risk" with narrower medial or lateral minimum JSW and higher WOMAC pain than the overall study population at baseline (n = 161) showed a significant improvement in WOMAC pain on 3-year follow-up (−8.8 (−22.4, 4.9]) in the 100-

µg Sprifermin group (n = 34) compared with the placebo (n = 33).[84] In another post hoc analysis using the cartilage thinning/thickening scores and ordered values on MRI over 24 months regardless of the location, 100-µg Sprifermin every 6 months causes cartilage thickening more than double and cartilage thinning almost reduced to that in healthy reference subjects from the Osteoarthritis Initiative data set (n = 82), supporting the structure-protective action of Sprifermin.[85]

Recently, a report on the 5-year efficacy and safety results from the FORWARD study (n = 494) revealed that sprifermin 100 µg every 6 months for 2 years maintained long-term structural protective effects on articular cartilage despite a treatment-free period of 3 years, with a good safety profile.[86] A recent meta-analysis published in 2021 included 8 reports from 3 original trials and confirmed the structure-protivive effects of sprifermin and safety profile, although symptomatic modifications were inconclusive.[87] The reasons for its nonsignificant effect on symptom alleviations are largely unclear, which might be attributed to the heterogeneity of patient populations with a high proportion of low-pain and/or high-cartilage thickness at baseline and to the placebo effect of IA saline injections, which improved symptoms in the placebo group.[7,88] These structure-protective findings together with the symptomatic improvement in the subgroup at risk could pave the way for future phase 3 clinical trials in the specific target OA endotype.

TRANSFORMING GROWTH FACTOR-β

Transforming growth factor-β (TGF-β) contributes to early cartilage development and maintains cartilage homeostasis in later life by stimulating the extracellular matrix protein synthesis.[89] Moreover, osteocyte TGF-β signaling may be associated with regulating subchondral bone remodeling in advanced OA.[90] TissueGene-C (TG-C) is retrovirally transduced to promote TGF-β1 transcription (hChonJb#7 cells).[91] A recent study in a monosodium iodoacetate model of OA rats showed that TG-C produces an M2 macrophage-dominant proanabolic microenvironment, promoting cartilage regeneration.[92]

In a phase 2 trial (NCT01221441), the IA TG-C administration (n = 57) had a positive effect on the progression of the cartilage damage and inflammation markers but not on BML and meniscal damage on MRI compared with the placebo (n = 29) over 12 months.[91] In a 2017 poster abstract, a single IA administration of the TG-C caused symptomatic improvement, but its effects on the cartilage were inconclusive at 12-month follow-up (n = 156).[93] These findings were confirmed by another study in 102 OA patients.[94] In a phase 3 trial (NCT02072070), improvement in pain and function was reported in 163 OA patients but with no significant structural benefits.[95] Despite clinical holds in April 2019 over the concerns of chemistry, manufacturing, and control issues related to the potential mislabeling of ingredients, this was lifted in April 2020.[96] In analysis of observational long-term safety follow-up data, there was no evidence showing the association of TG-C administration with increased risk of cancer or other major safety concerns over an average of 10 years.[97] The results of 2 pivotal phase 3 trials (NCT03203330, NCT03291470) are still awaited.

WNT SIGNALING INHIBITORS

Increased Wnt signaling in the chondrocytes results in degeneration of cartilage, whereas stimulation of the Wnt pathway in subchondral bone promotes bone formation and sclerosis.[98,99] Moreover, increased Wnt signaling in the synovium causes increased generation of MMPs and thus OA disease progression.[100] Lorecivivint (SM04690) is a small-molecule CLK/DYRK1A Wnt signaling inhibitor and reduced the cartilage damage in animal studies.[101] In a 52-week, multicenter, phase 2 trial (NCT02536833), IA injection of 0.07 mg revealed significant symptomatic and radiographic improvement compared with IA placebo saline injection starting from week 13 through to the 52-week follow-up in 455 patients with unilateral symptomatic knee OA,[102] although the primary symptomatic endpoints were not met. This was also confirmed by another phase 2 clinical trial (NCT03122860) (n = 700), and the lowest optimal dose was determined as 0.07 mg.[103] The analysis of safety data after combining the 2 trials (848 = Lorecivivint-treated and 360 = control subjects) exhibited the favorable safety profile.[104] Two small phase 2 (NCT03727022, NCT03706521) and 3 phase 3 (NCT03928184, NCT04385303, NCT04520607) trials are active.

SENOLYTIC THERAPIES

Senescence, in which cells cease dividing, is newly implicated in the aging-related OA pathogenesis[105] via the production of proinflammatory cytokines, chemokines, and dysfunction of neighboring cells.[106,107] Therefore, senotherapeutics are being investigated as an emerging therapy for treating aging-related diseases, such as OA. UBX0101 is a potent senolytic, a p53/MDM2 interaction inhibitor, and showed increased chondrogenesis in preclinical studies.[108] Despite its promising findings in a phase 1 study (n = 48),[109] there was no significant change in pain and function in a 12-week phase 2 clinical study (NCT04129944) (n = 183).[110] Failure to meet the primary and secondary endpoints lead to termination of a long-term follow-up study of the previous trial (NCT04349956). Future development for improving the specificity of senolytics to certain types of senescent cells, alternative senolytics with higher potency, or a combination of senolytic agents should be considered.[111]

PERSPECTIVES

The costs of commercial research and development from discovery through to phase 3 trials for a commercially viable product are estimated to have increased 9-fold from 1979 (US$92 million) to 2010 (US$883.6 million).[112] In a recent study, an estimated cost to bring a new therapeutic agent to market is averaged at US$1335.9 million (in 2018 US dollars).[113] Despite active research and immense investment, DMOAD development has been entangled with several challenges.

Regulatory approval of any drug requires the demonstration, in a relevant and defined study population, of the efficacy of the drug under investigation (intervention) determined on a few selected endpoints in comparison with either a placebo or an active comparator. Therefore, careful considerations should be given to each of these factors to tackle the challenges in the drug development process. These are discussed as the 4 sections in terms of the formulation of a research question known as *PICO approach*: (1) population, (2) interventions, (3) comparison or placebo, and (4) outcomes.

Osteoarthritis Population or Phenotypes in Clinical Trials

OA can be defined as a complex heterogeneous disease involving different tissue targets with differing severities in a slowly progressive manner,[3] with the "one-size-fits-all" approach unlikely to work. Because of marked interpatient variability in clinical and structural presentations in the OA disease process,[114] investigation of a targeted therapy in an appropriate patient/disease phenotype according to the targeted pathogenetic pathways would be required for successful drug development. However, the classification of the OA phenotypes is not straightforward, as, during different phases of the OA disease, more than 1 pathogenetic mechanism may contribute to OA in the same patient at varying degrees and that 1 phenotype rarely exists in isolation.[115] Therefore, a new model of classifying OA subtypes that is internationally accepted should be formulated for selecting appropriate study subtypes in clinical trials. For example, for clinical trials to examine the efficacy of anti-inflammatory pharmaceutical agents, the study population with effusion and synovial hypertrophy would be optimal for meeting the trial endpoints.

Advanced OA with extensive structural changes may preclude successful halting or reversal of the disease process, suggesting that the treatment strategy should be initiated as soon as possible to prevent disease progression.[116] Currently, most DMOAD therapies are investigated in the knee OA with KL grade 2 or 3 on plain radiograph. However, such degree of radiographic evidence of OA is a relatively late phenomenon in the process of structural evolution, as alterations in the periarticular bone changes often precede the radiographic OA evidence by 5 to 10 years.[117] There is a lack of consensus definition for identifying either an "early OA" or the prestages of OA, whereby effective cure would be more feasible, although draft classification criteria of "early OA" in the primary setting were recently proposed based on the Knee Injury and Osteoarthritis Outcome Score, clinical signs for joint line tenderness or crepitus, and KL grade 0 or 1.[118]

As the symptomatic improvement translated through the structural protection is essential for defining a DMOADs, the use of the "flare design" (selecting only patients whose pain worsens after withdrawal of their usual pharmacologic treatment) versus "no flare design" may be considered for recruiting nonsteroidal anti-inflammatory drug responders with a more "inflammatory" phenotype in clinical trials, as this may influence the effect sizes of the active treatment.[119] However, a meta-analysis published in 2016 revealed no such difference in effect sizes between the 2 designs.[120]

Interventions

Most phase 2/3 drug development programs failed to show adequate efficacy because of no validated animal models, insufficient linkage of the molecular target with the disease, and use in indications based on insufficient biological rationale.[121] The poor translation of preclinical research into clinical use may result from the fact that animal models are usually young, male mice with injured joints, whereas the human disease occurs mostly in older women with no recent injury.[122] In addition, the crucial factor for targeted therapy to work as expected is the selectivity and affinity of the agents to their receptors as in differential effects of aggrecan degradation in articular cartilage versus tendon. The ideal drug should be fulfilled with the attributes of receptor or functional selectivity, specificity, and potency.[123]

OA is a slowly progressive disease usually found in the obese elderly with multiple comorbidities [4] and so the ideal therapeutic drug should be not only efficacious but also extremely safe in the long-term treatment in such a fragile population. Therefore, systemic drug treatment is not preferred because of off-target effects and systemic toxicity, as in the case of broad-spectrum MMP inhibitors.[124] Another obstacle toward the successful development of DMOADs is their insufficient concentration in OA joints upon systemic administration, leading to low therapeutic efficacy and potential systemic effects.[125]

Local therapy, such as IA administration, will directly target the recognized pathogenetic tissues within the joint and may require lower doses because of increased bioavailability. Still, the IA route has several issues, such as the pain and swelling during procedures, rare cases of septic arthritis, and short half-life of residual times of the agents in the joints owing to rapid clearance by the body. To prolong the residence time in the joint, a variety of drug delivery systems (DDS) have been developed. An ideal DDS should provide controlled and/or sustained drug release for facilitating long-term treatment with a reduced number of injections[126] and possess adequate disease modification, biocompatibility, and biodegradability.[127] New smart drug delivery strategies, using nanoparticles, microparticles, and hydrogels methods, may increase the opportunity for detecting the therapeutic potential of IA agents.[128]

Comparison or Placebo

Administration of placebo in the control group in the RCT is essential in demonstrating the efficacy of active treatment. However, all the placebos are not equal in pain improvement, with greater effect sizes in the IA placebo [0.29 (95% credible interval, 0.09–0.49)] and topical placebo (0.20 [credible interval, 0.02–0.38]) compared with oral placebo.[129] IA saline is a commonly used placebo for control groups in RCTs of injective procedures with remarkable pain relief that is potentially clinically meaningful to patients based on minimal clinically important difference values.[130] This was supported by the finding of a recent meta-analysis in the placebo effects of IA saline at 6-month follow-up, which revealed a significant pain reduction on 0 to 100 VAS (−13.4 [−21.7/−5.1]), improvement in WOMAC function sub-score (−10.1 [−12.2,-8.0]), and 56% in the pooled responder rate in terms of the OMERACT-OARSI criteria.[131] Therefore, the placebo effects of IA saline should be accounted for in planning the trial design when pain and function endpoints are used as the primary measures.[132]

In addition, as the IA saline injection is more than a "mere" placebo owing to dilution effects,[133] future robust studies investigating the underlying mechanisms and the predictors of the placebo responses as well as the comparative effects of sham injections versus saline injections are recommended.[7] In the context of the DMOAD definition, which requires structure-protective effects leading to the clinical translation of symptomatic improvement, the failure of active agents to meet the primary clinical endpoint compared with the placebo should be interpreted in light of large placebo responses. In addition, no active drug comparator can be used currently for noninferiority trial design, as there is a lack of DMOADs approved by the regulatory bodies.[134,135]

Outcome Measures

The issues for measuring the efficacy of DMOAD candidates in clinical trials include the lack of responsiveness of plain radiographs required by the regulatory bodies for DMOAD approval,[7] the absence of biomarkers for structure modifying endpoints,[136] and the variation of definitions for long-term clinical outcomes.[137] Another well-established hurdle is the symptom-structure discordance in OA disease process,[138] suggesting that a structure-protective agent may require long-term follow-up to detect the symptomatic benefits[7] but with no consensus on the threshold of optimal follow-up duration sufficient for detecting DMOAD effects. The recent progress in these areas include the Food and Drug Administration's formal recognition of OA as a serious disease,[139] the validation studies and extensive utilization of MRI in the clinical studies,[140,141] and the OA Biomarkers effort contributed by the FNIH Biomarkers Consortium, a major public-private biomedical research partnership.[136] Therefore, new insight into and discovery of biomarkers with optimal predictive validity and responsiveness will enable the development of recommendations for using specific biomarkers in clinical trials and establishment of efficacy of future DMOAD agents.

SUMMARY

OA contributes to an immense disease burden with an intense unmet need for effective and safe therapies. Lessons have been learned from the failure to find a meaningful disease-modifying agent despite massive efforts and investments in research and development pipelines, providing the progression in developing new strategies for overcoming the barriers. By virtue of lessons learned from past clinical trials and insights gained through preclinical research, several agents are revealing some promising results in late-stage clinical trials. Further research should focus on the international consensuses on phenotype classification, appropriate selection criteria and trial design for each specific targeted therapy, the innovation of DDS for optimal drug residence in the joints, sufficient and appropriate procedures for target validation and linkage in preclinical research before progressing to clinical trials, and validation of imaging and biomarker outcomes.

ACKNOWLEDGMENTS

Dr WMO is supported by the Presidential Scholarship of Myanmar for his PhD course.

DISCLOSURE

Nothing to be disclosed.

REFERENCES

1. Cui A, Li H, Wang D, et al. Global, regional prevalence, incidence and risk factors of knee osteoarthritis in population-based studies. EClinicalMedicine. 2020; 29-30:100587.
2. Leifer VP, Katz JN, Losina E. The burden of OA-health services and economics. Osteoarthritis and Cartilage 2021.
3. Oo WM, Yu SP, Daniel MS, et al. Disease-modifying drugs in osteoarthritis: current understanding and future therapeutics. Expert Opin emerging Drugs 2018; 23(4):331–47.
4. Hunter DJ, Bierma-Zeinstra S. Osteoarthritis. The Lancet 2019;393(10182): 1745–59.
5. Castro-Domínguez F, Vargas-Negrín F, Pérez C, et al. Unmet needs in the osteoarthritis chronic moderate to severe pain management in Spain: a real word data study. Rheumatol Ther 2021;8(3):1113–27.
6. Malenfant JH, Batsis JA. Obesity in the geriatric population - a global health perspective. J Glob Health Rep 2019;3:e2019045.
7. Oo WM, Little C, Duong V, et al. The development of disease-modifying therapies for osteoarthritis (DMOADs): the evidence to date. Drug Des Devel Ther 2021;15:2921–45.
8. Felson DT. Identifying different osteoarthritis phenotypes through epidemiology. Osteoarthritis and cartilage. 2010;18(5):601–4.
9. Mobasheri A, van Spil WE, Budd E, et al. Molecular taxonomy of osteoarthritis for patient stratification, disease management and drug development: biochemical markers associated with emerging clinical phenotypes and molecular endotypes. Curr Opin Rheumatol 2019;31(1):80–9.
10. Prieto-Potin I, Largo R, Roman-Blas JA, et al. Characterization of multinucleated giant cells in synovium and subchondral bone in knee osteoarthritis and rheumatoid arthritis. BMC Musculoskelet Disord 2015;16:226.

11. Wojdasiewicz P, Poniatowski Ł A, Szukiewicz D. The role of inflammatory and anti-inflammatory cytokines in the pathogenesis of osteoarthritis. Mediators Inflamm 2014;2014:561459.
12. de Lange-Brokaar BJ, Ioan-Facsinay A, van Osch GJ, et al. Synovial inflammation, immune cells and their cytokines in osteoarthritis: a review. Osteoarthritis Cartilage. 2012;20(12):1484–99.
13. Oo WM, Linklater JM, Hunter DJ. Imaging in knee osteoarthritis. Curr Opin Rheumatol 2017;29(1):86–95.
14. Collins JE, Losina E, Nevitt MC, et al. Semiquantitative imaging biomarkers of knee osteoarthritis progression: data from the Foundation for the National Institutes of Health Osteoarthritis Biomarkers Consortium. Arthritis Rheumatol 2016; 68(10):2422–31.
15. Liacini A, Sylvester J, Li WQ, et al. Inhibition of interleukin-1-stimulated MAP kinases, activating protein-1 (AP-1) and nuclear factor kappa B (NF-κB) transcription factors down-regulates matrix metalloproteinase gene expression in articular chondrocytes. Matrix Biol 2002;21(3):251–62.
16. Hwang HS, Kim HA. Chondrocyte apoptosis in the pathogenesis of osteoarthritis. Int J Mol Sci 2015;16(11):26035–54.
17. Jenei-Lanzl Z, Meurer A, Zaucke F. Interleukin-1β signaling in osteoarthritis – chondrocytes in focus. Cell Signal 2019;53:212–23.
18. Kamath RV, Hart M, Conlon D, et al. 126 Simultaneous targeting OF IL-1A AND IL-1B by a dual-variable-domain immunoglobulin (DVD-IG(tm)) prevents cartilage degradation in preclinical models of osteoarthritis. Osteoarthritis and Cartilage. 2011;19:S64.
19. Fleischmann RM, Bliddal H, Blanco FJ, et al. A phase II trial of lutikizumab, an anti-interleukin-1α/β dual variable domain immunoglobulin, in knee osteoarthritis patients with synovitis. Arthritis Rheumatol 2019;71(7):1056–69.
20. Kloppenburg M, Peterfy C, Haugen IK, et al. Phase IIa, placebo-controlled, randomised study of lutikizumab, an anti-interleukin-1α and anti-interleukin-1β dual variable domain immunoglobulin, in patients with erosive hand osteoarthritis. 2019;78(3):413–420.
21. Gadotti VM, Martins DF, Pinto HF, et al. Diacerein decreases visceral pain through inhibition of glutamatergic neurotransmission and cytokine signaling in mice. Pharmacol Biochem Behav 2012;102(4):549–54.
22. Pelletier JP, Raynauld JP, Dorais M, et al. An international, multicentre, double-blind, randomized study (DISSCO): effect of diacerein vs celecoxib on symptoms in knee osteoarthritis. Rheumatology (Oxford). 2020;59(12):3858–68.
23. AgencyEM. PRAC re-examines diacerein and recommends that it remain available with restrictions. 2014.
24. Honvo G, Reginster J-Y, Rabenda V, et al. Safety of symptomatic slow-acting drugs for osteoarthritis: outcomes of a systematic review and meta-analysis. Drugs & Aging. 2019;36(1):65–99.
25. Wiegertjes R, van de Loo FAJ, Blaney Davidson EN. A roadmap to target interleukin-6 in osteoarthritis. Rheumatology (Oxford, England). 2020;59(10): 2681–94.
26. Latourte A, Cherifi C, Maillet J, et al. Systemic inhibition of IL-6/Stat3 signalling protects against experimental osteoarthritis. Ann Rheum Dis 2017;76(4):748–55.
27. Kamiya N, Kuroyanagi G, Aruwajoye O, et al. IL6 receptor blockade preserves articular cartilage and increases bone volume following ischemic osteonecrosis in immature mice. Osteoarthritis Cartilage. 2019;27(2):326–35.

28. Richette P, Latourte A, Sellam J, et al. Efficacy of tocilizumab in patients with hand osteoarthritis: double blind, randomised, placebo-controlled, multicentre trial. Ann Rheum Dis 2021;80(3):349–55.

29. Toyoda E, Maehara M, Watanabe M, et al. Candidates intra-articular adm ther therapies osteoarthritis. 2021;22(7):3594.

30. Broeren MGA, de Vries M, Bennink MB, et al. Suppression of the inflammatory response by disease-inducible interleukin-10 gene therapy in a three-dimensional micromass model of the human synovial membrane. Arthritis Res Ther 2016;18:186.

31. Watkins LR, Chavez RA, Landry R, et al. Targeted interleukin-10 plasmid DNA therapy in the treatment of osteoarthritis: toxicology and pain efficacy assessments. Brain Behav Immun 2020;90:155–66.

32. Cronstein BN, Aune TM. Methotrexate and its mechanisms of action in inflammatory arthritis. Nat Rev Rheumatol 2020;16(3):145–54.

33. Kingsbury SR, Tharmanathan P, Keding A, et al. Significant pain reduction with oral methotrexate in knee osteoarthritis; results from the promote randomised controlled phase iii trial of treatment effectiveness. Osteoarthritis and Cartilage. 2019;27:S84–5.

34. Hu W, Chen Y, Dou C, et al. Microenvironment in subchondral bone: predominant regulator for the treatment of osteoarthritis. Ann Rheum Dis 2020;80(4):413–22.

35. Nagae M, Hiraga T, Yoneda T. Acidic microenvironment created by osteoclasts causes bone pain associated with tumor colonization. J Bone Miner Metab 2007;25(2):99–104.

36. Zhu S, Zhu J, Zhen G, et al. Subchondral bone osteoclasts induce sensory innervation and osteoarthritis pain. The J Clin Invest 2019;129(3):1076–93.

37. Costa AG, Cusano NE, Silva BC, et al. Its skeletal actions and role as a therapeutic target in osteoporosis. Nat Rev Rheumatol 2011;7(8):447–56.

38. Hayami T, Zhuo Y, Wesolowski GA, et al. Inhibition of cathepsin K reduces cartilage degeneration in the anterior cruciate ligament transection rabbit and murine models of osteoarthritis. Bone. 2012;50(6):1250–9.

39. Lindström E, Rizoska B, Tunblad K, et al. The selective cathepsin K inhibitor MIV-711 attenuates joint pathology in experimental animal models of osteoarthritis. J translational Med 2018;16(1):56.

40. Conaghan PG, Bowes MA, Kingsbury SR, et al. Disease-modifying effects of a novel cathepsin K inhibitor in osteoarthritis: a randomized controlled trial. Ann Intern Med 2020;172(2):86–95.

41. Sampson ER, Hilton MJ, Tian Y, et al. Teriparatide as a chondroregenerative therapy for injury-induced osteoarthritis. Sci translational Med 2011;3(101). 101ra193-101ra193.

42. Cui C, Zheng L, Fan Y, et al. Parathyroid hormone ameliorates temporomandibular joint osteoarthritic-like changes related to age. Cell Prolif. 2020;53(4):e12755.

43. Chen C-H, Ho M-L, Chang L-H, et al. Parathyroid hormone-(1–34) ameliorated knee osteoarthritis in rats via autophagy. J Appl Physiol 2018;124(5):1177–85.

44. Sun Q, Zhen G, Li TP, et al. Parathyroid hormone attenuates osteoarthritis pain by remodeling subchondral bone in mice. eLife. 2021;10:e66532.

45. McGuire D, Lane N, Segal N, et al. TPX-100 leads to marked, sustained improvements in subjects with knee osteoarthritis: pre-clinical rationale and results of a controlled clinical trial. Osteoarthritis and Cartilage. 2018;26:S243.

46. McGuire D, Bowes M, Brett A, et al. Study TPX-100-5: significant reduction in femoral bone shape change 12 months after IA TPX-100 correlates with tibiofemoral cartilage stabilization. Osteoarthritis and Cartilage. 2020;28:S37–8.

47. Felson DT, Chaisson CE, Hill CL, et al. The association of bone marrow lesions with pain in knee osteoarthritis. Ann Intern Med 2001;134(7):541–9.

48. O'Neill TW, Felson DT. Mechanisms of osteoarthritis (OA) pain. Curr Osteoporos Rep 2018;16(5):611–6.

49. Zanetti M, Bruder E, Romero J, et al. Bone marrow edema pattern in osteoarthritic knees: correlation between MR imaging and histologic findings. Radiology 2000;215(3):835–40.

50. Singh V, Oliashirazi A, Tan T, et al. Clinical and pathophysiologic significance of MRI identified bone marrow lesions associated with knee osteoarthritis. Arch Bone Jt Surg 2019;7(3):211–9.

51. Fernández-Martín S, López-Peña M, Muñoz F, et al. Bisphosphonates as disease-modifying drugs in osteoarthritis preclinical studies: a systematic review from 2000 to 2020. Arthritis Res Ther 2021;23(1):60.

52. Moretti A, Paoletta M, Liguori S, et al. The rationale for the intra-articular administration of clodronate in osteoarthritis. Int J Mol Sci 2021;22(5):2693.

53. Vaysbrot EE, Osani MC, Musetti MC, et al. Are bisphosphonates efficacious in knee osteoarthritis? A meta-analysis of randomized controlled trials. Osteoarthritis Cartilage. 2018;26(2):154–64.

54. Eriksen EF, Shabestari M, Ghouri A, et al. Bisphosphonates as a treatment modality in osteoarthritis. Bone 2021;143:115352.

55. Deveza LA, Bierma-Zeinstra SMA, van Spil WE, et al. Efficacy of bisphosphonates in specific knee osteoarthritis subpopulations: protocol for an OA trial bank systematic review and individual patient data meta-analysis. BMJ open. 2018;8(12):e023889.

56. Frediani B, Toscano C, Falsetti P, et al. Intramuscular clodronate in long-term treatment of symptomatic knee osteoarthritis: a randomized controlled study. Drugs in R&D. 2020;20(1):39–45.

57. Hayes KN, Giannakeas V, Wong AKO. Bisphosphonate use is protective of radiographic knee osteoarthritis progression among those with low disease severity and being non-overweight: data from the Osteoarthritis Initiative. J Bone Mineral Res 2020;35(12):2318–26.

58. Cai G, Aitken D, Laslett LL, et al. Effect of intravenous zoledronic acid on tibiofemoral cartilage volume among patients with knee osteoarthritis with bone marrow lesions: a randomized clinical trial. JAMA. 2020;323(15):1456–66.

59. Kong C, Wang C, Shi Y, et al. Active vitamin D activates chondrocyte autophagy to reduce osteoarthritis via mediating the AMPK-mTOR signaling pathway. Biochem Cell Biol. 2020;98(3):434–42.

60. MacFarlane LA, Cook NR, Kim E, et al. The effects of vitamin D and marine omega-3 fatty acid supplementation on chronic knee pain in older US adults: results from a randomized trial. Arthritis Rheumatol 2020;72(11):1836–44.

61. Perry TA, Parkes MJ, Hodgson R, et al. Effect of vitamin D supplementation on synovial tissue volume and subchondral bone marrow lesion volume in symptomatic knee osteoarthritis. BMC Musculoskelet Disord 2019;20(1):76.

62. Tu L, Zheng S, Cicuttini F, et al. Effects of vitamin D supplementation on disabling foot pain in patients with symptomatic knee osteoarthritis. Arthritis Care Res 2021;73(6):781–7.

63. Zhao ZX, He Y, Peng LH, et al. Does vitamin D improve symptomatic and structural outcomes in knee osteoarthritis? A systematic review and meta-analysis. Aging Clin Exp Res 2021;33(9):2393–403.

64. Man GS, Mologhianu G. Osteoarthritis pathogenesis - a complex process that involves the entire joint. J Med Life 2014;7(1):37–41.

65. Yamamoto K, Wilkinson D, Bou-Gharios G. Targeting dysregulation of metalloproteinase activity in osteoarthritis. Calcif Tissue Int 2021;109(3):277–90.

66. Fields GB. The rebirth of matrix metalloproteinase inhibitors: moving beyond the dogma. Cells. 2019;8(9).

67. Wang M, Sampson ER, Jin H, et al. MMP13 is a critical target gene during the progression of osteoarthritis. Arthritis Res Ther 2013;15(1):R5.

68. Hu Q, Ecker M. Overview of MMP-13 as a promising target for the treatment of osteoarthritis. Int J Mol Sci 2021;22(4):1742.

69. Santamaria S. ADAMTS-5: a difficult teenager turning 20. Int J Exp Pathol 2020;101(1–2):4–20.

70. Brebion F, Gosmini R, Deprez P, et al. Discovery of GLPG1972/S201086, a potent, selective, and orally bioavailable ADAMTS-5 inhibitor for the treatment of osteoarthritis. J Med Chem 2021;64(6):2937–52.

71. Galapagos and Servier report topline results for ROCCELLA phase 2 clinical trial with GLPG1972/S201086 in knee osteoarthritis patients. 2020.

72. vanderAar E, Deckx H, Van Der Stoep M, et al. Study design of a phase 2 clinical trial with a disease-modifying osteoarthritis drug candidate GLPG1972/S201086: the Roccella trial. Osteoarthritis and Cartilage. 2020;28:S499–500.

73. Rose KWJ, Taye N, Karoulias SZ, et al. Regulation of ADAMTS proteases. Front Mol Biosciences. 2021;8(621).

74. Verma P, Dalal K. ADAMTS-4 and ADAMTS-5: key enzymes in osteoarthritis. J Cell Biochem. 2011;112(12):3507–14.

75. Wang VM, Bell RM, Thakore R, et al. Murine tendon function is adversely affected by aggrecan accumulation due to the knockout of ADAMTS5. J Orthopaedic Res 2012;30(4):620–6.

76. Cikach FS, Koch CD, Mead TJ, et al. Massive aggrecan and versican accumulation in thoracic aortic aneurysm and dissection. JCI Insight. 2018;3(5).

77. Song L, Huang Z, Chen Y, et al. High-efficiency production of bioactive recombinant human fibroblast growth factor 18 in Escherichia coli and its effects on hair follicle growth. Appl Microbiol Biotechnol 2014;98(2):695–704.

78. Hendesi H, Stewart S, Gibison ML, et al. Recombinant fibroblast growth factor-18 (sprifermin) enhances microfracture-induced cartilage healing. J orthopaedic Res : official Publ Orthopaedic Res Soc 2021.

79. Muurahainen N. Cartilage repair and the sprifermin story: mechanisms, preclinical and clinical study results, and lessons learned. Osteoarthritis and Cartilage. 2016;24:S4.

80. Lohmander LS, Hellot S, Dreher D, et al. Intraarticular sprifermin (recombinant human fibroblast growth factor 18) in knee osteoarthritis: a randomized, double-blind, placebo-controlled trial. Arthritis Rheumatol 2014;66(7):1820–31.

81. Roemer FW, Aydemir A, Lohmander S, et al. Structural effects of sprifermin in knee osteoarthritis: a post-hoc analysis on cartilage and non-cartilaginous tissue alterations in a randomized controlled trial. BMC Musculoskelet Disord 2016;17:267.

82. Eckstein F, Wirth W, Guermazi A, et al. Brief report: intraarticular sprifermin not only increases cartilage thickness, but also reduces cartilage loss: location-

independent post hoc analysis using magnetic resonance imaging. Arthritis Rheumatol 2015;67(11):2916–22.

83. Hochberg MC, Guermazi A, Guehring H, et al. Effect of intra-articular sprifermin vs placebo on femorotibial joint cartilage thickness in patients with osteoarthritis: the FORWARD randomized clinical trial. JAMA. 2019;322(14):1360–70.

84. Hans Guehring JK, Moreau Flavie, Daelken Benjamin, et al. Hochberg cartilage thickness modification with sprifermin in knee osteoarthritis patients translates into symptomatic improvement over placebo in patients at risk of further structural and symptomatic progression: post-hoc analysis of a phase II trial. Arthritis Rheumatol 2019;71(suppl 10).

85. Eckstein F, Kraines JL, Aydemir A, et al. Intra-articular sprifermin reduces cartilage loss in addition to increasing cartilage gain independent of location in the femorotibial joint: post-hoc analysis of a randomised, placebo-controlled phase II clinical trial. Ann Rheum Dis 2020;79(4):525–8.

86. Eckstein F, Hochberg MC, Guehring H, et al. Long-term structural and symptomatic effects of intra-articular sprifermin in patients with knee osteoarthritis: 5-year results from the FORWARD study. Ann Rheum Dis 2021;80(8):1062–9.

87. Zeng N, Chen X-Y, Yan Z-P, et al. Efficacy and safety of sprifermin injection for knee osteoarthritis treatment: a meta-analysis. Arthritis Res Ther 2021; 23(1):107.

88. Li J, Wang X, Ruan G, et al. Sprifermin: a recombinant human fibroblast growth factor 18 for the treatment of knee osteoarthritis. Expert Opin Investig Drugs 2021;30(9):923–30.

89. Zhai G, Dore J, Rahman P. TGF-beta signal transduction pathways and osteoarthritis. Rheumatol Int 2015;35(8):1283–92.

90. Dai G, Xiao H, Liao J, et al. Osteocyte TGFβ1-Smad2/3 is positively associated with bone turnover parameters in subchondral bone of advanced osteoarthritis. Int J Mol Med 2020;46(1):167–78.

91. Guermazi A, Kalsi G, Niu J, et al. Structural effects of intra-articular TGF-beta1 in moderate to advanced knee osteoarthritis: MRI-based assessment in a randomized controlled trial. BMC Musculoskelet Disord 2017;18(1):461.

92. Lee H, Kim H, Seo J, et al. TissueGene-C promotes an anti-inflammatory microenvironment in a rat monoiodoacetate model of osteoarthritis via polarization of M2 macrophages leading to pain relief and structural improvement. Inflammopharmacology. 2020;28(5):1237–52.

93. Cho J, Kim T, Shin J, et al. A phase III clinical results of INVOSSA™ (TissueGene C): a clues for the potential disease modifying OA drug. Cytotherapy. 2017; 19(5):S148.

94. Lee B, Parvizi J, Bramlet D, et al. Results of a phase II study to determine the efficacy and safety of genetically engineered allogeneic human chondrocytes expressing TGF-β1. The J knee Surg 2020;33(2):167–72.

95. Kim MK, Ha CW, In Y, et al. A multicenter, double-blind, phase III clinical trial to evaluate the efficacy and safety of a cell and gene therapy in knee osteoarthritis patients. Hum Gene Ther Clin Dev 2018.

96. Kolon TissueGene cleared to resume US phase III trial for Invossa. The pharma letter 2020.

97. DHunter RM Wang, M Noh. Overall safety of TG-C: safety analysis of phase-1, phase-2 and long-term safety trials [Abstract]. Osteoarthritis and Cartilage 2020;28.

98. Lories RJ, Monteagudo S. Review article: is Wnt signaling an attractive target for the treatment of osteoarthritis? Rheumatol Ther 2020;7(2):259–70.

99. Kovács B, Vajda E, Nagy EE. Regulatory effects and interactions of the Wnt and OPG-RANKL-RANK signaling at the bone-cartilage interface in osteoarthritis. Int J Mol Sci 2019;20(18):4653.

100. Cherifi C, Monteagudo S, Lories RJ. Promising targets for therapy of osteoarthritis: a review on the Wnt and TGF-β signalling pathways. Ther Adv Musculoskelet Dis 2021;13. 1759720X211006959.

101. Deshmukh V, O'Green AL, Bossard C, et al. Modulation of the Wnt pathway through inhibition of CLK2 and DYRK1A by lorecivivint as a novel, potentially disease-modifying approach for knee osteoarthritis treatment. Osteoarthritis Cartilage. 2019;27(9):1347–60.

102. Yazici Y, McAlindon TE, Gibofsky A, et al. Lorecivivint, a novel intraarticular CDC-like kinase 2 and dual-specificity tyrosine phosphorylation-regulated kinase 1A inhibitor and Wnt pathway modulator for the treatment of knee osteoarthritis: a phase II randomized trial. Arthritis Rheumatol (Hoboken, NJ). 2020; 72(10):1694–706.

103. Yazici Y, McAlindon TE, Gibofsky A, et al. A Phase 2b randomized trial of lorecivivint, a novel intra-articular CLK2/DYRK1A inhibitor and Wnt pathway modulator for knee osteoarthritis. Osteoarthritis Cartilage. 2021;29(5):654–66.

104. Simsek I, Swearingen C, Kennedy S, et al. OP0188 Integrated safety summary of the novel, intra-articular agent lorecivivint (SM04690), a CLK/DYRK1A inhibitor that modulates the WNT pathway, in subjects with knee osteoarthritis. Ann Rheum Dis 2020;79(Suppl 1):117.

105. Loeser RF. Aging and osteoarthritis: the role of chondrocyte senescence and aging changes in the cartilage matrix. Osteoarthritis Cartilage. 2009;17(8): 971–9.

106. Coppé JP, Patil CK, Rodier F, et al. Senescence-associated secretory phenotypes reveal cell-nonautonomous functions of oncogenic RAS and the p53 tumor suppressor. PLoS Biol 2008;6(12):2853–68.

107. Ferreira-Gonzalez S, Lu WY, Raven A, et al. Paracrine cellular senescence exacerbates biliary injury and impairs regeneration. Nat Commun 2018;9(1):1020.

108. Jeon OH, Kim C, Laberge R-M, et al. Local clearance of senescent cells attenuates the development of post-traumatic osteoarthritis and creates a pro-regenerative environment. Nat Med 2017;23(6):775–81.

109. Hsu B, Lane NE, Li L, et al. Safety, tolerability, pharmacokinetics, and clinical outcomes following single- dose IA administration of UBX0101, a senolytic MDM2/p53 interaction inhibitor, in patients with knee OA [abstract]. Osteoarthritis and Cartilage. 2020;28.

110. UnityBiotechnology I. UNITY biotechnology announces 12-week data from UBX0101 phase 2 clinical study in patients with painful osteoarthritis of the knee. 2020.

111. Zhang X-X, He S-H, Liang X, et al. Aging, cell senescence, the pathogenesis and targeted therapies of osteoarthritis. Front Pharmacol 2021;12(2200).

112. Morgan S, Grootendorst P, Lexchin J, et al. The cost of drug development: a systematic review. Health Pol (Amsterdam, Netherlands). 2011;100(1):4–17.

113. Wouters OJ, McKee M, Luyten J. Estimated research and development investment needed to bring a new medicine to market, 2009-2018. JAMA. 2020; 323(9):844–53.

114. Bierma-Zeinstra SM, Verhagen AP. Osteoarthritis subpopulations and implications for clinical trial design. Arthritis Res Ther 2011;13(2):213.

115. Karsdal MA, Michaelis M, Ladel C, et al. Disease-modifying treatments for oste-oarthritis (DMOADs) of the knee and hip: lessons learned from failures and op-portunities for the future. Osteoarthritis Cartilage. 2016;24(12):2013–21.

116. Felson DT, Hodgson R. Identifying and treating preclinical and early osteoar-thritis. Rheum Dis Clin North Am 2014;40(4):699–710.

117. Neogi T, Bowes MA, Niu J, et al. Magnetic resonance imaging-based three-dimensional bone shape of the knee predicts onset of knee osteoarthritis: data from the Osteoarthritis Initiative. Arthritis Rheum 2013;65(8):2048–58.

118. Luyten FP, Bierma-Zeinstra S, Dell'Accio F, et al. Toward classification criteria for early osteoarthritis of the knee. Semin Arthritis Rheum 2018;47(4):457–63.

119. Trijau S, Avouac J, Escalas C, et al. Influence of flare design on symptomatic efficacy of non-steroidal anti-inflammatory drugs in osteoarthritis: a meta-analysis of randomized placebo-controlled trials. Osteoarthritis Cartilage. 2010;18(8):1012–8.

120. Smith TO, Zou K, Abdullah N, et al. Does flare trial design affect the effect size of non-steroidal anti-inflammatory drugs in symptomatic osteoarthritis? A system-atic review and meta-analysis. Ann Rheum Dis 2016;75(11):1971–8.

121. Hunter DJ, Little CB. The great debate: should osteoarthritis research focus on "mice" or "men"? Osteoarthritis Cartilage. 2016;24(1):4–8.

122. Oo WM, Hunter DJ. Disease modification in osteoarthritis: are we there yet? Clin-ical & Experimental Rheumatology 2019;37 Suppl 120(5):135–40.

123. Berg KA, Clarke WP. Making sense of pharmacology: inverse agonism and functional selectivity. Int J Neuropsychopharmacol 2018;21(10):962–77.

124. Krzeski P, Buckland-Wright C, Balint G, et al. Development of musculoskeletal toxicity without clear benefit after administration of PG-116800, a matrix metal-loproteinase inhibitor, to patients with knee osteoarthritis: a randomized, 12-month, double-blind, placebo-controlled study. Arthritis Res Ther 2007;9(5): R109.

125. Oo WM, Liu X, Hunter DJ. Pharmacodynamics, efficacy, safety and administra-tion of intra-articular therapies for knee osteoarthritis. Expert Opin Drug Metab Toxicol 2019;15(12):1021–32.

126. Maudens P, Jordan O, Allémann E. Recent advances in intra-articular drug de-livery systems for osteoarthritis therapy. Drug Discov Today 2018;23(10): 1761–75.

127. Lima AC, Ferreira H, Reis RL, et al. Biodegradable polymers: an update on drug delivery in bone and cartilage diseases. Expert Opin Drug Deliv 2019;16(8): 795–813.

128. Gambaro FM, Ummarino A. Torres Andón F, Ronzoni F, Di Matteo B, Kon E. Drug delivery systems for the treatment of knee osteoarthritis: a systematic review of in vivo studies. Int J Mol Sci 2021;22(17).

129. Bannuru RR, McAlindon TE, Sullivan MC, et al. Effectiveness and implications of alternative placebo treatments: a systematic review and network meta-analysis of osteoarthritis trials. Ann Intern Med 2015;163(5):365–72.

130. Simsek I, Phalen T, Bedenbaugh A, et al. Adjusting for the intra-articular placebo effect in knee osteoarthritis therapies [Abstract]. 2018;77(Suppl 2):1135–1136.

131. Previtali D, Merli G. Di Laura Frattura G, Candrian C, Zaffagnini S, Filardo G. The long-lasting effects of "placebo injections" in knee osteoarthritis: a meta-anal-ysis. Cartilage 2020. 1947603520906597.

132. Enck P, Bingel U, Schedlowski M, et al. The placebo response in medicine: mini-mize, maximize or personalize? Nat Rev Drug Discov 2013;12(3):191–204.

133. Altman RD, Devji T, Bhandari M, et al. Clinical benefit of intra-articular saline as a comparator in clinical trials of knee osteoarthritis treatments: a systematic review and meta-analysis of randomized trials. Semin Arthritis Rheum 2016;46(2): 151–9.

134. Fleming TR. Design and interpretation of equivalence trials. Am Heart J 2000; 139(4):S171–6.

135. Greene CJ, Morland LA, Durkalski VL, et al. Noninferiority and equivalence designs: issues and implications for mental health research. J Trauma Stress 2008; 21(5):433–9.

136. Hunter DJ, Nevitt M, Losina E, et al. Biomarkers for osteoarthritis: current position and steps towards further validation. Best Pract Res Clin Rheumatol 2014; 28(1):61–71.

137. Kraus VB, Blanco FJ, Englund M, et al. Call for standardized definitions of osteoarthritis and risk stratification for clinical trials and clinical use. Osteoarthritis and cartilage. 2015;23(8):1233–41.

138. Hannan MT, Felson DT, Pincus T. Analysis of the discordance between radiographic changes and knee pain in osteoarthritis of the knee. J Rheumatol 2000;27(6):1513–7.

139. OARSI TP-cCfOPo. OARSI white paper- OA as a serious disease. 2016.

140. Roemer FW, Collins J, Kwoh CK, et al. MRI-based screening for structural definition of eligibility in clinical DMOAD trials: rapid OsteoArthritis MRI Eligibility Score (ROAMES). Osteoarthritis and Cartilage. 2020;28(1):71–81.

141. Roemer FW, Kwoh CK, Hayashi D, et al. The role of radiography and MRI for eligibility assessment in DMOAD trials of knee OA. Nat Rev Rheumatol 2018; 14(6):372–80.

Realizing Health and Well-being Outcomes for People with Osteoarthritis Beyond Health Service Delivery

Jocelyn L. Bowden, BLA, BHMSc, BSc(Hons), PhD[a,b],
Leigh F. Callahan, PhD[c], Jillian P. Eyles, BAppSc(Physiotherapy), PhD[a,b],
Jennifer L. Kent, BSc (Environmental Science), MEnvPl, PhD[d],
Andrew M. Briggs, BSc(Physiotherapy)Hons, PhD[e,*]

KEYWORDS

- Osteoarthritis • Chronic disease • Social determinants • Healthy built environment
- Healthy aging

KEY POINTS

- Social determinants of health cover a wide spectrum of contextual factors beyond direct health service delivery, including lifestyle, personal circumstances, psychosocial issues, and the built environment. These "extra-healthcare" factors influence health and well-being outcomes.
- Social determinants of health should be considered and incorporated into care planning and delivery to better support people with OA throughout their life-course.
- Understanding how social determinants of health impact health care is essential for all health care professionals delivering care to people with osteoarthritis.

INTRODUCTION AND BACKGROUND

Osteoarthritis (OA) is the leading cause of disability in people over 45 years and a recognized threat to healthy aging.[1] OA is associated with negative outcomes for well-being, health care utilization, and rising personal and societal costs.[2] OA can

[a] Institute of Bone and Joint Research, Kolling Institute, University of Sydney, Level 10, Kolling Building, Reserve Road, St Leonards, NSW, 2065, Australia; [b] Department of Rheumatology, Royal North Shore Hospital, St Leonards, New South Wales, Australia; [c] Division of Rheumatology, Allergy and Immunology, Thurston Arthritis Research Center, University of North Carolina, 3330 Thurston Building, CB 7280, Chapel Hill, NC 27599, USA; [d] School of Architecture, Design and Planning, The University of Sydney, Wilkinson Building, 148 City Road, Darlington, 2006, New South Wales, Australia; [e] Curtin School of Allied Health, Curtin University, GPO Box U1987, Perth, Western Australia 6845, Australia
* Corresponding author.
E-mail address: a.briggs@curtin.edu.au

Clin Geriatr Med 38 (2022) 433–448
https://doi.org/10.1016/j.cger.2021.11.011
0749-0690/22/© 2021 Elsevier Inc. All rights reserved.

geriatric.theclinics.com

have negative impacts on mobility, dexterity, physical function, social participation, mood, sleep, and quality of life.[3,4] Many people experience OA in multiple joints,[5] and live with multimorbidities, commonly hypertension, cardiovascular disease, diabetes, low back pain, and psychological distress.[6] People with OA report lower physical activity levels[7] and often struggle with their body weight.[8] They may report difficulty in undertaking their usual daily activities, including leaving the house for recreation or accessing care,[9] making social isolation and loneliness common.[10] According to international clinical practice guidelines, first-line treatments for OA include increasing physical activity, structured exercise and weight management, coupled with education, support for self-management, and appropriate use of medications[11] (**Table 1**). Yet, many people with OA do not receive first-line care,[12] and racial and socioeconomic disparities around OA care exist.[13]

Reducing the prevalence of OA and improving the well-being of people with the condition requires effective action beyond the traditional health service delivery paradigm.[14] Integration of health services with the different contexts and settings in which people work, live, play, and socialize,[15] also known as the social determinants of health (SDH), has long been accepted as essential to ensuring good health outcomes.[15] SDH are especially important for people with chronic, noncommunicable conditions such as OA, diabetes, heart disease, where multiple interacting factors influence the development, management, and progression across the life course.[16] Addressing the negative influences of SDH are essential to ensuring equity and equality in health service delivery[17] (**Box 1**). However, SDH concepts are poorly integrated into current OA health care,[16] where the focus remains on enabling access to disease therapies, often delivered with a biomedical paradigm in siloed health service delivery models. This article explores how SDH influence outcomes in people with OA, how factors may intersect at different levels of care (eg, individual, clinical practice, service delivery, and health systems levels), and potential opportunities to incorporate SDH into OA care (eg, **Fig. 1**). We will specifically consider the use of SDH to:

- identify people at high risk of developing OA to ensure they receive appropriate care,
- identify people at risk of having poor health and well-being outcomes related to OA to ensure they receive additional support, and

Table 1
Overview of key OA considerations for assessment, diagnosis, and management

Assessment and Diagnosis Considerations	Treatment and Management Strategies
Holistic assessment of: • Pain, functional limitations • Sleep and fatigue • Impact of multimorbidities • Social factors and supports (eg, family, culture, community) • Health beliefs (eg, negative beliefs, poor understanding of lifestyle interventions) • Psychological factors (eg, depression/ anxiety, fear of movement) • Support systems (eg, social, health) • Living location • Financial status	• Education and effective self-management of osteoarthritis[a] • Weight management and weight loss[a] • Exercise and physical activity[a] • Regular review of medications[a] • Mood and sleep management • Use of topical medications, heat/cold • Assistive devices and walking aids • Prudent use of pain-relieving medications

[a] Recommended first-line treatments.

> **Box 1**
> **Health equity versus health equality**[17]
>
> Health inequities and health equalities are shown to have significant impacts on health, and are linked to social determinants such as gender, race/ethnicity, education, income, occupation, and geography (rural, urban). These concepts have been defined as follows:
> *Health inequality*: Any measurable differences in health aspects across individuals or according to socially relevant groupings, without any moral judgment on whether the observed differences are fair or just.
> *Health inequity*: A specific type of health inequality that implies the differences in health is unjust or unfair.

- develop strategies to optimize the quality of life for people with OA, including participation in work and community.

DISCUSSION

What are SDH?

There is growing evidence that health outcomes (eg, mortality/life expectancy, quality of life, health status, functional limitations) are explained more by the context of people's lives, and less by the quality and availability of medical care.[18] Across all health conditions, the World Health Organization (WHO) estimates that SDH account 30% to 55% of health outcomes,[19] primarily from nonhealth sectors, such as work, transportation, education, and the built environment. In demographically adjusted models using data from the United States in 2015, health variance in health outcomes was explained by socioeconomic factors (45%), health behaviors (34%), clinical care (16%), and the physical environment (3%).[20] SDH can be considered as contexts,[21] or in terms of the settings and places that people use in daily life,[22] such as home, educational, environmental, geographic, organizational, or virtual settings (**Table 2**).

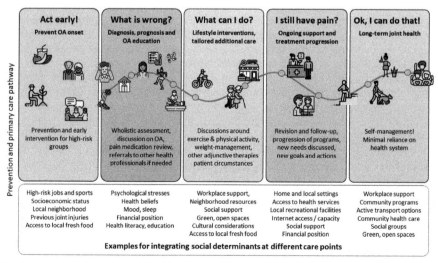

Fig. 1. Examples of SDH considerations in a primary care OA pathway. A broad range of interventions and treatments are recommended in a typical primary care OA pathway. There are many overlapping stages of care where SDH should be considered and integrated into care to ensure optional health outcomes are achieved.

Table 2
Examples of social determinants of health, context, and settings

Social Determinant[14]	Contextual Considerations Relevant to the Social Determinant[14]	Examples of Settings and Places[15]
Structural (individual) and socioeconomic position	Income, education, occupation, social class, gender, race/ethnicity, health literacy	Workplaces, home, health care, educational
Material circumstances	Living and working environment, food availability	Workplaces, neighborhoods,
Behavioral and biological contexts	Lifestyle factors (eg, diet, exercise)	Green spaces, sports facilities, neighborhoods, online
Socioenvironmental and psychosocial factors	Psychosocial stressors, lack of social support, stressful living conditions, coping styles	Home, workplaces, online/virtual settings
Social cohesion	Social relationships, social support	Faith and religious settings, community facilities, sports organizations
Socioeconomic and political contexts	Public, social, and economic policies; governance; cultural and societal values; epidemiologic conditions	Healthy cities, health services, community-based organizations

Relevance of SDH in OA Care

The biomedical considerations for OA care are well documented in international clinical guidelines and the individual psychosocial considerations (eg, social networks, mood) are becoming more widely recognized as necessary components of assessment and care (eg, see the American College of Rheumatology OA Clinical Guidelines[23]). Yet, within this biopsychosocial model, broader contexts relevant to SDHs are rarely addressed in guidelines and models of care. This may be partly due to a lack of high-quality OA clinical trials reporting SDH,[16,24] a poor societal understanding of the interdependency between SDH and health outcomes,[25] that health care and social care systems are often independent and nonintegrated across jurisdictions, and that measuring short-term outcomes associated with interventions in SDH is difficult.[26,27]

The relevance of SDH to OA care and health outcomes is reflected in evidence and global health reform for healthy aging. For example:

- A recent systemic review[25] examined the perceived needs of people with arthritis outside of health care, and identified 6 areas where SDH impacted life, particularly with regards to function. These included (i) needing assistance with activities of daily living, and lack of independence; (ii) social connectedness and social participation; (iii) financial security and costs of health-seeking; (iv) occupational needs and flexibility, including the desire/need to continue work for financial/social reasons; (v) exercise and leisure, including pain limitations; and (vi) transportation, including the inability to drive and/or take public transport because of restricted mobility.[25]

- The WHO defines healthy aging as the *"process of developing and maintaining the functional ability that enables wellbeing in older age"*.[28] Functional ability in older age is dependent on 2 factors: a person's intrinsic capacity (ie, composite physical and mental capacities) and their environment (ie, built environment, social support, services across their home, community and broader society). Health care is typically focused on arresting declines in intrinsic capacity (eg, musculoskeletal function) with less attention directed at environmental factors. The WHO model emphasizes the critical importance of acting on environmental factors to maintain functional ability by compensating for age-related losses in intrinsic capacity.[28] In this context promoting environments that optimize intrinsic capacity and remove barriers to participation become increasingly important, thereby highlighting the relevance of acting on SDH to support healthy aging.

SDH Considerations for OA Clinical Care

The following section will discuss potential SDH contexts and settings that should be considered in the OA clinical pathway (see **Fig. 1**), why they are important from the perspective of someone with OA, and how they could be used in clinical practice.

Individual demographic and socioeconomic factors

Age, sex, body mass index (BMI), and joint injury are important individual-level risk factors for both the development and progression of OA.[29] The prevalence of OA is higher in older populations, particularly women, and is consequently increasing as populations age. In 2019, the age-standardized OA prevalence was 6348 per 100,000 population.[30] Years lived with disability from OA were 18.9 million,[30] with an age-standardized increase of 9.6% since 1990.[31] OA affects all age groups with many individuals in prime working age[32]; incidence peaks at 55 to 64 years.[30,31] Consequently, OA can have a significant effect on work-life and socioeconomic prosperity, including reduced work productivity, increased risk of being jobless or taking early retirement,[33,34] and utilizing life-long rehabilitation services.[35]

A high BMI is a risk factor for OA development[36] and correlates with higher pain levels.[37] Obesity is a major contributor to increasing incidence of, and disability associated with OA. Maintaining a healthy weight can significantly reduce OA-related pain in the lower limb, and weight loss is recommended for people with a BMI ≥ 25 kg/m^2. There are significant overlaps between maintaining a healthy BMI and a range of SDH considerations, both in terms of diagnosis and management of the condition.

The social gradient in health, where people in lower socioeconomic positions experience worse health,[38] is also relevant to OA.[16,39] People with lower education, health literacy, unemployed, no life-partner, low income, and poor mental health are at higher risk for developing OA and multimorbidity[4,40] (**Box 2**). Socioeconomic position has been linked to inequity of health delivery and care disparities.[13] Poor access to rehabilitation, fewer referrals, lower health care utilization, and perceived bias in care (including lower rates of first-line care) have been reported for many communities with a lower socioeconomic status, including low-income and middle-income countries (LMIC).[41,42] For example, Odonkor and colleagues[41] reported black individuals in the United States were less likely to receive evidence-based care than other ethnic groups. Cultural backgrounds have also been reported to impact the uptake of OA care. Qualitative data from people with OA of Asian descent[43] highlighted the importance of family and peer assistance, culturally specific activities (eg, floor culture, such as where activities are undertaken while sitting or kneeling on the floor), a distrust in Western medicine, and the impact of positive coping mechanisms. Taking conscious

---

Box 2
Prevalence of OA in indigenous populations of high-income countries

Many high-income countries, such as Australia, New Zealand, the United States, and Canada, have vulnerable indigenous populations reporting high prevalence and impact OA, and many of whom live in remote and/or areas with poor health services. Several studies of remote indigenous communities in Australia estimated the prevalence of multijoint osteoarthritis as between 7% and 32%, and at the knee alone in 5% and 18%.[44] A recent systematic review identified the rate ratio of prevalence between Aboriginal and non-Aboriginal people in Australia of 1.2 to 1.5 for OA. Despite the higher rate, Aboriginal people accessed primary care for knee or hip OA at approximately half the rate of non-Aboriginal people, and were less than half as likely to have knee or hip arthroplasty.[45] Similarly, OA was reported in up to 17% of American Indian/Alaska Native women, 22% of Canadian First Nations people, and 6% of New Zealand Maori populations.[44]

---

action to identify and address these issues early in a care pathway is important to improving care for people at high risk of poor OA outcomes.

Psychosocial, socioenvironmental, and social cohesion considerations

Psychosocial, socioenvironmental, and social cohesion are major considerations for both planning and delivery of OA care. In addition to the functional impact of OA, the psychosocial and emotional impact can be high.[4,9,25] Family, social, and community participation are often negatively impacted, resulting in life adjustments, increased dependence on others, and lowered quality of life.[4,25,40,46] A recent systematic review found psychosocial impacts were a key factor in the lived experiences of people with knee OA. The authors concluded these should be a central consideration when planning and implementing care.[9] Furthermore, poor societal understanding about the impact of OA symptoms, particularly pain, can exacerbate the psychosocial and emotional sequelae.[47] People with OA report experiencing condition-related discrimination, stigmatism, and embarrassment, making them reluctant to participate in some aspects of recommended care (eg, public exercise).[25,48] Poor understanding of OA can also present as ageism, potentially leading to care inequities.[49] Joint pain is commonly ignored or passed off as "normal aging", or care options (eg, exercise) are either not adapted for older age groups or withheld.[50]

Friends, family, and caregivers have also been cited as important for social support, helping people with OA maintain their independence, and providing motivation to continue with meaningful activities[26,51] (**Box 3**). However, they are also commonly identified as sources of false or misleading OA information, and approaches to counter this influence may be needed.[48,52] For example, having family or friends who received opioids was associated with increased risk of opioid use and beliefs that opioids were low-risk.[52] Educating people with OA, their family, friends, and caregivers in first-line OA management has the potential to optimize social interaction and improve quality of life for all involved.[47,53]

Cultural and religious considerations can influence health care in many communities, with increasing calls for services and models of care that can be adapted to different cultural contexts.[43,46] Peer assistance programs, inclusion of cultural or religion-specific activities (eg, floor culture, prayer), or greater inclusion of traditional diets, medicines, and local healers are examples. Assistance with accessing and navigating health care (including health literacy programs), affordability of medications, and greater support for lifestyle interventions have also been suggested.[42,43,54] Codesign and codelivery of OA programs and services with the local community, and adopted at national, organizational, and professional levels are essential.[55]

Box 3
Addressing social isolation and loneliness

Limited social participation, social isolation, and loneliness can be a significant social consequence of having OA, and are linked to worse physical and mental health.[10] The European Project on OSteoArthritis (EPOSA) study[10] found having clinical OA at more than one site, increased the risk of social isolation even after adjusting for depression, cognitive impairment, and walking time. Changing social and familial structures also impact on the functional ability of older people. Isolation and lack of familial and community support may be particularly acute in rural and remote areas where migration of younger people to urban areas for work and other opportunities is increasingly common. Across some European nations, more than 40% of women aged more than 65 years live alone,[56] while dramatic social changes have been observed in the Asia-Pacific region.[57] These changing structures can further contribute to isolation, increase the risk of poverty, and reduce functional ability. Improved identification and use of local social networks and existing relationships is one way to support people at risk of social isolation.[58]

Occupational and work considerations

Occupation and work factors span many SDH domains (see **Table 2**), and should be explored when people present with joint pain. First, there is growing evidence on the role of occupational exposures on the development and progression of OA.[59–62] A recent umbrella review found high occupational physical activity was associated with developing OA, and in men, increased all-cause mortality, depression, anxiety, and poor-quality sleep.[60] Occupations that involve heavy physical workloads, such as heavy lifting, squatting, knee bending, and climbing, increased the risk of developing lower limb OA. High-risk occupations include agricultural and construction workers, tradespeople (eg, carpet layers),[59] and those with traumatic joint injuries at work or through other activities (eg, tendon ruptures, traffic accidents, high-impact sports).[29] Military personnel and firefighters are particularly high-risk groups[63] with knee OA a top cause of medical discharge. Traumatic or high-impact injuries are of particular concern in younger people who have a high probability of developing OA at a young age.[32,64] Identification of people with these high-risk exposures should be a priority to ensure appropriate prevention and early OA management strategies can be implemented.[62]

Workplace accommodations, supported by legislation or other policy processes, are important to enabling productivity at work and return to work after injury.[65] Lack of support and work flexibility from employers and work colleagues have been highlighted as concerns by people with OA in high-income countries.[66] Failure to provide this support may lead to changes in employment,[25] and is cited as a major contributor to being unemployed, or taking early retirement.[34,64] This is particularly problematic for younger people who want to work for financial and/or social reasons,[25] and who may experience pain and functional challenges at key stages of their careers.[67] Potential accommodations at the individual and employer level may include taking regular breaks, negotiating flexible working arrangements, environmental and task modification, supply and use of occupational aides, and enabling access to health services (eg, dietetics, physiotherapy).[68] Workplace support for OA may be more challenging in LMICs without social security or health "safety nets."[39] However, little is known in this area, and more research is needed to understand causality and prognostic pathways for all joints[62] and how workplaces can best support people with OA.

Built Environments and Neighborhoods

There are strong interconnections between the built environment, SDH and OA (**Fig. 2**[69]). The term "built environment" refers to all the elements of spaces that are

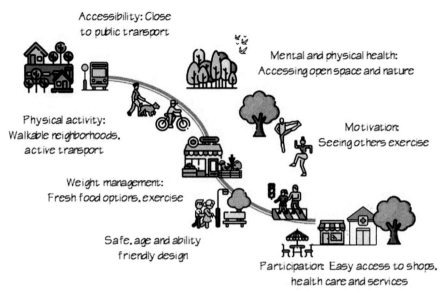

Fig. 2. Supportive neighborhoods for people with OA. There are many elements and in local neighborhoods that can support the mental and physical health of people with OA. *(From Bowden JL, Hunter DJ, Feng Y. Using neighbourhood environments to support osteoarthritis management - a scoping review. Osteoarthritis Cartilage. 2021;29:S377; with permission)*

modified by human intervention, including houses, streets, commercial spaces, green open spaces, and other uses that make a place urban rather than natural (**Box 4**). It comprises all the spaces where people live, work, and socialize and the way people travel between these spaces.[70]

Box 4
Utilizing the built environment at different scales

The way built environments shape health, including the prevention and treatment of OA, needs to be conceptualized at different scales. At the scale of the city, healthy built environments require connectivity through active and public transport infrastructure, dense networks of green and public spaces, and a diversity of housing choices. Healthy cities aspire to the strategic location of services and employment in centers close to where people live, so that the things people need to be healthy can be accessed easily and safely. They typically discourage over-reliance on the private car. At the scale of the neighborhood, healthy built environments contain intuitive street networks that are safe, and public and open spaces that are responsive to context and well maintained. Healthy neighborhoods provide infrastructure for community interaction and physical activity, such as playgrounds, public squares, community facilities, and parks. They offer a diversity of densities and uses, catering to the needs of different populations. At the scale of the building, healthy built environments are designed to provide protection from harms, including noise and air pollution, and extremes of heat and cold. They are well constructed to ensure longevity and resilience. Healthy buildings are open to the streets on which they sit. They encourage social interactions, but also provide spaces of privacy and retreat. At all scales, healthy built environments are planned and managed to be inclusive and responsive to diverse spatial, temporal, and cultural contexts. Planning for healthy built environments aspires to equity and balance in built, social, and economic outcomes.[71]

Healthy built environments can enhance OA care by providing opportunities for physical activity through active transport and recreational walking (see **Fig. 2**). For example, built environments with higher population densities and access to a variety of commercial destinations, where streets are grid-like and easy to navigate, sidewalk and cycleway provision is prolific and of high quality, and public transit is available, encourage transport by alternative modes, including those using physical activity such as walking and cycling. Access to prolific and well-designed green open spaces can encourage recreational physical activity, including recreational walking. By getting people out and about in the neighborhood, well-designed neighborhood environments that are safe and inviting can also facilitate social interactions, which are important in fostering resilience to mental health conditions, as well as preventing loneliness.[72] By providing greater accessibility to shops and services, healthy built environments can also facilitate regular access to fresh and healthy food by ensuring all the ingredients for a fresh meal can be purchased at a reasonable price within walking distance. Environments that reserve space for community gardens and other forms of urban agriculture can provide opportunities for communities to engage in the process of growing fresh produce for the enjoyment of communities.

The critical link between built environments and health has been recognized globally and reflected in the Sustainable Development Goals. Many countries now integrate health within the urban planning reform through legislative and policy mechanisms,[73] which can help combat barriers to better use of the built environment (**Box 5**). Argentina, for example, has developed a guidance framework for local municipalities to implement components of the National Health Plan.[74] The actions target healthy eating, physical activity, and combatting tobacco use by outlining suggested actions

---

Box 5
Barriers to the use of the built environments in OA care

Although the evidence linking the way built environments are structured and managed to the SDH is clear and prolific, there are several barriers to the use of built environments for the prevention and treatment of OA, specifically:

1. although built environments relate to an array of chronic noncommunicable and communicable health conditions, the research and practice agenda has generally directed focus on several specific diseases, in particular cardiovascular diseases (eg, Ref. [81]).
2. built environments that characterize urban spaces and cities around the world are, notoriously if unintentionally, only designed for people who do not experience impairments in physical function. Built environments are often blind to the needs of the diversity of ages, stages, and abilities that is the community in reality.[82] People with specific health conditions, older people, or those with limited mobility experience unique barriers to the everyday use of neighborhood-built environments for physical activity and social interaction.[83] For example, areas with poor walkability, where curb cuts (ramps) and connectivity are sporadic, as well as inaccessible public transport services, significantly limit social participation for people with OA.[9,72] This is not just limited to people with lower limb OA, but also hand OA, where the use of public transport and active transport requiring hand dexterity is limited by an inability to hold straps or poles, open doors, or use the brakes on a conventional bicycle.[25] These details are rarely considered in even the most comprehensive efforts to promote the provision of healthy built environments, creating major barriers to participation in the day-to-day activities that support good OA health and management.
3. mobilizing change in built environments requires a deep and broad engagement with institutions not generally considered within the remit of health. Achieving the scale of change required demands not only reform at the level of service delivery, but also policy reform at the system level across health, industry, transportation, education, and urban planning portfolios.[84] Often such change is dependent on political will, which can be notoriously unpredictable.

for improving health in schools, universities, and workplaces, including the option of certification as a health-promoting institution. Within a municipality, there is guidance on enabling safe and active transport, healthy squares and parks, and creating smoke-free environments.

There is, therefore, untapped potential to address built environments in OA prevention and care plans, and this is increasingly recognized by professions working in this space. A recent study of international key informants in health systems strengthening for musculoskeletal conditions stressed the importance of attention to the built environment, among other SDH, to realize health and well-being outcomes.[14] One avenue to better incorporate OA considerations in built environment planning would be to leverage existing ground forged by other conditions such as diabetes[75] and cardiovascular disease,[76] particularly in justifying interventions that promote physical activity.[77] Aging in place interventions, the walkable cities movement, and age-friendly cities are also examples of strategies with existing programs and support that could focus attention on built environments supportive of OA treatment.[78,79] Although acknowledging OA is relevant from younger adulthood and disability peaks at 55 to 69 years, the WHO Healthy Ageing model provides helpful guidance to health and social care systems on supporting functional ability. Specifically, integration between health care (ie, across multiple domains of intrinsic capacity) and social care (ie, long-term care services) are advocated.[80] Although integrated health care and long-term care are oriented toward healthy aging, the principles apply to optimizing outcomes in older people with OA.

Broader socioeconomic and political considerations of OA care

SDH have been recognized internationally as requiring priority attention, both as general public health initiatives[15] and more specifically in the context of OA[85,86] (eg, **Box 6**). Whole-of-government and whole-of-society approaches are required to ensure cross-sector actions are coordinated to facilitate the necessary sociocultural shifts.[85] The recently released OA Agenda 2020,[86] coauthored by a range of US OA stakeholders, endorsed the SDH section of the Healthy People 2020[87] as important to creating social and physical environments that promote good health across multiple sectors, including housing, education, parks, recreation, fitness, and transportation.

Although effective partnerships among public health, community-based organizations, social services, and medical care could improve population health outcomes, it has been challenging to develop sustainable payment models to support such

---

Box 6
Integration of social and medical care delivery

While recognizing that public health initiatives to improve social conditions occur outside of health care settings, health professional organizations have recommended better integration of social and medical care delivery systems as part of a comprehensive strategy to identify and address the social determinants of health.[91,92] Recommendations are being made for an expanded social history at the point-of-care,[93] yet most health care systems lack the infrastructure required. Systems need to develop comprehensive, systematic screening protocols that take into consideration patients' extra-personal, socioeconomic, or educational circumstances or responsibilities that may compromise their care, such as sole income provider, or childcare.[25,39,47,48] The training of health care professionals to address the SDH within their scope of practice is key for ensuring more equitable health outcomes for people with OA, their families, and communities.[92] In addition, referral protocols and relationships need to be developed between the health care systems and the various community service providers to address the health-related social needs of patients.

partnerships.[88,89] Several innovation projects in the United States have provided some valuable insights regarding addressing SDH.[89] These include: (i) the importance of establishing cross-sector partnerships; (ii) building data systems that bridge health and community services, and (iii) developing a workforce to deliver interventions to vulnerable populations.[89] In the United States, the Centers for Medicare and Medicaid Services has a program designed to accelerate the development of a scalable delivery model called the Accountable Health Communities (AHC) to assess whether systematically identifying and addressing health-related social needs can improve health and reduce costs and utilization among community-dwelling Medicare and Medicaid beneficiaries.[89,90] Evaluation of the AHC may provide valuable insights for ways to develop models around the world.

SUMMARY

Integration of the different contexts and settings in which people live, work, and socialize has the potential to improve the health and well-being of people with OA. Yet, many of these SDH are poorly integrated into current OA care. Exploring and integrating factors such as work, education, psychosocial issues, and the built environment when discussing OA care with patients has the potential to enrich the management of OA across the life course. Having these factors accepted and implemented at all levels of health care delivery is essential to ensuring everyone can live well with OA.

CLINICS CARE POINTS

- Greater consideration and integration of social determinants of health are needed to ensure people with OA can continue to work and live well with their communities.
- Successful integration of social determinants of health requires a comprehensive assessment of an individual's circumstances, including socioeconomic and psychosocial factors, and the settings in which they live, work, play, and socialize.
- Building linkages to local health care, community, and cultural services is an effective way to support people with their care, within their local neighborhoods.

DISCLOSURE

This research did not receive any specific grant from any funding agency. Dr Kent is funded by the Australian Research Council Discovery Early Career Researcher Award (DE190100211).

REFERENCES

1. Hunter DJ, Bierma-Zeinstra S. Osteoarthritis. Lancet 2019;393(10182):1745–59.
2. Callander EJ, Schofield DJ. Arthritis and the risk of falling into poverty: a survival analysis using Australian data. Arthritis Rheumatol 2016;68(1):255–62.
3. Hawker GA, Stewart L, French MR, et al. Understanding the pain experience in hip and knee osteoarthritis - an OARSI/OMERACT initiative. Osteoarthritis Cartilage 2008;16(4):415–22.
4. Vitaloni M, Botto-van Bemden A, Sciortino Contreras RM, et al. Global management of patients with knee osteoarthritis begins with quality of life assessment: a systematic review. BMC Musculoskelet Disord 2019;20(1):493.
5. Nelson AE, Smith MW, Golightly YM, et al. Generalized osteoarthritis: a systematic review. Semin Arthritis Rheum 2014;43(6):713–20.

6. Muckelt PE, Roos EM, Stokes M, et al. Comorbidities and their link with individual health status: a cross-sectional analysis of 23,892 people with knee and hip osteoarthritis from primary care. J Comorb 2020;10:1–11.

7. Wallis JA, Webster KE, Levinger P, et al. What proportion of people with hip and knee osteoarthritis meet physical activity guidelines? A systematic review and meta-analysis. Osteoarthritis Cartilage 2013;21(11):1648–59.

8. Herbolsheimer F, Schaap LA, Edwards MH, et al. Physical activity patterns among older adults with and without knee osteoarthritis in six European countries. Arthritis Care Res (Hoboken) 2016;68(2):228–36.

9. Wallis JA, Taylor NF, Bunzli S, et al. Experience of living with knee osteoarthritis: a systematic review of qualitative studies. BMJ Open 2019;9(9):e030060.

10. Siviero P, Veronese N, Smith T, et al. Association between osteoarthritis and social isolation: data from the EPOSA study. J Am Geriatr Soc 2020;68(1):87–95.

11. Bowden JL, Hunter DJ, Deveza LA, et al. Core and adjunctive interventions for osteoarthritis: efficacy and models for implementation. Nat Rev Rheumatol 2020;16(8):434–47.

12. Hagen KB, Smedslund G, Osteras N, et al. Quality of community-based osteoarthritis care: a systematic review and meta-analysis. Arthritis Care Res (Hoboken) 2016;68(10):1443–52.

13. Reyes AM, Katz JN. Racial/ethnic and socioeconomic disparities in osteoarthritis management. Rheum Dis Clin North Am 2021;47(1):21–40.

14. Briggs AM, Jordan JE, Kopansky-Giles D, et al. The need for adaptable global guidance in health systems strengthening for musculoskeletal health: a qualitative study of international key informants. Glob Health Res Policy 2021;6(1):24.

15. World Health Organization. Equity, social determinants and public health programmes. Geneva (Switzerland): WHO; 2010.

16. Luong ML, Cleveland RJ, Nyrop KA, et al. Social determinants and osteoarthritis outcomes. Aging health 2012;8(4):413–37.

17. Whitehead M. The concepts and principles of equity and health. Int J Health Serv 1992;22(3):429–45.

18. Daniel H, Bornstein SS, Kane GC, et al. Addressing social determinants to improve patient care and promote health equity: an American College of Physicians position paper. Ann Intern Med 2018;168(8):577–8.

19. World Health Organization. About social determinants of health. Health Topics Web site. 2020. Available at: https://www.who.int/health-topics/social-determinants-of-health. Accessed August 1, 2021.

20. Hood CM, Gennuso KP, Swain GR, et al. County health rankings: relationships between determinant factors and health outcomes. Am J Prev Med 2016;50(2): 129–35.

21. Solar O, Irwin A. A conceptual framework for action on the social determinants of health. Social determinants of health discussion paper 2. Geneva (Switzerland): WHO; 2018. p. 1–75.

22. Newman L, Baum F, Javanparast S, et al. Addressing social determinants of health inequities through settings: a rapid review. Health Promot Int 2015; 30(Suppl 2):ii126–43.

23. Kolasinski SL, Neogi T, Hochberg MC, et al. 2019 American College of Rheumatology/Arthritis Foundation guideline for the management of osteoarthritis of the hand, hip, and knee. Arthritis Rheumatol 2020;72(2):220–33.

24. Smith TO, Kamper SJ, Williams CM, et al. Reporting of social deprivation in musculoskeletal trials: an analysis of 402 randomised controlled trials. Musculoskeletal Care 2021;19(2):180–5.

25. Fairley JL, Seneviwickrama M, Yeh S, et al. Person-centred care in osteoarthritis and inflammatory arthritis: a scoping review of people's needs outside of health-care. BMC Musculoskelet Disord 2021;22(1):341.
26. Ali SA, Lee K, MacDermid JC. Applying the International Classification of Func-tioning, Disability and Health to understand osteoarthritis management in urban and rural community-dwelling seniors. Osteoarthritis and Cartilage Open 2021; 3(1):100132.
27. Lee J, Schram A, Riley E, et al. Addressing health equity through action on the social determinants of health: a global review of policy outcome evaluation methods. Int J Health Policy Manag 2018;7(7):581–92.
28. World Health Organization. World report on ageing and health. Geneva (Switzerland): WHO; 2015.
29. O'Neill TW, McCabe PS, McBeth J. Update on the epidemiology, risk factors and disease outcomes of osteoarthritis. Best Pract Res Clin Rheumatol 2018;32(2): 312–26.
30. Institute for Health Metrics and Evaluation (IHME). GBD 2019 cause and risk sum-mary: osteoarthritis level 3 causes. Seattle (USA): IMHE, University of Washing-ton; 2020.
31. Safiri S, Kolahi AA, Smith E, et al. Global, regional and national burden of osteo-arthritis 1990-2017: a systematic analysis of the Global Burden of Disease Study 2017. Ann Rheum Dis 2020;79(6):819–28.
32. Driban JB, Harkey MS, Liu S-H, et al. Osteoarthritis and aging: young adults with osteoarthritis. Curr Epidemiol Rep 2020;7(1):9–15.
33. Schofield DJ, Callander EJ, Shrestha RN, et al. Labour force participation and the influence of having arthritis on financial status. Rheumatol Int 2015;35(7): 1175–81.
34. Schofield D, Cunich M, Shrestha RN, et al. The long-term economic impacts of arthritis through lost productive life years: results from an Australian microsimula-tion model. BMC Public Health 2018;18(1):654.
35. Cieza A, Causey K, Kamenov K, et al. Global estimates of the need for rehabili-tation based on the global burden of disease study 2019: a systematic analysis for the global burden of disease study 2019. Lancet 2020;396(10267):2006–17.
36. Reyes C, Leyland KM, Peat G, et al. Association between overweight and obesity and risk of clinically diagnosed knee, hip, and hand osteoarthritis: a population-based cohort study. Arthritis Rheumatol 2016;68(8):1869–75.
37. Christensen R, Bartels EM, Astrup A, et al. Effect of weight reduction in obese pa-tients diagnosed with knee osteoarthritis: a systematic review and meta-analysis. Ann Rheum Dis 2007;66(4):433–9.
38. Marmot M. The health gap: the challenge of an unequal world. Lancet 2015; 386(10011):2442–4.
39. Brennan-Olsen SL, Cook S, Leech MT, et al. Prevalence of arthritis according to age, sex and socioeconomic status in six low and middle income countries: anal-ysis of data from the World Health Organization study on global AGEing and adult health (SAGE). BMC Musculoskelet Disord 2017;18(1):271.
40. Vennu V, Abdulrahman TA, Alenazi AM, et al. Associations between social deter-minants and the presence of chronic diseases: data from the osteoarthritis Initia-tive. BMC Public Health 2020;20(1):1323.
41. Odonkor CA, Esparza R, Flores LE, et al. Disparities in health care for black pa-tients in physical medicine and rehabilitation in the United States: a narrative re-view. PM R 2021;13(2):180–203.

42. Coetzee M, Giljam-Enright M, Morris LD. Rehabilitation needs in individuals with knee OA in rural Western Cape, South Africa: an exploratory qualitative study. Prim Health Care Res Dev 2020;21:e7.

43. Sathiyamoorthy T, Ali SA, Kloseck M. Cultural factors influencing osteoarthritis care in Asian communities: a review of the evidence. J Community Health 2018;43(4):816–26.

44. McDougall C, Hurd K, Barnabe C. Systematic review of rheumatic disease epidemiology in the indigenous populations of Canada, the United States, Australia, and New Zealand. Semin Arthritis Rheum 2017;46(5):675–86.

45. Lin IB, Bunzli S, Mak DB, et al. Unmet needs of Aboriginal Australians with musculoskeletal pain: a mixed-method systematic review. Arthritis Care Res 2018;70(9):1335–47.

46. Al-Khlaifat L, Okasheh R, Muhaidat J, et al. Knowledge of knee osteoarthritis and Its impact on health in the Middle East: are they different to countries in the developed world? a qualitative study. Rehabil Res Pract 2020;2020:9829825.

47. Briggs AM, Houlding E, Hinman RS, et al. Health professionals and students encounter multi-level barriers to implementing high-value osteoarthritis care: a multi-national study. Osteoarthritis Cartilage 2019;27(5):788–804.

48. Spitaels D, Vankrunkelsven P, Desfosses J, et al. Barriers for guideline adherence in knee osteoarthritis care: a qualitative study from the patients' perspective. J Eval Clin Pract 2017;23(1):165–72.

49. Chang ES, Kannoth S, Levy S, et al. Global reach of ageism on older persons' health: a systematic review. PLoS One 2020;15(1):e0220857.

50. Stone RC, Baker J. Painful choices: a qualitative exploration of facilitators and barriers to active lifestyles among adults with osteoarthritis. J Appl Gerontol 2017;36(9):1091–116.

51. Willett M, Greig C, Fenton S, et al. Utilising the perspectives of patients with lower-limb osteoarthritis on prescribed physical activity to develop a theoretically informed physiotherapy intervention. BMC Musculoskelet Disord 2021;22(1):155.

52. Vina ER, Quinones C, Hausmann LRM, et al. Association of patients' familiarity and perceptions of efficacy and risks with the use of opioid medications in the management of osteoarthritis. J Rheumatol 2021;48(12):1863–70.

53. Callahan LF, Ambrose KR, Albright AL, et al. Public health interventions for osteoarthritis - updates on the osteoarthritis action alliance's efforts to address the 2010 OA public health agenda recommendations. Clin Exp Rheumatol 2019; 37:31–9. Suppl 120(5).

54. Booker S, Herr K. Voices of African American older adults on the implications of social and healthcare-related policies for osteoarthritis pain care. Pain Management Nurs 2021;22(1):50–7.

55. Briggs AM, Slater H, Jordan JE, et al. Towards a global strategy to improve musculoskeletal health. Sydney (Australia): Global Alliance for Musculoskeletal Health; 2021.

56. Central Statistics Office. Ageing in Ireland. Dublin (Ireland): The Stationery Office; 2007.

57. Phillips DR, Cheng KHC. The impact of changing value systems on social inclusion: an Asia-Pacific perspective. In: Scharf T, Keating NC, editors. From exclusion to inclusion in old age: a global challenge. Bristol (UK): Policy Press; 2012. p. 109–24.

58. University of Kansas. Community Tool Box, Chapter 2. Other models for promoting community health and development, addressing social determinants of health in your community. 2021. Available at: https://ctb.ku.edu/en/table-of-

contents/overview/models-for-community-health-and-development/social-determinants-of-health. Accessed September 27, 2021.

59. Wang X, Perry TA, Arden N, et al. Occupational risk in knee osteoarthritis: a systematic review and meta-analysis of observational studies. Arthritis Care Res 2020;72(9):1213–23.

60. Cillekens B, Lang M, van Mechelen W, et al. How does occupational physical activity influence health? An umbrella review of 23 health outcomes across 158 observational studies. Br J Sports Med 2020;54(24):1474–81.

61. Schram B, Orr R, Pope R, et al. Risk factors for development of lower limb osteoarthritis in physically demanding occupations: a narrative umbrella review. J Occup Health 2020;62(1):e12103.

62. Gignac MAM, Irvin E, Cullen K, et al. Men and women's occupational activities and the risk of developing osteoarthritis of the knee, hip, or hands: a systematic review and recommendations for future research. Arthritis Care Res 2020;72(3):378–96.

63. Cameron KL, Driban JB, Svoboda SJ. Osteoarthritis and the tactical athlete: a systematic review. J Athl Train 2016;51(11):952–61.

64. Ackerman IN, Kemp JL, Crossley KM, et al. Hip and knee osteoarthritis affects younger people, too. J Orthop Sports Phys Ther 2017;47(2):67–79.

65. Crawford JO, Berkovic D, Erwin J, et al. Musculoskeletal health in the workplace. Best Pract Res Clin Rheumatol 2020;34(5):101558.

66. van Duijn M, Miedema H, Elders L, et al. Barriers for early return-to-work of workers with musculoskeletal disorders according to occupational health physicians and human resource managers. J Occup Rehabil 2004;14(1):31–41.

67. Berkovic D, Ayton D, Briggs AM, et al. "I Would be More of a Liability than an Asset": navigating the workplace as a younger person with arthritis. J Occup Rehabil 2020;30(1):125–34.

68. Oakman J, Keegel T, Kinsman N, et al. Persistent musculoskeletal pain and productive employment; a systematic review of interventions. Occup Environ Med 2016;73(3):206–14.

69. Bowden JL, Hunter DJ, Feng Y. Using neighbourhood environments to support osteoarthritis management - a scoping review. Osteoarthr Cartil 2021.

70. Barton H, Thompson S, Burgess S, et al. The routledge handbook of planning for health and well-being shaping a sustainable and healthy future. Hoboken (NJ): Taylor and Francis; 2015.

71. Kent J, Thompson S. Planning Australia's healthy built environments. New York: Routledge; 2019.

72. Bowden JL, Hunter DJ, Feng Y. How can neighborhood environments facilitate management of osteoarthritis: a scoping review. Semin Arthritis Rheum 2021; 51(1):253–65.

73. World Health Organization. Integrating health in urban and territorial planning: a sourcebook. Geneva (Switzerland): WHO; 2020.

74. Dirección de Promoción de la Salud y Control de Enfermedades No Transmisibles. Estrategia Nacional de Prevención y Control de Enfermedades no Transmisibles., 2013, Promoción de la Salud. Minestro de Salud; Buenos Aires.

75. Hill-Briggs F, Adler NE, Berkowitz SA, et al. Social determinants of health and diabetes: a scientific review. Diabetes Care 2020;44(1):258–79.

76. Koohsari MJ, McCormack GR, Nakaya T, et al. Neighbourhood built environment and cardiovascular disease: knowledge and future directions. Nat Rev Cardiol 2020;17(5):261–3.

77. Bonaccorsi G, Manzi F, Del Riccio M, et al. Impact of the built environment and the neighborhood in promoting the physical activity and healthy aging in older people: an umbrella review. Int J Environ Res Public Health 2020;17(17):6127.

78. McCue P. Walking policy steps – the policy development process for the first state walking target in NSW, vol. 9. Australia (Bingley): Emerald Publishing Limited; 2017. p. 233–48.

79. van Hoof J, Marston HR. Age-friendly cities and communities: state of the art and future perspectives. Int J Environ Res Public Health 2021;18(4).

80. Briggs AM, Araujo de Carvalho I. Actions required to implement integrated care for older people in the community using the World Health Organization's ICOPE approach: a global Delphi consensus study. PLoS One 2018;13(10):e0205533.

81. Crist K, Benmarhnia T, Zamora S, et al. Device-measured and self-reported active travel associations with cardiovascular disease risk factors in an ethnically diverse sample of adults. Int J Environ Res Public Health 2021;18(8).

82. Doi K, Sunagawa T, Inoi H, et al. Transitioning to safer streets through an integrated and inclusive design. IATSS Res 2016;39(2):87–94.

83. Kerr J, Rosenberg D, Frank L. The role of the built environment in healthy aging. J Plan Lit 2012;27(1):43–60.

84. Briggs AM, Huckel Schneider C, Slater H, et al. Health systems strengthening to arrest the global disability burden: empirical development of prioritised components for a global strategy for improving musculoskeletal health. BMJ Glob Health 2021;6(6):e006045.

85. National Osteoarthritis Strategy Project Group. National osteoarthritis strategy. Institute of Bone and Joint Research, University of Sydney; 2018.

86. Osteoarthritis (OA) Action Alliance, US Centre for Disease Control and Prevention, The Arthritis Foundation. A national public health agenda for osteoarthritis: 2020 update 2020.

87. U.S. Department of Health and Human Services. Healthy people. 2020. Available at: https://www.healthypeople.gov/2020/topics-objectives/topic/Arthritis-Osteoporosis-and-Chronic-Back-Conditions. Accessed September 2, 2021.

88. Eggleston EM, Finkelstein JA. Finding the role of health care in population health. JAMA 2014;311(8):797–8.

89. Alley DE, Asomugha CN, Conway PH, et al. Accountable health communities-addressing social needs through Medicare and Medicaid. N Engl J Med 2016; 374(1):8–11.

90. Gottlieb L, Colvin JD, Fleegler E, et al. Evaluating the accountable health communities demonstration project. J Gen Intern Med 2017;32(3):345–9.

91. Institute of medicine of the National Academies Committee on the Recommended Social and Behavioral Domains and Measures for Electronic Health Records. Capturing social and behavioral domains and measures in electronic health records: phase 2. Washington, DC: The National Academies Press; 2014.

92. Canadian Medical Association. Health equity and the social determinants of health: a role for the medical profession. CMAJ 2013;1–10.

93. Adler NE, Stead WW. Patients in context–EHR capture of social and behavioral determinants of health. N Engl J Med 2015;372(8):698–701.

Moving?

Make sure your subscription moves with you!

To notify us of your new address, find your **Clinics Account Number** (located on your mailing label above your name), and contact customer service at:

Email: journalscustomerservice-usa@elsevier.com

800-654-2452 (subscribers in the U.S. & Canada)
314-447-8871 (subscribers outside of the U.S. & Canada)

Fax number: 314-447-8029

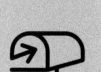

Elsevier Health Sciences Division
Subscription Customer Service
3251 Riverport Lane
Maryland Heights, MO 63043